**Springer Series in Cognitive Development**

*Series Editor*
Charles J. Brainerd

## Springer Series in Cognitive Development

*Series Editor:* Charles J. Brainerd
(recent titles)

---

Adult Cognition: An Experimental Psychology of Human Aging
*Timothy A. Salthouse*

Recent Advances in Cognitive-Development Theory: Progress in Cognitive Development Research
*Charles J. Brainerd (Ed.)*

Learning in Children: Progress in Cognitive Development Research
*Jeffrey Bisanz/Gay L. Bisanz/Robert Kail (Eds.)*

Cognitive Strategy Research: Psychological Foundations
*Michael Pressley/Joel R. Levin (Eds.)*

Cognitive Strategy Research: Educational Applications
*Michael Pressley/Joel R. Levin (Eds.)*

Equilibrium in the Balance: A Study of Psychological Explanation
*Sophie Haroutunian*

Crib Speech and Language Play
*Stan A. Kuczaj, II*

Discourse Development: Progress in Cognitive Development Research
*Stan A. Kuczaj, II*

Cognitive Development in Atypical Children: Progress in Cognitive Development Research
*Linda S. Siegel/Frederick J. Morrison (Eds.)*

Basic Processes in Memory Development: Progress in Cognitive Development Research
*Charles J. Brainerd/Michael Pressley (Eds.)*

Cognitive Learning and Memory in Children: Progress in Cognitive Development Research
*Michael Pressley/Charles J. Brainerd (Eds.)*

The Development of Word Meaning
*Stan A. Kuczaj, II/Martyn D. Barrett (Eds.)*

Formal Methods in Development Psychology: Progress in Cognitive Development Research
*Jeffrey Bisanz/Charles J. Brainerd/Robert Kail (Eds.)*

Children's Counting and Concepts of Number
*Karen C. Fuson*

Memory Development Between 2 and 20
*Karen C. Fuson*

Cognitive Development in Adulthood: Progress in Cognitive Development Research
*Mark L. Howe/Charles J. Brainerd (Eds.)*

Mark L. Howe and Charles J. Brainerd
Editors

# Cognitive Development in Adulthood

## Progress in Cognitive Development Research

With 20 Illustrations

Springer-Verlag
New York Berlin Heidelberg
London Paris Tokyo

**Mark L. Howe**
Department of Psychology
Memorial University
St. John's, Newfoundland
Canada A1B 3X9

**Charles J. Brainerd**
Program in Educational
Psychology
University of Arizona
Tuscon, AZ 85721
USA

*Series Editor:* Charles J. Brainerd

Library of Congress Cataloging in Publication Data
Cognitive development in adulthood.
(Springer series in cognitive development)
Includes bibliographies and indexes.
1. Aging—Psychological aspects. 2. Cognition.
3. Memory. 4. Adulthood—Psychological aspects.
I. Howe, Mark L. II. Brainerd, Charles J. III. Series.
BF724.85.C64C64 1988 155.6 88-4604


Softcover reprint of the hardcover 1st edition 1988


Typeset by Ampersand Publisher Services, Inc., Rutland, Vermont.

9 8 7 6 5 4 3 2 1

ISBN-13: 978-1-4612-8377-5 e-ISBN-13: 978-1-4612-3852-2
DOI: 10.1007/ 978-1-4612-3852-2

For Mabel Gertrude Le Bas (nee Glover),
1892–1986 (MLH)

# Series Preface

For some time now, the study of cognitive development has been far and away the most active discipline within developmental psychology. Although there would be much disagreement as to the exact proportion of papers published in developmental journals that could be considered cognitive, 50% seems like a conservative estimate. Hence, a series of scholarly books devoted to work in cognitive development is especially appropriate at this time.

The Springer Series in Cognitive Developmemt contains two basic types of books, namely, edited collections of original chapters by several authors, and original volumes written by one author or a small group of authors. The flagship for the Springer Series is a serial publication of the "advances" type, carrying the subtitle *Progress in Cognitive Development Research.* Each volume in the *Progress* sequence is strongly thematic, in that it is limited to some well-defined domain of cognitive-developmental research (e.g., logical and mathematical development, development of learning). All *Progress* volumes will be edited collections. Editors of such collections, upon consultation with the Series Editor, may elect to have their books published either as contributions to the *Progress* sequence or as separate volumes. All books written by one author or a small group of authors are being published as separate volumes within the series.

A fairly broad definition of cognitive development is being used in the selection of books for this series. The classic topics of concept development, children's thinking and reasoning, the development of learning, language development, and memory development will, of course, be included. So, however, will newer areas such as social-cognitive development, educational applications, formal modeling, and philosophical implications of cognitive-developmental theory. Although it is anticipated that most books in the series will be empirical in orientation, theoretical and philosophical works are also welcome. With books of the latter sort, heterogeneity of theoretical perspective is encouraged, and no attempt will be made to foster some specific theoretical perspective at the expense of others (e.g., Piagetian versus behavioral or behavioral versus information processing).

C. J. Brainerd

# Preface

When we speak of cognitive development, we normally mean the changes in functioning that occur between birth and physical maturity. This general tendency is reflected in many of the preceding volumes in the Springer Series in Cognitive Development, where the primary focus has been upon the advancement of knowledge in areas such as learning, memory, and cognition throughout childhood and early adolescence. As we are all aware, however, cognitive development does not end with adolescence, but, rather, continues over the life course. Although the study of development in adulthood has a rich history, the past few years have witnessed a dramatic increase in research activity, particularly in the area of changes in cognitive functioning that occur during late adulthood. This intensification of interest has led to an extensive literature, one that has even warranted the establishment of a new journal, *Psychology and Aging*, devoted to issues involved in understanding the nature of developmental changes that occur in adulthood.

In surveying this expanding literature, it became clear to us that an advances volume was needed, one that captured the diversity of both the content and the methodological/analytical procedures that typify the study of cognitive development in adulthood. Although a number of "handbooks" exist, some of which are excellent, the motivation for the present volume was to present chapters that not only review and discuss topics that are central to cognitive development in adulthood, but also integrate theory, analytical techniques, and new empirical findings, thereby providing a state-of-the-art snapshot of the study of cognitive aging. In soliciting chapters, we asked authors to prepare their contributions so as to weave their theoretical positions together with discussions of methodological considerations and the presentation of new empirical findings. It is this blend of theory, data, and methodology, as well as the willingness of the authors to include original data and analyses, that should help make this volume a useful resource.

This volume is divided into two sections. The first section contains chapters that are concerned with the contributions of memory factors to cognitive aging. The second section contains chapters that are concerned with cognitive and performance factors. The first section begins with two chapters that focus on problems associated with the measurement of age changes in memory. In Chapter 1, Darlene Howard examines the use of explicit and implicit measures to assess memory changes in adulthood. The research reviewed in this chapter clearly shows that implicit memory measures yield different patterns of age variation than do explicit measures. It is argued that the reliance on explicit measures in most previous research has led to an overly pessimistic view of memory in the aged, and that a complete picture must incorporate both implicit and explicit aspects of memory. A second, classical problem in studies of memory and memory development concerns how we can obtain independent ratio-scale measures of basic processes such as storage and retrieval. In Chapter 2, Mark Howe discusses measurement problems arising from attempts to dissever storage and retrieval processes in developmental studies of long-term memory, and describes one resolution, namely, the use of Markov models. A recent identifiable implementation of a two-stage Markov model is then applied to a series of eight experiments. Here, it is shown that although the magnitude of age differences at retrieval exceed those at storage, both age invariances and age differences occur in these factors. In line with the arguments presented by Howard, Howe concludes that theories positing a unitary decline in memory functioning with age are at odds with the data and that a complete theory of memory aging must consider age changes as well as age invariances.

In Chapter 3, David Hultsch, Christopher Hertzog, Roger Dixon, and Heather Davidson describe their research on metamemory in adulthood. Using metamemory questionnaires, these authors have not only established the reliability and factorial validity of these measures, but have also shown consistent age differences in metamemory, particularly in relationship to measures of self-efficacy. In Chapter 4, Donald Kausler and Wemara Lichty discuss a program of research on memory for activities and the implications of this research for the study of both rehearsal-independent and rehearsal-dependent memory. They describe a two-stage model of activity/action memory in which age deficits in recall are attributed to differences in encoding contextual information. In the last chapter in this section, Chapter 5, Elizabeth Zelinski and Michael Gilewski present a meta-analysis of studies of the aging of prose memory. The results of this analysis, like those of other chapters, argue for both age differences and age invariances in memory for discourse.

The second section begins with an analysis of problem solving in adulthood. In Chapter 6, David Arenberg discusses two components of problem solving, namely, analysis, and synthesis. Although individual differences are evident, both longitudinal and cross-sectional analyses reveal that older adults have more difficulty than younger adults at identifying the relevant information needed for the problem solution (analysis) and at putting the information together (synthesis). In Chapter 7, Timothy Salthouse provides a critical analysis of the concept of processing resources. Following a more formal articulation of this construct, he proceeds to examine the role of processing resources in a programmatic series of studies. He concludes that although the notion of processing resources should not be abandoned, neither should it be considered a true explanation of cognitive aging until it has been properly operationalized.

In Chapter 8, K. Warner Schaie outlines some further methodological problems in the study of cognitive aging that fall under the general heading of internal validity. After reviewing the nature of these problems and proposing relevant solutions, he provides a new analysis of some recent data from the Seattle Longitudinal Study. Schaie concludes that when the appropriate correction procedures for internal validity threats are in place, longitudinal parameter estimates are a preferred source of information in the study of cognitive aging. Finally, in the last chapter in this section, Chapter 9, Michael Stones and Albert Kozma provide a unique look at the relationship between activity levels and the aging of cognitive/motor performance. Following a review of both the empirical and theoretical literature, they propose a functional age model that is subsequently investigated in a series of studies. They conclude that (chronically) increased activity levels do indeed appear to influence cognitive performance, perhaps through a reduction in hypoxia. Importantly, these results suggest that physiological measures play a critical role in our understanding of cognitive aging.

Despite the diversity of topics and research methods contained in this book, when taken together the chapters paint an optimistic picture of the aging of memory and cognition. The different contributions in both sections illustrate an important point about the study of cognitive development in adulthood: While there are clear circumstances in which older adults do not perform as well as younger adults (instances that tell us much about the decline of functioning with age), there are many other circumstances in which age differences are absent (or favor older adults). It is only when both age differences and age invariances are considered in concert that a satisfactory theory of the aging of memory and cognition will emerge.

*Acknowledgment.* Preparation of this volume was facilitated by a research grant from the Natural Sciences and Engineering Research Council of Canada (No. A3334) to Mark L. Howe.

M.L. Howe
C.J. Brainerd

# Contents

## Part II Cognitive and Performance Factors

# Contributors

*David Arenberg* Gerontology Research Center, National Institute on Aging, Baltimore, Maryland 21224, USA.

*Heather Davidson* Department of Psychology, University of Victoria, Victoria, British Columbia V8W 2Y2, Canada.

*Roger A. Dixon* Department of Psychology, University of Victoria, Victoria, British Columbia V8W 2Y2, Canada.

*Michael J. Gilewski* Veterans Administration Outpatient Clinic, Los Angeles, California 90013, USA.

*Christopher Hertzog* School of Psychology, Georgia Institute of Technology, Atlanta, Georgia 30332, USA.

*Darlene V. Howard* Department of Psychology, Georgetown University, Washington, D.C. 20057, USA.

*Mark L. Howe* Department of Psychology, Memorial University, St. John's, Newfoundland A1B 3X9, Canada.

*David F. Hultsch* Department of Psychology, University of Victoria, Victoria, British Columbia V8W 2Y2, Canada.

*Donald H. Kausler* Department of Psychology, University of Missouri, Columbia, Missouri 65211, USA.

*Albert Kozma* Department of Psychology, Memorial University, St. John's, Newfoundland A1B 3X9, Canada.

*Wemara Lichty* Department of Psychology, Washington University, St. Louis, Missouri 63130, USA.

*Timothy A. Salthouse* School of Psychology, Georgia Institute of Technology, Atlanta, Georgia 30332, USA.

*K. Warner Schaie* Department of Individual and Family Studies, Pennsylvania State University, University Park, Pennsylvania 16802, USA.

*Michael J. Stones* Department of Psychology, Memorial University, St. John's, Newfoundland A1B 3X9, Canada.

*Elizabeth M. Zelinski* Leonard Davis School of Gerontology, University of Southern California, Los Angeles, California 90089, USA.

# Part I Memory Factors

# 1. Implicit and Explicit Assessment of Cognitive Aging

*Darlene V. Howard*

When we speak of memory, it is usually of conscious recollection. I conclude that I remember someone's name if I am able to recall it when we meet or, failing that, am able to recognize that the name is familiar when the person announces it. Psychologists and other scholars have not limited their definition of memory solely to such *explicit* measures, as Schacter's (1987) historical review outlines, but explicit measures have, nonetheless, dominated the study of memory. The laboratory tests most frequently used require that the person report a conscious recollection of the tested event. This is true both for recall tests (e.g., "What words were in the list you just studied?" "Tell me everything you remember of the paragraph you just read.") and for recognition tests (e.g., "Was the word ABODE in the list you just studied?" "Did the paragraph you read state that Fred was a carpenter?").

But memory is also revealed by *implicit* means. A prior event may be shown to influence subsequent performance in the absence of any conscious memory for its occurrence. Even though I am not aware of either recognizing or recalling someone's name, I might be able to understand it more readily now in a noisy environment than if I had not encountered it before. Similarly, if the reader attempts to complete the word stem ABO ______ with the first word that comes to mind, chances are that ABODE will be the outcome, thanks to the example in the preceding paragraph. In the absence of that recent encounter, the completion ABOUT would have been more likely, given frequency of occurrence in the language. Such *priming* of word stem completion, then, reveals implicit memory for the previous occurrence, regardless of whether the reader recognizes explicitly that ABODE had occurred earlier.

The fact that the memory tapped by implicit means is often outside of the rememberer's awareness and control does not mean that it is unimportant. Indeed, this characteristic unawareness probably leads us to underestimate the role of implicit memory in everyday life. Research suggests that the memories tapped by implicit tests influence the ease and accuracy with which we perceive external stimuli, (Jacoby & Dallas, 1981), the meaning we assign to them (Eich, 1984), the likelihood that particular ideas will come to mind (Graf, Shimamura, & Squire, 1985), and even our preferences (Zajonc, 1984).

Despite the importance of implicit memory, the study of cognitive aging has, until very recently, been limited almost exclusively to performance on explicit tests. The purposes of this chapter are (1) to review what is known about the aging of implicit memory, (2) to consider the implications of the distinction between implicit and explicit means of assessment for our understanding of aspects of cognition other than memory, and (3) to advocate the more extensive use of implicit measures to gain a more balanced view of cognitive aging.

I begin with a discussion of the distinction between implicit and explicit memory. I then review what is known and what is not known about the aging of implicit memory by summarizing the findings of other investigators and by outlining the results of three series of studies conducted in my laboratory. Finally, I discuss the implications of the implicit/explicit distinction for other domains of cognitive gerontology.

## Implicit Versus Explicit Memory

### Definitions and Distinctions

The dichotomy of interest here goes by several names, including: "knowing that" versus "knowing how" (Cohen & Squire, 1980), "autobiographical memory" versus 'perceptual recognition" (Jacoby & Dallas, 1981), "memory with awareness" versus "memory without awareness" (Jacoby & Witherspoon, 1982), "declarative" versus "procedural knowledge" (Cohen, 1984), "memories" versus "habits" (Mishkin & Petri, 1984), and "explicit" versus "implicit memory" (e.g., Graf & Schacter, 1985). At this time, it is by no means clear that these various names are synonymous. They are accompanied by slightly different definitions, at least in part because the researchers are using different tasks and subject populations.

This chapter follows Graf and Schacter (1985) and Schacter (1987) in adopting the terms explicit and implicit memory and in using them in a descriptive way. I will refer to *explicit* tasks (and memories) as those in which the memory test requires an introspective report of remembering, that is, an intention to recollect, and *implicit* tasks (and memories) as those in which conscious recollection does not occur.

The tasks used to assess implicit and explicit memory differ in the *instructions* given to the subject; in explicit tests, but not implicit ones, the person is asked to attempt to remember the tested material. As used here, then, the implicit/explicit distinction forms a *test instruction* parallel of the incidental/intentional *study instruction* distinction. In both cases, the critical variable refers to the intent of the subject, although the implicit/explicit distinction refers to intent at time of test, whereas the incidental/intentional distinction refers to intent at the time of study. In both cases, too, the experimenter attempts to vary the subject's intent, but can do so only by varying instructions in the hope that the subject will both believe and obey. To the extent that the subject does not (using conscious recollection on an implicit test), then the task will not be assessing the aspect of memory intended by the experimenter; this is a complication other researchers have noted (e.g., Cohen & Squire, 1980; Jacoby, 1983; Light & Singh, 1987; Moscovitch, Winocur, & McLachlan, 1986) and one to which I shall return often.

## Qualitative Differences Between Explicit and Implicit Memory

Whether implicit and explicit memories reflect the operation of two different memory systems or whether both depend on a single underlying system is a question of some debate (cf. Schacter, 1987; Tulving, 1984), and one about which this chapter makes no claims. Regardless of whether two different systems are involved, it is clear that explicit and implicit tests often yield qualitatively different patterns of results. At least three kinds of differences have been found both in earlier research and in our work as described here.

*First,* implicit and explicit memory can be influenced differently by the same independent variables and thus can show functional independence (Tulving, 1984). For example, despite the fact that proactive and retroactive interference have large effects on explicit memory, Graf and Schacter (1987) have shown that they do not influence implicit memory. In contrast, switches in modality of presentation between study and test usually have little, if any, effect on explicit memory, but do influence implicit memory (Jacoby & Dallas, 1981).

*Second,* within an individual, explicit memory may be impaired while implicit memory remains intact. For example, amnesia patients who have such severely impaired explicit memory that they cannot remember having studied any list at all often show implicit memory for the content of the list that is indistinguishable from that of normal controls (Schacter, 1985). Even within a normal population, we have found that a person's relative skill at explicit memory tasks is often unrelated to his or her skill at implicit memory, as assessed by correlations between the tasks, using subjects as units of analysis (e.g., Howard, in press; Howard, Heisey, & Shaw, 1986). This second kind of difference may be viewed, of course, as a form of the first, i.e., as a form of functional independence in which the "independent" variable is that of the individual or of brain damage (in the case of certain forms of amnesia).

*Third,* implicit and explicit measures are sometimes stochastically independent (Tulving, 1984) in that whether or not a person remembers a given item according to one measure is unrelated to whether or not it is remembered according to the other (e.g., Jacoby & Witherspoon, 1982; Tulving, Schacter, & Stark, 1982). As Tulving (1984) has noted, such stochastic independence provides strong evidence that implicit memory tests are not simply easier versions of explicit ones.

## Item Versus Associative Memory

It is also important to distinguish between at least two kinds of implicit memory, item and associative (Graf & Schacter, 1985). *Implicit item memory* is memory for the occurrence of an already well-known unit, whereas *implicit associative memory* is memory for a new association between previously unrelated items. One way to envision the distinction is to adopt a network theory of long-term memory (Anderson, 1983; Collins & Loftus, 1975; discussed in Howard, in press), which assumes that memory consists of a set of concept nodes interconnected by labeled, directed associative links. It is further assumed that these nodes vary in level of activation (and hence accessibility) and that activation spreads along links in the network. In this light, then, implicit *item* memory reflects activation of an already established concept node or a set of previously related nodes. In contrast, implicit *associative* memory requires establishment of a new association between previously unrelated nodes.

These two kinds of implicit memory differ on several counts. *First,* associative memory is more subject to disruption by clinical conditions. Implicit item memory has been shown to remain intact in virtually all clinical populations tested (although Shimamura, Salmon, Squire, & Butters, 1987 reported evidence for one exception). Implicit associative memory also remains intact in many clinical populations that show severe deficits on explicit counterparts, but it is absent (or at least severely impaired) in some severe forms of amnesia and in some Alzheimer's disease patients (Knopman & Nissen, 1987; Schacter, 1985).

*Second,* implicit item and associative memories sometimes show functional independence in that a given variable can affect one but not the other. In particular, implicit item memory is unaffected by strategies used to encode the stimulus, such as semantic processing strategies (Graf & Mandler, 1984; Jacoby & Dallas, 1981). In contrast, in order to reveal implicit associative memory for a pairing between previously unassociated words, people must have encoded some meaningful relation between them. although implicit associative memory is much less influenced by the *degree* of such elaboration than its explicit counterpart (Schacter & Graf, 1986).

A *third* difference concerns the role of attention in establishing implicit memory. Using a spelling bias measure of implicit memory (discussed in more detail later), Eich (1984) showed that establishment of an implicit memory for items does not require attention to the study stimulus at all; mere exposure in an unattended ear while shadowing an attended ear is sufficient. In contrast, using a very different procedure, Nissen and Bullemer (1987) showed that forming a new association does require processing capacity. They found no implicit memory for a repetitive pattern in a visually presented sequence when the subject had to perform a simultaneous attention-demanding task during exposure to the pattern. It is important, however, that *awareness* is not required for establishing implicit associative memories; in the absence of the simultaneous task, Korsakoff's patients who showed no awareness at all of the sequence pattern still showed implicit learning of it that was indistinguishable from that of normals (Nissen & Bullemer, 1987). Thus, even though establishing implicit associative memory does not require awareness, it should not be classified as an "automatic" activity in the sense used by Hasher & Zacks, 1979), because it draws on limited processing capacity.

## Hypotheses About Aging

The fact that there are qualitative differences between the results obtained using implicit as opposed to explicit measures of memory suggests that the picture of memory aging is likely to differ substantially, depending on which type of measure is used. Further, the differences between implicit item and implicit associative memory outlined previously suggest that these two types of implicit memory might be differentially spared in normal aging. Implicit associative, but not implicit item, memory (1) requires attention in the sense of drawing on limited processing resources, and (2) in the case of verbal material, at least, requires that the person encode some meaningful relationship between the items to be associated. One popular hypothesis about aging is that it is characterized by a decrease in processing resources [although the exact nature of any such decline is far from settled (Light & Burke, in press; Salthouse, 1985, and this volume)]. There is also evidence of an age-related decline in the degree to which people engage in semantic elaboration of material to be memorized (Craik, 1985; Kausler, 1985; Poon, 1985).

Therefore, what is known of cognitive aging, coupled with the characteristics of implicit and explicit memory outlined previously, suggest two general hypotheses. The first is that implicit item memory, unlike its explicit counterpart, does not decline with normal aging. In terms of network theories, this hypothesis assumes that the activation of already established nodes and the spread of activation along established nodes is not age sensitive. This hypothesis predicts that as long as acquisition conditions permit adequate sensory processing *and* as long as the contributions of explicit memory are eliminated, tests of implicit item memory will yield no age differences.

The second hypothesis is that, unlike its explicit counterpart, implicit associative memory does not decline with normal aging, *except* under conditions in which the processing capacity of older people is either exceeded, or fails to be allocated to memorization-enhancing processes, such as semantic elaboration. In terms of network theory, this hypothesis assumes that establishing a new link or association in long-term memory calls on limited processing capacity and hence is age-sensitive under certain demanding acquisition conditions. The rest of this chapter considers the evidence pertaining to both of these hypotheses.

## Previous Research on the Aging of Implicit Memory

### Implicit Item Memory

Within the last 5 years, the aging of implicit item memory has been investigated using several different methods. All have yielded reasonably consistent results.

#### Repetition Priming of Judgments

In one of the earliest studies, Moscovitch (1982) examined *repetition priming of lexical decisions* by asking people to make speeded "yes/no" judgments about whether each item of a series was a word. Moscovitch found the same pattern for both younger and older participants; response times were faster on the second than on the first presentation of a given word (i.e., a repetition-priming effect), and the magnitude of this effect did not vary with lag between the two tests, being just as great after 29 as after 0 intervening items. Further, the magnitude of the priming effect did not vary with age, suggesting no age differences in implicit item memory. In contrast, explicit recognition of the items declined significantly with both age and lag.

Rabbitt (1982) reported similar results using *repetition priming of category judgments and letter detection.* For each of a series of words, people made a speeded category judgment (Is this a mammal or a fish?) or letter-detection judgment (Does this word have an A or an E?), with a given word (and judgment) being repeated after a variable lag. As in Moscovitch (1982), the magnitude of repetition priming and its persistence (as revealed by lag effects) did not vary with age. (It should be noted that Rabbitt reported a second experiment that did yield age differences in priming, but the processing required for this task does not seem to tap either item or associative memory in any direct way and thus is not relevant to the present discussion.)

#### Repetition Priming of Word Completion

Light and her colleagues reported three experiments using word completion priming to tap implicit item memory. In Light, Singh, and Capps (1986), people were given 5 seconds to study each of a list of words (e.g., BEHAVIOR) for a later memory test of unspecified nature. Implicit memory was tapped immediately and again 7 days later in a *fragment completion test* in which people were asked to complete a series of word fragments (e.g., BE___VI___; C_O___RA), each having only one possible completion. The magnitude of implicit memory was assessed by subtracting correct completions of words not studied earlier from those for words that were studied earlier. The magnitude of this priming effect did not vary significantly with age, and although it did decline over the 7-day delay, the amount of decline was the same for both ages. In contrast, on a test of explicit recognition there was a significant age difference favoring the younger on the delayed, although not the immediate, test.

Light and Singh (1987) reported similar results in two experiments using a *word-stem completion* measure of implicit memory. In both experiments people first were given 5 seconds per word to make either a pleasantness judgment (Experiments 1 and 2) or a vowel comparison (Experiment 1) about each of a series of words. For the completion test, they were given word stems consisting of three letters and asked to complete the stem with the first word that came to mind. In keeping with the previous findings, in both experiments both younger and older people who had encountered the word during the earlier rating task had higher completion scores than in a baseline condition in which the words had not been studied earlier, and the magnitude of this advantage did not vary significantly with age. In contrast, there were significant age differences favoring the younger on both word-stem-cued recall and forced-choice recognition of the same words.

### Repetition Priming of Perceptual Identification and Reading Speed

Light and Singh (1987; Experiment 3) demonstrated a similar dissociation between the aging of implicit and explicit memory when the dependent variable that taps implicit memory is the probability of correct identification of perceptually degraded words. Both their younger and older subjects were better at identifying perceptually degraded words that had been presented during an earlier acquisition phase than control words, and the magnitude of this priming effect did not vary significantly with age. The older and younger groups differed significantly, however, on both free recall and forced-choice recognition of these same items.

Moscovitch et al. (1986; Experiment 3, Table 8) obtained a similar pattern of findings, showing that even when nondegraded stimuli are presented people read previously studied words more quickly than new ones; this advantage is actually greater for older people than for younger whether absolute or percent improvement is considered.

### Priming of Category-Exemplar Generation

All the foregoing studies are similar in that some stimulus is perceived visually during an acquisition phase, and implicit memory for it is then inferred from faster (or more accurate) reperception of it. An additional study reported by Light (1987) makes it clear, however, that the opportunity for such facilitation of reperception is not a *necessary* condition for obtaining age similarity in implicit memory. During an acquisition phase, people first rated 50 words for pleasantness; embedded in this list were three relatively low-dominance members of each of six categories (the category names, however, were *not* presented). Later, to test implicit memory, people were asked to generate exemplars for a list of category names. Both younger and older participants were more likely to produce the exemplars they had encountered earlier than in a baseline condition in which they had not encountered the items previously, and the magnitude of this priming did not vary significantly with age. Thus, having previously encountered a *word* influenced the likelihood that it would come to mind later when the name of its *category* was encountered, and there was no significant diminution in this influence with age. In contrast, when people were asked explicitly to recall the exemplers of each category that they had heard earlier, a significant advantage for the younger people appeared.

## Summary

The studies of item memory just discussed support the hypothesis that there are no significant age differences in implicit item memory, in sharp contrast to explicit item memory, which almost always yields large and significant age differences. When viewed in light of activation models, these results suggest that there is no decline with normal aging in the activation (and hence heightened accessibility) of a concept node that accompanies perception of its referent, although there is an age deficit in the ability to engage in conscious, deliberate retrieval. In addition, the few studies that have varied retention interval (Light et al., 1986; Moscovitch, 1982; Rabbitt, 1982) indicate that the duration of activation is also immune to the effects of normal aging.

I know of only one published finding that contradicts this hypothesis concerning the stability of implicit item memory; this is a study of spelling bias by Rose, Yesavage, Hill, and Bower (1986), which will be considered in more detail later when our similar studies are outlined. However, one possible caveat has been pointed out by Light and her colleagues. Light and Burke (in press) and Light and Singh (1987) noted that although they have never obtained *statistically significant* age differences in repetition priming, there is a nonsignificant advantage for the younger participants in all their studies. As they indicated, this could either result from actual, although small, age differences in implicit memory *or* from subjects calling on explicit memory in so-called implicit tasks, which would then give an advantage to the younger participants. At present there is no conclusive evidence supporting one of these interpretations rather than the other. Nonetheless, I favor the explicit memory contamination interpretation for two reasons. First, some studies discussed (e.g., Moscovitch et al., 1986, Experiment 3: Rabbitt, 1982, Table 1) and some of our own reported here show nonsignificant age differences in priming that favor the older. In addition, there is considerable evidence in both our work and that of other researchers that subjects often do call on explicit recollection in implicit tests.

## Implicit Associative Memory

Less is known about implicit associative memory than about implicit item memory. In the memory literature at large, not only have fewer experiments been reported, but fewer methods have been developed for its assessment. The only published studies of the aging of implicit associative memory appear to be the following.

### Reading Speed

Moscovitch and his colleagues (e.g., Moscovitch, 1982; Moscovitch et al., 1986) reported several experiments using a reading speed measure. For example, in Moscovitch et al. (1986; Experiment 3), groups of younger, older, and memory-disordered adults first saw randomly paired words (e.g., ANGER-PATTERN, MERCHANT-TRIBUTE). The younger were allowed 3 seconds of study per pair, and the other two groups 5 seconds, with the instruction to read the pair aloud and commit it to memory. To test implicit memory, people were asked to read lists of words as quickly as possible. The results showed clear evidence of implicit associative memory for all three groups; all read a list of old pairs (e.g., ANGER-PATTERN), significantly more rapidly than a list of recombined pairs (e.g., ANGER-TRIBUTE), indicating that they had retained information about the original pairing. The absolute magnitude of this effect appears (in Table 6 of Moscovitch et al., 1986) to be slightly greater for the older than for the younger participants, although the proportional effect is in the direction of being smaller for the older, given their longer baseline reading times. Moscovitch et al (1986; Experiment 2) obtained a similar finding when the study materials were sentences. In both experiments, explicit recognition, in contrast, yielded significant age differences favoring the younger participants.

### Cognitive and Perceptual Motor Skills

Implicit tests of the acquisition of perceptual motor and cognitive skills, such as speed in solving the Tower of Hanoi puzzle (Cohen, 1984) or reading geometrically transformed print (Moscovitch et al., 1986; Experiment 1) would seem to rest, at least in part, on implicit associative memory. And so would acquisition of the conditioned eye-blink response (Woodruff-Pak, 1987). But as Light and Burke (in press) argued in a brief review of research on the aging of such skills, it is not at all clear that such acquisition remains unchanged in the course of aging. Although older adults certainly improve with practice, there are ofen age differences in either the rate of acquisition or the asymptotic skill level. In any event, for present purposes such tasks would seem to provide impure tests of implicit associative memory at best, because they likely call heavily on both explicit strategies (particularly for the cognitive skills) and on sensory motor speed and motor dexterity.

### Summary

Given that the studies of cognitive and perceptual-motor skill acquisition that sometimes show age differences are impure indices, and given that the experiments of Moscovitch et al. (1986) showed no age deficits at all, it might appear that implicit associative memory remains intact in old age. This conclusion would also gain support from an item-recognition priming study by Rabinowitz (1986) and from one of our own studies (Howard, Heisey, & Shaw, 1986; Experiment 1), both of which are discussed in more detail later. In what follows I present evidence that even though implicit associative memory is relatively spared compared to explicit, there are instances nonetheless in which clear age differences emerge.

## Our Studies of the Aging of Implicit Memory

We have completed studies using three different ways of assessing implicit memory: spelling bias, item recognition, and word-stem completion. We have used these different methods to establish the generality of any age differences or similarities revealed and to enable us to examine both item and associative memory.

In all the studies discussed here, the subjects were groups of younger and older people similar in number of years of education completed and in WAIS vocabulary score. The younger people averaged approximately 20 years of age and were typically undergraduate students at Georgetown University. The older subjects were noninstitutionalized people, healthy by their own report, who live in the surrounding community. Most range in age from 65 to 85 years (mean, approximately 70). In all our studies, stimulus counterbalancing is such that individual test items occur equally often in both control and primed conditions, so that each item serves as its own control.

### Studies of Spelling Bias

This series of studies, which investigate implicit *item* memory, was suggested by the work of Jacoby and Witherspoon (1982). They first asked five Korsakoff's patients and five university students to listen to and answer a series of questions. A critical subset of these contained homophones in contexts biasing their less frequent meaning and hence spelling (e.g., "Name a musical instrument that employs a *reed.*"). A few minutes later, implicit memory was tested by giving an auditory list of isolated words that included the previously biased homophones as well as control homophones that had not been in the questions. People were to write down each item as it was presented. This task was described to the participants as a spelling test, in the hope that only implicit memory would be tapped. Finally, explicit recognition memory was tested by giving an auditory presentation of the words in isolation and asking the participant to judge whether each word had occurred in the earlier questions.

There were three important findings. First, as expected, Korsakoff's patients were significantly poorer at explicit recognition than were the students. Second, both groups of people were more likely to produce the less frequent spelling for homophones that had been presented earlier in the biasing context than for control homophones that had not been presented before. Moreover, this *spelling bias effect,* and by inference implicit item memory, was at least as large for the Korsakoff's patients as for the students. The spelling bias effect (percentage of biased minus percentage of control homophones given the infrequent spelling) was 42 for the patients and 29 for the students. Third, both groups of subjects exhibited stochastic independence between the spelling bias and explicit recognition measures.

The spelling bias effect seems to track the influence of context on the activation of memory. The fact that a person assigns a biased meaning to a homophone a few minutes after hearing it in a biased context indicates that the context biased the interpretation initially *and* that this activation continues for at least several minutes. Given that so many individual words are potentially ambiguous out of context, this continuing activation of a contextually appropriate meaning would facilitate language comprehension and production, making it likely that during a conversation or story the contextually appropriate meaning will come to mind.

The fact that spelling bias reflects the immediate and lingering effects of context on semantic processing, makes it particularly interesting for the study of aging because there is some debate regarding the nature and extent of any age-related declines in semantic processing. On the one hand, some views of aging (Craik & Simon, 1980; Eysenck, 1974) have not only proposed that there is a decline in semantic processing, but have also used such a decline to account for age differences in explicit memory. On the other hand, there is evidence for substantial age constancy in at least some aspects of semantic processing, both in our own work (Howard, 1983; Howard, Lasaga, & McAndrews, 1980; Howard, McAndrews & Lasaga, 1981; summarized in Howard, in press) and that of others (Balota & Duchek, 1988; Bowles & Poon, 1985; Burke & Yee, 1984; Burke, White, & Diaz, 1987; Cerella & Fozard, 1984; Chiarello, Church, & Hoyer, 1985; Cohen & Faulkner, 1983; Madden, 1986). All these studies assessed semantic priming and found that it does not decline in old age. That is, a given word is processed more rapidly (i.e., primed) when it follows a semantically related word than when it does not, and the magnitude of this effect does not decline in old age.

Another reason for using the spelling bias procedure was that although findings from it are cited widely in the literature on implicit memory, it has been used in only a few studies (Britton, 1976; Eich, 1984; Jacoby & Witherspoon, 1982). The Britton study was not designed to investigate implicit memory per se, and tested only college students; the Eich experiment focused primarily on memory for unattended material (again using only college students), and the condition testing implicit memory for attended material was described only briefly as a subsidiary study; and the Jacoby and Witherspoon study (1982) is reported in only scant detail in fewer than three pages. Therefore, it seemed useful to establish the replicability and generality of the effect.

In the first of our spelling bias studies, 12 younger and 12 older adults first answered 64 aurally presented questions, 16 of which contained homophones biased to the less frequent meaning; e.g., "If you were making a pizza, which kind of cheese would you grate?" We then gave implicit and explicit memory tests simultaneously by playing a tape-recorded list of 128 words and asking the person to circle a "Y" or "N" depending on whether or not the word had occurred in the earlier sentences (the explicit recognition test) and then to write the word down in the blank provided so that we could be sure that the person had understood the spoken word (the implicit spelling bias test). Of the 128 test words, 16 were the previously biased homophones and 16 others were control homophones that had not been presented during study.

Row (a) of Table 1.1 shows the mean spelling bias scores and the mean percent correct recognition of homophones in the experiment. These scores show that, as expected, explicit recognition is significantly better for younger than older participants. More importantly, although both age groups show a significant spelling bias, the effect is larger for the younger than the older participants. Thus, *if* spelling bias is providing a pure test of implicit memory, then this experiment would indicate there are age deficits in implicit item memory. However, several aspects of the data suggested that spelling bias was reflecting explicit memory as well for subjects of both ages. Correlations between spelling bias and recognition accuracy across subjects revealed that individuals who were good at one task tended to be good at the other. Further, analyses of stochastic independence indicated that, for participants of both ages, items that were recognized explicitly were more likely to be given the infrequent spelling than those that were not. Therefore, although this study revealed clearly that both younger and older participants show a spelling bias, it suggested that at least some of the bias (and perhaps the age difference in its magnitude) reflected explicit rather than implicit memory.

In a second experiment (Howard, 1986a), we followed a procedure that was closer to that of Eich (1984) than of Jacoby and Witherspoon (1982). People

Table 1.1. Spelling Bias Experiments: Mean Spelling Bias Percent Difference Scores, Percent Correct Recognition, and Percent Correct Recall

| | Implicit Test | | | Explicit Tests | | | | | | |
|---|---|---|---|---|---|---|---|---|---|---|
| | Spelling Bias[a] | | | Recognition[b] | | | Recall[c] | | | |
| Time of Test | Younger | Older | Age Diff? | Younger | Older | Age Diff? | Younger | Older | Age[d] Diff? | Row |
| *Experiment 1* | | | | | | | | | | |
| Study: answer questions | | | | | | | | | | |
| Test: spelling | | | | | | | | | | |
| Immediate | 45* | 27* | Yes | 81 | 70 | Yes | — | — | — | (a) |
| *Experiment 2* | | | | | | | | | | |
| Study: learn word pairs | | | | | | | | | | |
| Test: spelling | | | | | | | | | | |
| Immediate | 30* | 34* | No | 74 | 72 | No | 60 | 39 | Yes | (b) |
| Two-day delay | 33* | 16* | Yes | 65 | 61 | No | 55 | 31 | Yes | (c) |
| *Experiment 3* | | | | | | | | | | |
| Study: answer questions | | | | | | | | | | |
| Test: sentence generation | | | | | | | | | | |
| Immediate | 13* | 9* | No | 74 | 58 | Yes | — | — | — | (d) |
| Two-day delay | 5 | 13* | No | 58 | 51 | Yes | — | — | — | (e) |

[a] Spelling bias equals percent less frequent spelling produced for biased minus that for control homophones. *indicates this effect is significantly different from 0 at $p < .05$.
[b] Recognition is percent correct recognition of homophones.
[c] Recall is percent correct recall of homophones.
[d] Age diff? indicates whether or not there was a significant ($p < .05$) age difference.

listened to and were instructed to try to memorize a list of 32 related stimulus–response word pairs. Of these, 16 contained homophones as response items paired with a stimulus word biasing the homophone's less frequent meaning (e.g., CHEESE–GRATE). The implicit and explicit tests were similar to those in Experiment 1 above, except that the recognition test was conducted on all the response words first (stimulus words never appeared) and the tape was then replayed for the spelling test [the procedure adopted by both Jacoby and Witherspoon (1982) and Eich (1984)]. At the end of the session, we added a second test of explicit memory, a cued recall test in which the first word in each pair was presented as a cue for recall of the second. A final addition was motivated by the observation that all previous work has tested for a spelling bias within an hour of the original presentation of the words. In order to examine the duration of the bias, we tested half the participants immediately and the other half after 2 days.

As rows (b) and (c) of Table 1.1 indicate, this experiment (unexpectedly) revealed no age differences in explicit recognition for either the immediate or the delayed groups, although scores were slightly higher for the younger participants. There were, nonetheless, large age differences in explicit cued recall for both immediate and delayed tests, despite the fact that the cue in each case was a word highly related to the sought-after item. With regard to the implicit test, when study and test occurred on the same day, the magnitude of the spelling bias was at least as large for the older as the younger participants. On the 2-day delay test, however, an age difference favoring the younger appeared; the younger groups, but not the older, showed equal spelling bias for immediate and delayed tests. Even for the older people, however, there was still a highly significant spelling bias 2 days after original study of the pairs.

The age difference in spelling bias seen on the delayed tests *could* reflect an age difference in the persistence of implicit memory. However, there was evidence that, as in Experiment 1, the spelling bias measure was not providing a pure test of implicit memory. During the spelling test, many participants of both ages asked, "Do you want me to give the same spelling I heard earlier?" Correlations and anlayses of stochastic independence also supported this explicit contamination interpretation.

In our third experiment (Howard, 1986b), we changed the spelling test in the hope of making its memory demands less transparent. Participants first answered the same series of questions as in Experiment 1. (We returned to this incidental memory procedure in the hope of further masking the memory nature of the experiment.) Then, as in Experiment 2, people were given explicit recognition and implicit tests either immediately or 2 days later. For the implicit task, people were presented with a list of isolated words, but rather than being asked to spell them were told to "write down a novel sentence using the word." We then noted the spelling used in this sentence-generation task.

Spontaneous comments and postexperimental questionnaire responses suggested that the sentence-generation test had the desired effect. For example, *none* of the 48 participants asked which meaning (or spelling) to use when they were asked to create novel sentences. There was support for this conclusion in the analyses of functional and stochastic independence as well. For example, correlations between an individual's spelling bias and recognition accuracy failed to reach significance for either group under either immediate or delayed tests. Therefore, it appears that the sentence-generation version of the spelling test offers a relatively pure measure of implicit memory. It is thus of particular interest that, as rows (d) and (e) of Table 1.1 show, there were no effects of either age or delay on spelling bias. In contrast, the explicit recognition measure yields significant effects of both variables.

## Summary

Taken together, our spelling bias experiments lead to several conclusions. First, the spontaneous comments of our subjects, our postexperimental questionnaire responses, and the patterns of intertask correlations in our Experiments 1 and 2 all suggest that spelling bias effects represent a combination of both implicit and explicit memory, under some conditions. Our results in Experiment 3 suggest that a purer measure of implicit memory is obtained when sentence-generation instructions, rather than the typical spelling instructions, are used.

Second, the spelling bias effect is obtained across a range of conditions, including both incidental and intentional study, and this bias is long lived, lasting for at least 2 days even when (as in Experiment 3) incidental learning instructions are given and the contribution of explicit recollection at testing appears to be eliminated. This suggests that the activation of a contextually appropriate concept that occurs during language processing is surprisingly long lived. The mechanisms underlying this longevity are worth further investigation.

Third, a significant spelling bias effect was obtained for the older participants in all conditions in all three experiments. In fact, the spelling bias is obtained as reliably in older as younger people. Of the 60 participants of each age tested when our three spelling bias experiments are combined, 51 of the older and 50 of the younger participants showed a positive spelling bias. This finding stands in sharp contrast with those of a study by Rose et al. (1986) that was published after we had conducted the experiments just described. Using a procedure very similar to the original Jacoby and Witherspoon (1982) experiment and a subject population comparable to ours, Rose et al. obtained a significant spelling bias effect of 12% for their younger participants, but a nonsignificant −4% for the older. (In fact, the findings of Rose et al. with younger adults differ substantially from those of Jacoby and

Witherspoon, since the latter obtained a spelling effect of 29% for their younger participants.) We can find no obvious explanation for the discrepancy between the Rose et al. findings on age differences and ours, although there are a number of procedural differences between the studies.

Fourth, we find that when the contribution of explicit memory to spelling bias is reduced (as in Experiment 3), age differences in spelling bias disappear. This suggests that there are, in fact, no age differences in the implicit item memory (i.e., the continuing memory activation) that underlies the spelling bias effect, and that the age differences we observed under some conditions result from the contributions of explicit memory.

## Studies of Item-Recognition Priming

In another series, we used McKoon and Ratcliff's item-recognition priming method (McKoon & Ratcliff, 1979; Ratcliff & McKoon, 1978) to study the aging of implicit *associative* memory. In all our studies using this method, people are first shown a series of sentences containing unrelated and unassociated nouns (e.g., the sentence THE SCARECROW WORE SILK or the sentence THE BATH OVERFLOWED ON THE CARPET). Then, in a series of item-recognition trials, they are shown individual nouns and, for each, are to respond as quickly as possible, pushing a button labeled "yes" if the item was in the sentences encountered earlier and "no" if it was not. We measure both accuracy and response time from onset of the test noun.

From the subject's point of view, this item-recognition test is a series of isolated trials, a feature that has the advantage of making it less likely that the person will notice that we are measuring memory for associations between words. For purposes of analysis, however, we break down the series of trials into prime–target pairs. *Primed trials* are those in which the prime and target nouns are from the same studied sentence (e.g., a test of SILK following a test of SCARECROW). *Control trials* are those in which the prime and target are from different studied sentences (e.g., a test of SILK following a test of BATH).

We infer the degree of *implicit memory* for the *association* between the nouns in each sentence by calculating a *prime effect* in which correct response time (or alternatively error rate) on primed trials is subtracted from that on control trials. The prime effect taps *implicit* associative memory in that people are not asked explicitly whether they remember that SILK and SCARECROW occurred in the same sentence; such memory is inferred from the fact that, as a result of the earlier exposure, processing one of these words now facilitates processing of the other.

In addition to the item-recognition trials, all of our experiments using this method include one or two *explicit* tests of associative memory. Some include an *explicit paired recognition* test immediately following the item-recognition series. On each trial, two nouns from the studied sentences are presented and the participant is asked to push a button labeled "yes" if both had occurred in the *same* studied sentence and a button labeled "no" otherwise. In addition, all of these experiments include a final *explicit cued recall* task in which a word from each sentence is presented and the subject is asked to recall the noun(s) that occurred in that sentence.

There is an important characteristic of the item-recognition procedure that affects the conclusions that can be drawn about implicit memory. Typically (and in the data reported here in Tables 1.2 and 1.3), the only response-time data included in the calculation of priming are those of correct recognition responses immediately following correct recognition responses. Thus, the assessment of implicit associative memory is limited to those nouns for which there is explicit item memory. Strictly speaking, then, conclusions about implicit associative memory can be made only about associations between individual items that are recollected (or responded to correctly by chance). If item-recognition error rates are very low for both age groups, then this restriction has little effect on conclusions. The restriction is of most concern when error rates are high and are greater for older than younger participants, since this means that associative memory for many sentences is not being tapped at all *and* that the data from the older group are based on a smaller proportion of the material studied. Thus, it is important to keep item-recognition error rates in mind when interpreting the priming results. For this reason the column on the far right of Table 1.2 displays the percentage of misses (old items that were not recognized and hence were excluded from the priming analysis) for each of the experiments discussed later.

Table 1.2 also shows both the absolute and percent prime effects for each age group, as well as the percent correct cued recall and paired recognition for all our item-recognition studies. Rows (a) through (c) are from our first two experiments using this method (Howard, Heisey, & Shaw, 1986). Subjects first saw 36 one-propositional sentences like the examples given above, with the instruction to memorize the sentences for later testing of an unspecified nature. Some subjects [row (a)] had several opportunities to study each sentence with recall tests interspersed; others [row (b)] received two presentations of each sentence, for a total of 25 seconds of study per sentence, and still others [row (c)] received one 15-second presentation of each sentence.

As expected, the cued recall test tapping explicit associative memory yielded large and significant age differences favoring the younger for all three degrees of study, and particularly in the several presentations condition [row (a)], but there were no significant age differences in the prime effect for either the several or the two-presentation conditions [rows (a) and (b)]. Thus, after two or more study presentations, we find age equivalence in implicit associative memory for the nouns within the studied sentences.

In contrast, after a single study [row (c)] we found a large prime effect for our younger participants, but none at all among our older participants. This lack of priming in the older group is particularly striking in that it occurs even for those sentences in which the subject explicitly recognized both of

TABLE 1.2. Item-Recognition Priming Experiments: Prime Effects, Percent Correct Recall, Percent Correct Paired Recognition, and Percent Errors for Old Items Only in Item Recognition

| | | | Implicit | | Explicit | | | | | | |
|---|---|---|---|---|---|---|---|---|---|---|---|
| | | Test | Prime Effect[a] | | Cued Recall | | Paired Recognition | | Item Error Rates | | |
| Study | Number of Presentations | Delay (days) | Younger | Older | Younger | Older | Younger | Older | Younger | Older | Row |
| *One-proposition* | Several | 0 | 88 (12) | 101 (10) | 90 | 56* | — | — | 4 | 7* | (a) |
| Howard et al. (1986) | 2 | 0 | 86 (13) | 61 (7) | 60 | 37* | — | — | 11 | 9 | (b) |
| | 1 | 0 | 122 (15) | 2 (0)* | 36 | 25* | — | — | 17 | 17 | (c) |
| *Word pairs* Rabinowitz (1986)[b] | 1 | 0 | 150 (17) | 140 (13) | 55 | 18* | — | — | 23 | 34* | (d) |
| *Study variation* | 1—Read | 0 | 120 (13) | 250 (23) | 39 | 21* | 79 | 70* | 37 | 40 | (e) |
| Howard (in preparation) | 1—Continue | 0 | 151 (16) | 116 (11) | 62 | 44* | 90 | 83* | 32 | 29 | (f) |
| *Two-proposition* Howard (1985) | 2 | 0 | 96 (11) | 74 (6) | 52 | 28* | 94 | 84* | 21 | 17* | (g) |
| *Delay* | 3 | 0 | 63 (8) | 96 (9) | 83 | 57* | — | — | 10 | 13 | (h) |
| Howard (in preparation) | 3 | 3 | 153 (18) | 73 (7)* | 79 | 36* | — | — | 15 | 24* | (i) |

[a]*Prime effect* equals control response time minus primed response time. *Percent prime effect* (in parentheses) equals prime effect divided by control response time. *indicates a significant ($p < .05$) age difference.
[b]Data from Rabinowitz (1986) are based on unrelated trials only (item recognition only on his "A" items), and most values are extrapolated from graphs and thus approximate.

the nouns within the sentence, suggesting that the older people had difficulty in forming a new associative link after only one presentation of each sentence. In fact, the item-recognition error rates, which tap explicit *item* memory, were identical for younger people and older, indicating that the difficulty the older people encountered was not in remembering individual items, but in learning new associations among them.

The priming results in our single study condition above differ from those of Moscovitch et al. (1986; Experiment 3) discussed earlier, in which a speeded reading measure of implicit associative memory was used. Our findings in this condition also differ from those of Rabinowitz (1986) obtained in an item-recognition experiment similar to our own. Rabinowitz's subjects were given 5 seconds each to study word pairs, some related (e.g., STRING–GUITAR) and others unrelated (e.g., CARD–GUITAR), and were told that in a later test they would be required to recall the right-hand member of the pair when presented with the left. Rabinowitz found the same pattern of results for both related and unrelated pairs, but I will consider only the latter here, since it is these that tap implicit memory for *new* associations. Rabinowitz's data from unrelated trials are shown in row (d) of Table 1.2. They are similar to ours in showing large age deficits in explicit cued recall and in showing a prime effect among the younger people similar to that we obtained. However, his single-presentation results were in contrast to ours; he found a prime effect that was just as large among his older as his younger participants. This age similarity in priming must be interpreted with some caution, because Rabinowitz's analyses of item-recognition misses revealed high error rates for both groups as well as significant differences favoring the younger people. Nonetheless, it is highly unlikely that these differences in error rates account for the difference between his priming results and ours, particularly in light of the similarity between Rabinowitz's findings and those of Moscovitch et al. (1986; Experiment 3).

A more reasonable explanation of the different findings is that the conditions of study in our experiment were such that the older people failed to form the meaningful relation between the nouns that Graf and Schacter (1985; Schacter & Graf, 1986) have shown to be necessary for implicit associative memory. Perhaps our nonspecific study instructions, combined with a single presentation of sometimes difficult-to-interpret sentences led our older subjects to be uneasy and thus to process the sentences superficially. This explanation is consistent with our subjects' comments as they encountered the sentences for the first time (e.g., "I'm not learning a thing. I don't know what to do.")

This explanation gains credence from an experiment we conducted subsequently in which each person encountered a total of 72 sentences like the examples given previously with a single 10-second presentation of each. For a random one-half of sentences, the person received a "Read Aloud" cue that indicated that the sentence should simply be read aloud during the 10 seconds. For the other half, there was a "Continue" cue that indicated the person should read the sentence aloud and then provide a logical continuation of it. People were told that it was important to follow the instruction given "because we want to see how the way in which you respond to each sentence affects your performance in later tasks." The results of this study variation experiment are shown in rows (e) and (f) of Table 1.2. The most important finding is that both our younger and our older participants showed significant priming for both study conditions, and there was no overall age difference in the magnitude of the priming. Apparently both the read-aloud and the continue conditions enabled both age groups to establish a meaningful relation among the words in the sentences. This was sufficient to lead the groups to have equivalent implicit associative memory.

This study also demonstrates functional independence of implicit and explicit associative memory. Study condition affected explicit memory just as expected; for both ages, continue instructions led to significantly better *explicit* memory than did read-aloud instructions for cued recall, paired recognition, and item-recognition accuracy. In contrast, for the younger people the magnitude of priming did not vary with study condition, and for the older, there was actually more priming for Read-Aloud sentences than Continue ones.

We have completed two other item-recognition experiments in which we find age similarity in priming when more than one opportunity to study each sentence is given, despite large age differences in explicit associative memory for the same sentences. In one of these (Howard, 1985), the difficulty of the memory task was increased by showing people a list of 36 two-propositional sentences (e.g., THE MEAT FRIED IN THE SKILLET WHILE THE AUTHOR RUBBED HIS STOMACH). Each sentence was presented twice for a total of 30 seconds of study, and participants were instructed to try to understand each sentence for later testing of an unspecified nature. Despite the fact that these sentences are relatively difficult to understand, the results [shown in row (g) of Table 1.2] revealed significant priming for both younger and older people; although the younger people are in the direction of showing more priming than the older, the age difference does not approach significance.

In yet another study, we investigated the longevity of the prime effect over days. Participants were first given three presentations (for a total of 30 seconds) of each of 36 one-proposition sentences of the sort used in our earlier experiments. Then they were given the item-recognition series and an explicit cued-recall test (without feedback) both immediately and after a 3-day delay. The results, which are shown in rows (h) and (i) of Table 1.2, show that on the immediate test there were no age differences in priming. Three days later, both groups still showed significant prime effects, and although there was an age difference favoring the younger, it resulted from, not a decline in priming over days for the older group (who, in fact, showed no significant decline), but instead from an *increase* over days in the effect for the younger.

This increase appears to be because some of the subjects adopted explicit memory strategies (i.e., expecting words from the same sentence to be tested next to each other) during their second day of item-recognition testing.

So far only overall prime effects have been considered, but by breaking down the data further it is also possible to make inferences about the memory structure of what is retained. For example, if a subject has studied the sentence "THE SCARECROW WORE SILK," we can examine directionality of priming by comparing forward priming in which the first noun in a sentence occurs as a prime for the second (e.g., SCARECROW priming SILK) with backward priming, in which the second noun in a sentence occurs as a prime for the first (e.g., SILK priming SCARECROW).

Table 1.3 displays forward and backward priming separately for younger and older participants in our studies. For the most part, the younger people we have tested, like Ratcliff and McKoon's college students (1978) have shown approximately equal forward and backward priming. Our older participants reveal similar results for all the conditions in which there are two or more study opportunities *and* in which the priming test is on the same day as the study of the sentences [i.e., rows (a), (b), (f), and (g)]. However, when either there is only one study of each sentence [rows (c), (d), and (e)] *or* when 3 days elapse between study and testing [row (h)], older people show substantially larger forward than backward priming. The relevant interaction between direction and age is not significant in the one-proposition (Howard et al., 1986) experiment [rows (a) through (c)]. However, it approaches significance ($p = .10$) in the delay study [rows (g) and (h)] and is significant ($p < .02$) in the study variation experiment [rows (d) and (e)]. This age difference in the directional symmetry of priming after minimal study is likely contributing to the differences mentioned earlier between our findings in our original single-presentation study [row (c) of Table 1.2] and those of Rabinowitz (1986) [row (d) of Table 1.2] and of Moscovitch et al. (1986; Experiment 3). We tested forward and backward priming equally often across trials, whereas the other researchers tested only forward priming.

Our two-proposition experiment [row (f) of Table 1.3] is in keeping with the above pattern in revealing equivalent forward and backward priming for both age groups when two studies of each sentence are allowed, but points to another kind of age difference in memory structure. Our younger subjects, like those of Ratcliff and McKoon (1978), were in the direction of showing greater within- than between-proposition priming, whereas our older were not. That is, having studied THE DRAGON SNIFFED THE FUDGE WHILE THE NOOSE CIRCLED HIS NECK, Ratcliff and McKoon's subjects and our own younger subjects revealed greater priming between DRAGON and FUDGE than between NOOSE and FUDGE, but our older subjects did not (see Howard, in press, Table 3, for a summary of the relevant data). Thus our younger subjects appear to be more sensitive than our older to the propositional structure of studied sentences.

TABLE 1.3. Item-Recognition Priming Experiments: Forward Versus Backward Prime Effects

| Study | Number of Presentations | Test Delay (days) | Prime Effects[a] Younger Forward | Younger Backward | Older Forward | Older Backward | Row |
|---|---|---|---|---|---|---|---|
| *One-proposition* | Several | 0 | 82 (11) | 95 (13) | 86 (9) | 116 (12) | (a) |
| Howard et al. (1986) | 2 | 0 | 114 (16) | 59 (9) | 60 (7) | 62 (7) | (b) |
| | 1 | 0 | 133 (16) | 112 (14) | 69 (7) | −64 (−7) | (c) |
| *Study variation* | 1—Read | 0 | 75 (8) | 166 (17) | 374 (36) | 127 (12) | (d) |
| Howard (in preparation) | 1—Continue | 0 | 128 (14) | 174 (19) | 173 (15) | 59 (6) | (e) |
| *Two-proposition* | 2 | 0 | 93 (10) | 103 (11) | 73 (6) | 73 (6) | (f) |
| Howard (1985) | | | | | | | |
| *Delay* | 3 | 0 | 65 (8) | 60 (8) | 85 (8) | 107 (11) | (g) |
| Howard (in preparation) | 3 | 3 | 155 (18) | 151 (18) | 164 (14) | −19 (−2) | (h) |

[a]Prime effect equals control response time minus primed response time. Percent prime effect (in parentheses) equals prime effect divided by control response time.

### Summary

Our studies, using item-recognition priming as a measure of implicit associative memory, led to the following conclusions. First, age differences are less pronounced when implicit rather than explicit tests of associative memory are given. This is based on the fact that we obtained significant age differences in explicit associative memory in *all* our experiments, whereas we obtained significant age differences in associative priming of item recognition in only two experiments [and in one of these, the 3-day delay condition shown in row (i) of Table 1.2, it appeared that explicit memory strategies were contaminating the implicit measure].

Second, associative priming of item recognition is not always age constant. After certain difficult study conditions, the parameters of which have yet to be specified precisely, we find age differences favoring the younger in implicit associative memory.

Third, at least after such low levels of study, the item-recognition priming measure suggests that there are age differences in the structure of what is stored, with the younger people retaining a more abstract (in being nondirectional) representation of the underlying propositional structure of the sentence.

Fourth, the associative priming seen in item recognition is long lived, lasting as long as 3 days for both younger and older people. In fact, in an additional condition in which only younger people were tested (summarized in Howard, in press) we have found priming undiminished after 7 days.

## Studies of Word-Stem Completion

The spelling bias series of studies investigated only implicit item memory, and the item-recognition series focused only on implicit associative memory. For the present series, we adopted a task developed by Graf and Schacter (1985) that makes it possible to assess both types of implicit memory simultaneously. In addition, the measure of implicit associative memory gained from Graf and Schacter's task is based on *all* items presented, not just those correctly recognized, as had been the case for the item-recognition series, and so makes it possible to test the generality of the item-recognition results.

In our experiments using this method (Fry and Howard, 1987), people are first exposed to new associations among normatively unrelated word pairs (e.g., QUEEN–STAIRS, MOLD–HANDLE). We then give several unrelated filler tasks (e.g., WAIS digit/symbol) in order to provide a retention interval of several minutes and also to mask the nature of the implicit memory test to follow. *Implicit memory* is tapped in a word-stem completion task in which participants are asked to complete a word stem, preceded by a stimulus word, with the first word that comes to mind. This task contains four kinds of test trials. In Same-Context-Presented trials (QUEEN–STA_____; MOLD–

HAN______), the word stem is tested with the word with which it was paired during study. In Different-Context-Presented trials (QUEEN–HAN______: MOLD–STA______), the word stem is tested with a stimulus from a different studied pair. On Same-Context-Not-Presented and Different-Context-Not-Presented trials, the test items had not been presented at all during study. We assess the degree of *implicit item memory* by subtracting the percent of correct word-stem completions on Different-Context-Not-Presented trials from that on Different-Context-Presented, since this reflects the advantage conferred by previous study of the item. We assess the degree of *implicit associative memory* by subtracting the percent of completions on Different-Context-Presented trials from that on Same-Context-Presented trials, since this reflects the advantage conferred by testing the word stem in the same context in which it was studied.

Following the word-stem completion test of implicit memory, there are two tests of explicit associative memory. The first is *stimulus-cued recall* in which the stimulus items are presented alone (e.g., QUEEN-____________: MOLD-____________), and the subject is asked to complete the blank with the word that had been paired with the stimulus during study. The second explicit test is *word-stem-cued recall,* in which the stimulus word and the word stem with which it had been studied are presented (e.g., QUEEN-STA______; MOLD-HAN______), and the participant is instructed to complete the word stem with the word with which it had been studied earlier. This measure of explicit memory is of particular interest, because it differs from the test of implicit memory *only* in the instructions given the subject; the test stimuli are identical for the two tests

In our first experiment using this task, during the study phase 20 younger and 20 older participants were shown word pairs printed in all capitals (as in the example), and were given as much time as they liked to make a sentence out of each pair and then to rate (on a scale of 1 to 5) how difficult it was to do so. The main results of the experiment are shown in rows (a) through (c) of Table 1.4. As the columns on the far right indicate, the younger group performed significantly (and substantially) better than the older on both explicit cued recall tests. In contrast, however, there were no significant age differences in either implicit item *or* implicit associative memory.

The study conditions of the first word-stem completion experiment would be likely to maximize learning; not only was the study self-paced, but the sentence-generation task required people to form a meaninglful relation between the words within a pair and to reflect on how difficult it was to do so. Given that we found age differences in associative priming in our item-recognition studies under less optimal study conditions, we wondered whether such an age deficit would also appear with the word-stem completion measure. Therefore, we conducted a second word-stem completion experiment in which the testing conditions were identical to those in the first; however, during study people were presented with sentences containing the nouns (e.g., THE QUEEN FELL DOWN THE STAIRS). Each sentence was

TABLE 1.4. Word-Stem Completion Experiments: Percent Difference Scores Assessing Implicit-Item and Implicit Associative Memory, and Percent Correct Recall for Stimulus-Cued Recall and Word-Stem-Cued Recall

| | Implicit Tests | | Explicit Tests | | |
|---|---|---|---|---|---|
| Age Group | Implicit Item Memory Score[a] | Implicit Associative Memory Score[b] | Stimulus-Cued Recall[c] | Word-Stem-Cued Recall[c] | Row |
| *Experiment 1* | | | | | |
| Younger | 7.5*[d] | 17.0***[d] | 82.2 | 89.7 | (a) |
| Older | 7.5* | 14.0*** | 43.0 | 66.0 | (b) |
| Age diff? | No | No | Yes | Yes | (c) |
| *Experiment 2* | | | | | |
| Younger | 0.0 | 19.5*** | 41.5 | 62.5 | (d) |
| Older | 7.5**[d] | 4.5 | 13.7 | 39.5 | (e) |
| Age diff? | Yes | Yes | Yes | Yes | (f) |

[a]Implicit item memory score equals percent correct completion on Different-Context-Presented trials minus that on Different-Context-Not-Presented in the completion task.
[b]Implicit associative memory score equals percent correct completion on Same-Context-Presented trials minus that on Different-Context-Presented in the completion task.
[c]Cued recall scores indicate percent correct completion on the recall tasks.
[d]Significance levels: *, $p \leq .10$; **, $p < .05$; ***, $p < .01$.

presented in all capitals on an index card, and the critical nouns were not highlighted in any way. While the card was shown, the participant heard the sentence read aloud on a tape and then was given 8 seconds to provide a logical expansion of the sentence.

These study conditions might appear to differ little from those in the first experiment, but the data in rows (d) through (f) of Table 1.4 show that the change in study task did make a difference. Looking first only at the younger participants, we find that explicit recall is much poorer in Experiment 2 than in Experiment 1, particularly for the stimulus-cued recall task (scores of 41.5% and 82.2%, respectively). This is consistent with the notion that the study conditions of Experiment 2 led to less elaborative processing than those of Experiment 1, and hence to poorer explicit associative memory. In contrast, however, the degree of *implicit* associative memory is almost identical for the younger people in the two experiments (scores of 17.0 and 19.5 for Experiments 1 and 2, respectively). This is consistent with Schacter and Graf's (1986) findings; there is functional independence between the implicit and explicit measures of associative memory in that *degree* of semantic elaboration influences them differently.

The data from the older participants showed that the change in study conditions from Experiment 1 to Experiment 2 influenced their *explicit* associative memory much as it affected that of the younger people. However, unlike their younger counterparts, the change influenced their *implicit* associative memory as well. In fact, in Experiment 2 the older group did not show significant implicit associative memory.

There are several potentially important differences between the study conditions in Experiments 1 and 2, and so it will only be possible to isolate the important one(s) by conducting further studies. It appears that, in Experiment 1, the requirement to make a sentence out of the two critical words without a time constraint encouraged participants of both ages to form a meaningful relation between the two words, thus leading both groups to establish a new association in memory. In contrast, in Experiment 2 in which study time was constrained and the to-be-critical words were embedded in a sentence, the younger people were still able to process the meaningful relation (albeit not as well as in Experiment 1), but the older people did not do so. Instead, the older people usually focused on reading the sentence shown them and did not establish a relation between the critical words. This resulted in the older people having (1) unimpaired implicit item memory, which does not require semantic processing, (2) extremely poor explicit cued recall, and (3) poor implicit associative memory. This explanation gains some support from our observation that the actual sentence continuations our older participants produced were poorer than those of the younger people.

The foregoing explanation assumes that the study conditions of Experiment 2 were demanding and that this led our older subjects to allow semantic processing to take second place to superficial physical processing of the stimulus. There is, in fact, one otherwise anomalous aspect of our data that suggests that the conditions were also demanding for the younger people, but that in the semantic-versus-superficial tradeoff they opted for the former. This is the finding that in Experiment 2 our younger people showed no evidence at all of implicit *item* memory. Since such memory is known to be sensitive to physical similarity between study and test (Jacoby & Dallas, 1981), this suggests that the younger people spent little time looking at the words shown (it being possible to simply listen to them), and instead concentrated their energies on processing the meaning.

### Summary

First, in keeping with our studies of spelling bias described above and with the findings of other researchers using other tasks, we find no decline with age in implicit item memory in our studies of word-stem completion. Second, age differences are less pronounced on the word-stem completion test of implicit memory than on explicit tests of associative memory. In our first experiment there was age equivalence on the implicit word-stem completion test even though there were large age differences on an explicit word-stem-cued recall test containing test stimuli identical to those in the implicit test. Third, in keeping with our studies of item recognition, the second word-stem completion experiment shows that age equivalence in implicit associative memory is not always obtained.

## Summary of the Aging of Implicit Memory

The following summary should be viewed as more or less informed speculation, since it is based on a relatively modest number of studies. The purpose is to propose reasonable hypotheses.

In the case of *item memory,* the research reviewed here indicates that the age differences that are usually seen on explicit tests are either reduced or eliminated when memory is tapped using implicit means. This conclusion holds across a wide range of measures of implicit memory, and it suggests that, in the course of normal aging, there is no notable decline either in the likelihood that a familiar external stimulus will activate its relevant concept node or in the longevity of the resulting activation.

The evidence reviewed here indicates that, in the case of *memory for new associations* as well, the age differences that almost always appear on explicit tests are often reduced or eliminated when implicit tests are used. However, under certain study conditions that need to be specified more precisely, there are age deficits in implicit associative memory. We propose that this is because establishing a new associative link requires that some minimal processing capacity be allocated to establishing a relation between the to-be-associated items (Nissen & Bullemer, 1987; Schacter & Graf, 1986). Often, then, the study conditions wil make it likely that adults of all ages will meet this minimal criterion, and it is in these cases that no age differences in implicit associative memory appear. But under some more challenging study conditions, older people will not meet even this minimal criterion, possibly because of an age-related decline either in processing capacity itself, or in the efficiency with which capacity is allocated. It is under these conditions that age differences in implicit associative memory appear.

Research on the aging of implicit memory, like that on the aging of explicit memory (see, for example, the reviews by Burke and Light, 1981; Kausler, 1982), indicates that old age is characterized by increases in both retrieval *and* acquisition (encoding) difficulties. Studies of implicit memory have, however, helped to characterize these deficits more fully. With regard to *acquisition,* the age-related deficit appears to be limited to the formation of *new* associations, perhaps because such formation is capacity-demanding. Thus, it is important to do research on the acquisition (and developing structure) of new traces using implicit measures of associative memory.

With regard to *retrieval,* comparisons of implicit and explicit memory indicate that older people have particular difficulties with deliberate, intentional retrieval of a specific sought-after item (see also Howard, 1987). As Light and Singh (1987) have pointed out, the pattern of age differences and similarities in memory tasks cannot be accounted for simply by assuming that older people need more retrieval support (i.e., retrieval cues containing components of the sought-after item) than younger. In Light and Singh's Experiment 2 and in our first word-stem completion experiment (Fry and Howard, 1987), the implicit and explicit associative memory tests gave identical retrieval cues. The tasks differed only in whether or not instructions for *deliberate* retrieval of a particular earlier stimulus was requested. When such deliberate retrieval was not requested, younger and older performed equally well, but when it was requested, age differences appeared.

Thus, increasing age seems to bring with it a decline in the *conscious control* of retrieval. This decline is not limited to retrieving new material. In fact, one common complaint voiced by the aged (Burke & Harrold, in press; Burke, Worthley, & Martin, 1987; Cowley, 1982; Hebb, 1978; Skinner, 1983) is of an increase in word-finding difficulties for long-known words, the familiar tip-of-the-tongue experience. Such age deficits in word finding are also apparent in standardized tests of naming (e.g., Obler & Albert, 1985). That the sought-after words have not been erased from memory is witnessed by the fact that they later pop to mind spontaneously at least as often for older as for younger people (Burke & Harrold, in press; Burke et al., 1987), and that providing the first few letters of the word enables the older person to produce it as accurately as the younger (Bowles & Poon, 1985).

Thus, comparisons of implicit and explicit memory lead to the hypothesis that the memory deficits of old age are limited to establishing new associations, and, even more, to engaging in conscious, deliberate retrieval of both old and newly learned material. It should be noted that since most of the relevant research on the aging of implicit memory has used verbal materials, it is not yet clear whether this characterization will hold for nonverbal memory as well. It is also of theoretical and practical importance to determine the extent to which this same characterization holds for the memory disorders seen in various clinical populations (see Light and Burke, in press, for a recent review of the relevant evidence).

## Implications for Cognitive Aging

The fact that implicit tests of memory yield patterns of aging that differ from explicit ones, coupled with the fact that the overwhelming majority of studies in cognitive gerontology have relied only on explicit measures, leads to the conclusion that our current picture of cognitive aging is not only incomplete, but distorted. The findings on implicit and explicit memory suggest that we must rethink conclusions we have drawn about many aspects of cognitive aging. Some examples follow.

### Memory

The research reviewed here has demonstrated that whether an implicit or an explicit test is given is a critical determinant of whether or not age differences emerge, perhaps an even *more* critical determinant than the more widely recognized variable of intentional versus incidental study. In fact, comparisons across the studies reviewed here suggest that whether intentional or incidental study instructions were given had little, if any, effect on the patterns of age differences on explicit and implicit memory tests. Therefore, it is at least as important to consider this type-of-test variable as the type-of-study variable. One area in which this might be beneficial concerns the study of memory for noncontent attributes of events, such as their frequency, modality, or spatial location (see review by Kausler, 1985). Appropriate emphasis has been placed on how intentional versus incidental study instructions influence such memory, but the influence of the test type (which is almost always explicit) has not. Indeed, the small age differences found in the memory for such attributes might disappear completely if implicit tests were used.

### Perception

What is known of the aging of perceptual processes is also based primarily on explicit measures. For example, with age there appears to be an increase in the interstimulus interval that is necessary to overcome the effects of backward masking (see reviews by Kline & Schieber, 1985; Plude & Hoyer, 1985), and this is usually taken to indicate that there is an age-related slowing in visual pattern recognition processes, with readout from iconic memory taking longer with advanced age. It is potentially important, however, that the measure of whether the person has avoided the effects of backward masking is typically an *explicit* one; e.g., people are required to report the letters in the original display and if they cannot do so, it is *assumed* that the letters were not recognized. Research with college students using semantic priming as an implicit measure calls this assumption into question, because it shows that explicit detection and recognition measures underestimate what is actually processed. Even when a prime word is pattern-masked such that the observer fails to identify or even detect it, the prime facilitates processing of a subsequent semantically related word (see Holender, 1986, for review). Therefore, it is possible that using such implicit measures in studies of aging would alter some widely accepted conclusions about the time course of perceptual processing.

## Language

Analyses of the aging of language comprehension have, for the most part, depended on explicit measures, in that people are asked to report what they recall or recognize or understand of a paragraph or story. Yet it is clear already from studies of semantic priming (e.g., Burke & Harrold, in press; Burke & Yee, 1984; Cohen & Faulkner, 1983; Howard, in press; Howard et al., 1981) that using implicit measures as well will give a fuller, and perhaps quite different, picure of age differences and similarities in language processes, a point made recently by Light and Burke (in press). Implicit measures are proving useful both for tracking moment-to-moment changes in on-line language comprehension (e.g., Burke & Yee, 1984), and for assessing the subsequent structure of what is stored in memory (e.g., our item-recognition studies above; Howard, in press).

## Thinking

The implicit/explicit distinction is also potentially useful for expanding our understanding of the relatively understudied topic of thinking, a domain again dominated by explicit measures. One area in which a beginning has been made is that of conceptual thinking. Hess and his colleagues (Hess 1982; Hess & Slaughter, 1986a, 1986b) have domonstrated that the large age differences that appear in explicit concept acquisition tasks are reduced or eliminated when implicit acquisition is studied.

## Compensation and Intervention

Attempts at helping older people to reverse or compensate for troublesome cognitive declines have also focused on explicit techniques, since the emphasis has been on teaching explicit strategies for remembering or solving problems (see reviews by Poon, 1985; Poon, Walsh-Sweeney, & Fozard,

1980). These approaches have met with some success, but intervention might be even more effective if it were supplemented by methods that exploit implicit memory and acquisition processes. For example, Schacter and Glisky (in press; Glisky, Schacter, & Tulving, 1986) have demonstrated that remediation techniques (such as a method of vanishing cues) that call on amnesic patients' preserved implicit memory abilities enable them to learn relatively complex computer skills.

### Summary

The foregoing examples are only that. They are meant to illustrate that the dissociations between implicit and explicit measures should lead us to take a new look at virtually all of what we *think* we know about the nature of cognitive aging.

*Acknowledgments.* This research was supported by Grants R23 AG00713 and R01 AG02751 awarded by the National Institute on Aging. I am happy to acknowledge the contributions of the following undergraduate research assistants: Maria Acosta, Lisa Conomy, Martha Farmelo, Astrid Fry, Christina Emanuel, Holly Gomes, Jane Gillette Heisey, Mary Beth Quig, Raymond Shaw, Cathy Stanger, Tom Steif, Lisa Swartz, Paige Wilhite, and Bob Zozus. I am also grateful to Jim Howard for many suggestions on this research and for comments on the manuscript.

## References

Anderson, J.R. (1983). A spreading activation theory of memory. *Journal of Verbal Learning and Verbal Behavior, 22,* 261–295.

Balota, D.A., & Duchek, J.M. (1988). Age-related differences in lexical access, spreading activation and simple pronunciation. *Psychology and Aging, 3,* 84–93.

Bowles, N.L., & Poon, L.W. (1985). Aging and retrieval of words in semantic memory. *Journal of Gerontology, 40,* 71–77.

Britton, B.K. (1976). Semantic encoding stability and context. *Journal of Experimental Psychology: Human Learning and Memory, 2,* 69–75.

Burke, D.M., & Harrold, R.M. (in press). Approaches to the study of language and memory in old age. To appear in L.L. Light & D.M. Burke (Eds.), *Language, memory, and aging.* New York: Cambridge University Press.

Burke, D.M., & Light, L.L. (1981). Memory and aging: The role of retrieval processes. *Psychological Bulletin, 90,* 513–546.

Burke, D.M., White, H., & Diaz, D.L. (1987). Semantic priming in young and older adults: Evidence for age constancy in automatic and attentional processes. *Journal of Experimental Psychology: Human Perception and Performance, 13,* 79–88.

Burke, D.M., Worthley, J., & Martin, J. (1987). *I'll never forget what's-her-name: Aging and tip of the tongue experiences in everyday life.* Presented at the Second International Conference on Practical Aspects of Memory, Swansea, Wales.

Burke, D.M., & Yee, P.L. (1984). Semantic priming during sentence processing by young and older adults. *Developmental Psychology, 20,* 903–910.
Cerella, J., & Fozard, J.L. (1984). Lexical access and age. *Developmental Psychology, 20,* 235–243.
Chiarello, C., Church, K.L., & Hoyer, W.J. (1985). Automatic and controlled semantic priming: Accuracy, response bias, and aging. *Journal of Gerontology, 40,* 593–600.
Cohen, G., & Faulkner, D. (1983). Word recognition: Age differences in contextual facilitation effects. *British Journal of Psychology, 74,* 239–251.
Cohen, N.J. (1984). Preserved learning capacity in amnesia: Evidence for multiple memory systems. In L.R. Squire & N. Butters (Eds.), *Neuropsychology of memory* (pp. 83–103). New York: Guilford Press.
Cohen, N.J., & Squire, L.R. (1980). Preserved learning and retention of pattern-analyzing skill in amnesia: Dissociation of "knowing how" and "knowing that." *Science, 210,* 207–209.
Collins, A.M., & Loftus, E.F. (1975). A spreading-activation theory of semantic processing. *Psychological Review, 82,* 407–428.
Cowley, M. (1982). *The view from 80.* New York: Penguin Books.
Craik, F.I.M. (1985). Paradigms in human memory research. In L.G. Nilsson & T. Archer (Eds.), *Perspectives on learning and memory* (pp. 197–221). Hillsdale, NJ: Erlbaum.
Craik, F.I.M., & Simon, E. (1980). Age differences in memory: The roles of attention and depth of processing. In L.W. Poon, J.L. Fozard, L.S. Cermak, D. Arenberg, & L.W. Thompson (Eds.), *New directions in memory and aging: Proceedings of the George A. Talland Memorial Conference* (pp. 95–112). Hillsdale, NJ: Erlbaum.
Eich, E. (1984). Memory for unattended events: Remembering with and without awareness. *Memory & Cognition, 12,* 105–111.
Eysenck, M.W. (1974). Age differences in incidental learning. *Developmental Psychology, 10,* 936–941.
Fry, A., & Howard, D.V. (1987). *Adult age differences in implicit and explicit memory for printed material.* Presented at the Second International Congress of Applied Psycholinguistics, Kassel, Federal Republic of Germany.
Glisky, E.L., Schacter, D.L., & Tulving, E. (1986). Computer learning by memory-impaired patients: Acquisition and retention of complex knowledge. *Neuropsychologia, 24,* 313–328.
Graf, P., & Mandler, G. (1984). Activation makes words more accessible, but not necessarily more retrievable. *Journal of Verbal Learning and Verbal Behavior, 23,* 553–568.
Graf, P., & Schacter, D.L. (1985). Implicit and explicit memory for new associations in normal and amnesic subjects. *Journal of Experimental Psychology: Learning, Memory, and Cognition, 11,* 501–518.
Graf, P., & Schacter, D.L. (1987). Selective effects of interference on implicit and explicit memory for new associations. *Journal of Experimental Psychology: Learning, Memory, and Cognition, 13,* 45–53.
Graf, P., Shimamura, A.P., & Squire, L.R. (1985). Priming across modalities and priming across category levels: Extending the domain of preserved function in amnesia. *Journal of Experimental Psychology: Learning, Memory, and Cognition, 11,* 386–396.
Hasher, L., & Zacks, R.T. (1979). Automatic and effortful processes in memory. *Journal of Experimental Psychology: General, 108,* 356–388.

Hebb, D.O. (1978). On watching myself get old. *Psychology Today,* 15-23.

Hess, T.M. (1982). Visual abstraction processes in young and old adults. *Developmental Psychology, 18,* 473-484.

Hess, T.M., & Slaughter, S.J. (1986a). Aging effects of prototype abstraction and concept identification. *Journal of Gerontology, 41,* 214-221.

Hess, T.M., & Slaughter, S.J. (1986b). Specific exemplar retention and prototype abstraction in young and old adults. *Psychology and Aging, 1,* 202-207.

Holender, D. (1986). Semantic activation without conscious identification in dichotic listening, parafoveal vision, and visual masking: A survey and appraisal. *The Behavioral and Brain Sciences, 9,* 1-66.

Howard, D.V. (1983). The effects of aging and degree of association on the semantic priming of lexical decisions. *Experimental Aging Research, 9,* 145-151.

Howard, D.V. (1985). *Aging and episodic priming: The propositional structure of sentences.* Presented at the meetings of the American Psychological Association, Los Angeles, CA.

Howard, D.V. (1986a). *Implicit memory and aging: Effects of delay on spelling bias.* Presented at the meetings of the American Psychological Association, Washington, D.C.

Howard, D.V. (1986b). *The aging of implicit memory.* Presented at the meetings of the Psychonomic Society, New Orleans, LA.

Howard, D.V. (1987). *Semantic organization: Overview and theoretical issues.* Paper presented at the First Annual Meeting of the Cognitive Aging Conference, Atlanta, GA.

Howard, D.V. (in press). Aging and memory activation: The priming of semantic and episodic memories. To appear in L.L. Light & D.M. Burke (Eds.), *Language, memory, and aging.* New York: Cambridge University Press.

Howard, D.V., Heisey, J.G., & Shaw, R.J. (1986). Aging and the priming of newly learned associations. *Developmental Psychology, 22,* 78-85.

Howard, D.V., Lasaga, M.I., & McAndrews, M.P. (1980). Semantic activation during memory encoding across the adult lifespan. *Journal of Gerontology, 35,* 884-890.

Howard, D.V., McAndrews, M.P., & Lasaga, M.I. (1981). Semantic priming of lexical decisions in young and old adults. *Journal of Gerontology, 36,* 707-714.

Jacoby, L.L. (1983). Perceptual enhancement: Persistent effects of an experience. *Journal of Experimental Psychology: Learning, Memory, and Cognition, 9,* 23-38.

Jacoby, L.L., & Dallas, M. (1981). On the relationship between autobiographical memory and perceptual learning. *Journal of Experimental Psychology: General, 110,* 306-340.

Jacoby, L.L., & Witherspoon, D. (1982). Remembering without awareness. *Canadian Journal of Psychology, 36,* 300-324.

Kausler, D.H. (1982). *Experimental psychology and human aging.* New York: Wiley.

Kausler, D.H. (1985). Episodic memory: Memorizing performance. In N. Charness (Ed.), *Aging and human performance* (pp. 101-141). New York: Wiley.

Kline, D.W., & Schieber, F. (1985). Vision and aging. In J.E. Birren & K.W. Schaie (Eds.), *Handbook of the psychology of aging* (2nd ed., pp. 296-331). New York: Van Nostrand Reinhold.

Knopman, D.S., & Nissen, M.J. (1987). Implicit learning in patients with probable Alzheimer's Disease. *Neurology, 37,* 784-788.

Light, L.L. (1987) *Preserved implicit memory in old age.* Presented at the Second International Conference on Practical Aspects of Memory, Swansea, Wales.

Light, L.L., & Burke, D.M. (in press). Patterns of language and memory in old age. To

appear in L.L. Light & D.M. Burke (Eds.), *Language, memory, and aging.* New York: Cambridge University Press.
Light, L.L., & Singh, A. (1987). Implicit and explicit memory in young and older adults. *Journal of Experimental Psychology: Learning, Memory, and Cognition, 13,* 531–541.
Light, L.L., Singh, A., & Capps, J.L. (1986). The dissociation of memory and awareness in young and older adults. *Journal of Clinical Neuropsychology, 8,* 62–74.
Madden, D.J. (1986). Adult age differences in visual word recognition: Semantic encoding and episodic retention. *Experimental Aging Research, 12,* 71–78.
McKoon, G., & Ratcliff, R. (1979). Priming in episodic and semantic memory. *Journal of Verbal Learning and Verbal Behavior, 18,* 463–480.
Mishkin, M., & Petri, H.L. (1984). Memories and habits: Some implications for the analysis of learning and retention. In L.R. Squire & N. Butters (Eds.), *Neuropsychology of memory* (pp. 287–296). New York: Guidford Press.
Moscovitch, M. (1982). A neuropsychological approach to perception and memory in normal and pathological aging. In F.I.M. Craik & S. Trehub (Eds.), *Aging and cognitive processes* (pp. 55–78). New York: Plenum Press.
Moscovitch, M., Winocur, G., & McLachlan, D. (1986). Memory as assessed by recognition and reading time in normal and memory-impaired people with Alzheimer's disease and other neurological disorders. *Journal of Experimental Psycology: General, 115,* 331–347.
Nissen, M.J., & Bullemer, P. (1987). Attentional requirements of learning: Evidence from performance measures. *Cognitive Psychology, 19,* 1–32.
Obler, L.K., & Albert, M.L. (1985). Language skills across adulthood. In J.E. Birren & K.W. Schaie (Eds.), *Handbook of the psychology of aging* (2nd ed., pp. 463–473). New York: Van Nostrand Reinhold.
Plude, D.J., & Hoyer, W.J. (1985). Attention and performance: Identifying and localizing age deficits. In N. Charness (Ed.), *Aging and human performance* (pp. 47–99). New York: Wiley.
Poon, L.W. (1985). Differences in human memory with aging: Nature, causes, and clinical implications. In J.E. Birren & K.W. Schaie (Eds.), *Handbook of the psychology of aging* (2nd ed., pp. 427–462). New York: Van Nostrand Reinhold.
Poon, L.W., Walsh-Sweeney, L., & Fozard, J.L. (1980). Memory skill training for the elderly: Salient issues on the use of imagery mnemonics. In L.W. Poon, J.L. Fozard, L.S. Cermak, D. Arenberg, & L.W. Thompson (Eds.), *New directions in memory and aging: Proceedings of the George A. Talland Memorial Conference.* (pp. 461–484) Hillsdale, NJ: Erlbaum.
Rabinowitz, J.C. (1986). Priming in episodic memory. *Journal of Gerontology, 41,* 204–213.
Rabbitt, P.M.A. (1982). How do old people know what to do next? In F.I.M. Craik & S. Trehub (Eds.), *Aging and cognitive processes* (pp. 79–98). New York: Plenum Press.
Ratcliff, R., & McKoon, G. (1978). Priming in item recognition: Evidence for the propositional structure of sentences. *Journal of Verbal Learning and Verbal Behavior, 17,* 403–417.
Rose, T.L., Yesavage, J.A., Hill, R.D., & Bower, G.H. (1986). Priming effects and recognition memory in young and elderly adults. *Experimental Aging Research, 12,* 31–37.
Salthouse, T.A. (1985). *A theory of cognitive aging.* Amsterdam: North-Holland.

Schacter, D.L. (1985). Priming of old and new knowledge in amnesic patients and normal subjects. *Annals of the New York Academy of Sciences, 444,* 41–53.
Schacter, D.L. (1987). Implicit memory: History and current status. *Journal of Experimental Psychology: Learning, Memory, and Cognition, 13,* 501–518.
Schacter, D.L., & Glisky, E.L. (in press). Memory remediation: Restoration, alleviation and the acquisition of domain-specific knowledge. In B. Uzzell & Y. Gross (Eds.), *Clinical neuropsychology of intervention.* Boston: Martinus Nijhoff.
Schacter, D.L., & Graf, P. (1986). Effects of elaborative processing on implicit and explicit memory for new associations. *Journal of Experimental Psychology: Learning, Memory, and Cognition, 12,* 432–444.
Skinner, B.F. (1983). Intellectual self-management in old age. *American Psychologist, 38,* 239–244.
Shimamura, A.P., Salmon, D.P., Squire, L.R., & Butters, N. (1987). Memory dysfunction and word priming in dementia and amnesia. *Behavioral Neuroscience, 101,* 347–351.
Tulving, E. (1984). How many memory systems are there? *American Psychologist, 40,* 385–398.
Tulving, E., Schacter, D.L., & Stark, H.A. (1982). Priming effects in word-fragment completion are independent of recognition memory. *Journal of Experimental Psychology: Learning, Memory, and Cognition, 8,* 336–342.
Woodruff-Pak, D.S. (1987). *Parallel studies of classical conditioning and aging in rabbits and humans.* Paper presented at the First Annual Meeting of the Cognitive Aging Conference, Atlanta, GA.
Zajonc, R.B. (1984). On the primacy of affect. *American Psychologist, 39,* 117–123.

# 2. Measuring Memory Development in Adulthood: A Model-Based Approach to Disentangling Storage–Retrieval Contributions

*Mark L. Howe*

As everyone knows, and as this volume clearly attests, the ability to process information undergoes substantial change throughout adulthood. Although considerable variability exists in the rates at which these cognitive functions develop in adulthood (e.g., Baltes & Willis, 1982; Denney, 1984), a number of writers have speculated that changes observed on specific cognitive tasks (e.g., episodic memory, speeded classification, problem solving, decision making, etc.) are actually the consequence of changes in some general or common component that uniformly alters information-processing abilities (e.g., slows, produces more errors, etc.) (cf. Cerella, 1985; Hasher & Zacks, 1979; Salthouse, 1982, and this volume). Others have suggested that these developments may be brought about by age-related changes in a number of different factors (e.g., spontaneous strategic processing [Perlmutter & Mitchell, 1982], attentional resources [Craik & Byrd, 1982], etc.).

Although it is by no means clear whether a single- or multifactor theory will provide an adequate explanation of the aging of cognitive functioning, it is clear that most if not all intellectual and cognitive functions depend heavily on processes that control the availability and accessibility of information in long-term memory. Indeed, it has been argued that the changes in general cognitive functioning may derive, at least in part, from corresponding changes in the underlying input and output mechanisms of memory (cf. Botwinick, 1977; Horn, 1982; Howe & Hunter, 1986). It would appear, therefore, that a comprehensive theory about the development of general cognitive abilities in adulthood should include some understanding of parallel developments that occur in long-term memory.

In the literature on memory development in adulthood, it is common knowledge that aging is associated with marked declines in performance on many if not all memory tasks. Although a considerable body of research has documented these developmental decrements in memorization (see reviews in Burke & Light, 1981; Craik, 1977; Craik & Byrd, 1982; Craik & Rabinowitz, 1984; Howe & Hunter, 1986; Kausler, 1982, 1985; Poon, 1985; Salthouse, 1982; Smith, 1980), there is little concensus concerning the source(s) of these age-related changes in memory. Agreement does exist, however, concerning the importance of measuring the relative contribution of storage and retrieval processes to overall memory development in adulthood. Indeed, one of the dominant themes in current theorizing about memory development, both in childhood and adulthood, concerns the extent to which age differences in memory are primarily the result changes in storage processes, changes in retrieval processes, or both (Brainerd, 1985a; Burke & Light, 1981; Howe & Hunter, 1985, 1986; Poon, 1985).

The distinction between processes that lead to the formation of long-term memory traces, known collectively as storage, and processes that mediate recovery of such traces, known collectively as retrieval, has a long tradition and is central to current theories of memory. Consistent with information-processing views of memory, a number of investigators have suggested that the aging of memory can be best understood in terms of some form of reduction in the execution of the basic memory processes of storage and retrieval (e.g., Burke & Light, 1981; Craik & Rabinowitz, 1984; Duchek, 1984; Howe & Hunter, 1985, 1986; Smith, 1980). Unfortunately, tests of specific hypotheses about these processing declines have remained somewhat elusive. This is because it has often proved difficult to disentangle the storage and retrieval components of long-term memory (see discussions in Howe & Hunter, 1985, 1986; Poon, 1985).

In the present chapter, I discuss the importance of the storage–retrieval distinction in understanding memory development in adulthood. As the chapter unfolds, the discussion focuses on some of the difficulties that are encountered when attempting to segregate storage and retrieval processes in recall data, and a recently developed model-based approach to disentangling these processes is presented. Finally, the extent to which developmental differences in adult memory functioning can be attributed to decrements in storage processes, retrieval processes, or both is examined in a series of eight previously unreported experiments that examined developmental differences in free and cued recall of verbal material in young and old adult long-term memory.

## On the Measurement of Storage and Retrieval Processes

The importance of the storage–retrieval distinction in both memory data and theory has been recognized for some time. Indeed, it is generally accepted that contemporary explanations of developmental changes in memory must, at the very least, account for developmental variations in storage and retrieval processes. The one issue that has not been adequately addressed, and which serves as the focus of this chapter, concerns the manner in which these changes are measured. In particular, a procedure is required that permits the segregation of storage and retrieval processes on equally sensitive, but independent, scales of measurement. In this way, precise quantitative estimates of the extent (magnitude) to which the development of these processes is differentially accelerated can be obtained.

The disentangling of storage and retrieval processes has presented an enigma for some time. Traditionally, the separation of these process variables has been considered a problem in experimental design. To illustrate, consider a standard episodic memory task in which subjects are given an opportunity to study the to-be-remembered material followed by a test (e.g., recognition, recall) of that material. Here, it is assumed that storage factors are relatively more important on study trials than test trials and, conversely, that retrieval factors are relatively more important on test trials than study trials. According to this logic, the effects of some variable on the storage and retrieval components of long-term memory can be isolated by independently manipulating it on study and test trials in some factorial design. If the manipulated variable has a larger effect on study trials than on test trials, it is concluded that this factor predominantly affects storage, whereas if this manipulation has a larger effect on test trials than study trials, it is concluded that the manipulated factor primarily affects retrieval.

Design-based approaches to disentangling storage and retrieval effects in long-term memory have tended to dominate the memory literature. It is not surprising, therefore, that this approach is also the mainstay in the literature on memory development. Indeed, the adult literature is replete with examples of attempts to isolate storage and retrieval effects using design-based strategies. For example, list-learning studies that have examined age differences in organized memory have factorially varied the presence or absence of category labels on study and test trials (e.g., Hultsch & Craig, 1976; Smith, 1977). Although age differences do not disappear completely, they are considerably reduced in the presence of retrieval cues. The bulk of these studies report greater reductions when cues were presented on test trials, although others have reported reductions when cues were presented on study trials. The general conclusion from this line of research is that there is a considerable retrieval deficit for elderly adults, although retrieval alone may not account for the entire decline observed in aging memory (for review, see Burke & Light, 1981; Guttentag, 1985; Poon, 1985).

Some memory researchers recently pointed out that the logic underlying this design-based strategy of separating storage and retrieval effects is intrinsically flawed. Specifically, it appears that a number of unresolved measurement and scaling issues complicate the interpretation of storage and retrieval effects when isolated in this manner (e.g., Brainerd, 1985a; Chechile, Richman, Topinka, & Ehrensbeck, 1981). In general, these problems arise because differentiating storage and retrieval processes is tantamount to differentiating theoretical constructs, not empirical variables. What is critical, therefore, is knowledge about the scale of measurement that is associated with the memory task. More particularly, it does not suffice to simply assume that performance measures are monotonically related to theoretical constructs of storage and retrieval by some function whose properties and structure are unknown. Rather, what is needed is knowledge of the precise nature of the scaling assumptions that are permitted in order that the rule(s) that maps changes in performance (empirical data) onto changes in storage and retrieval (theoretical constructs) can be determined.

When these rules have not been explicitly specified, it is impossible to know, for example, whether a smaller effect on study than test trials (performance outcome) is really caused by a corresponding smaller impact of this variable on storage than retrieval (theoretical conclusion). This is because, depending on one's scaling assumptions, it is entirely possible to obtain this result under conditions in which the impact of this variable is actually larger at retrieval than at storage (see examples in Brainerd, 1985a). The critical point is that when the functional rules that map theoretical constructs onto performance outcomes are unknown (or unspecified), it is essentially impossible to determine how a particular outcome is related to these underlying theoretical constructs. Because it is the set of theoretical constructs that provide the impetus for research, failures to specify how they are to be measured surely defeats the primary purpose of any study. Clearly, then, design-based approaches to disentangling storage–retrieval contributions to memory development tend to be inadequate in the absence of serious scaling considerations.[1]

In light of these concerns, it would seem prudent when studying memory development to secure a technique in which the nature of the mapping function is well known. It is perhaps obvious that model-based approaches to separating storage and retrieval factors are a natural choice because models contain precise mathematical statements concerning the assumed underlying scale of measurement. That is, observable outcomes are mapped onto theoretical constructs (in this case storage and retrieval) by well-defined algebraic functions. This permits the precise measurement of theoretical processes on a common ratio scale (Brainerd, 1985a; Chechile et al., 1981). Recent advances in mathematical modeling techniques have provided a

[1]These measurement and scaling problems refer not only to the study-test example given here, but apply equally to other familiar techniques (e.g., comparing performance on recognition-recall tasks) thought to isolate storage and retrieval. In general, these problems are common in any design-based paradigm in which the scale of measurement and rules governing the relationship between theoretical memory constructs and empirical performance variables remain unspecified. Readers interested in a more detailed discussion of this problem, including several worked examples in the area of children's memory development, should consult Brainerd (1985a).

number of useful procedures, each of which is uniquely suited to the study of different (developmental) aspects of human memory. For example, there are procedures for studying short-term memory (Chechile & Meyer, 1976; Chechile & Richman, 1982), procedures for studying repeated recall and forgetting (e.g., Brainerd, Kingma, & Howe, 1985; Howe & Hunter, 1986; Wilkinson & Koestler, 1983, 1984), and procedures for studying long-term memory (Brainerd, Howe, & Kingma, 1982; Howe & Hunter, 1985, 1986). Because these different models have recently been reviewed (Brainerd, 1985a), and because this chapter focuses on the contribution of storage and retrieval to the development of long-term memory in adulthood, the remainder of the chapter considers the explication of the latter two-stage model of long-term memory as a method of factoring storage and retrieval processes.

Before turning to a description of this model, it is important to note that modeling approaches contain a number of specific assumptions, as does the design-based approach. However, these assumptions are algebraic in nature, thus more tractable, and unlike the assumptions in design-based approaches are subject to disconfirmation. Specifically, assumptions concerning the appropriateness of a particular mathematical model can be examined empirically either through validity or goodness-of-fit tests. It is only when a model is found to provide an acceptable account of the set of observable outcomes under study that it can be used to dissect performance according to the relevant theoretical constructs. Thus, although it is often difficult to rule out qualitative theories that rely on design-based separations of theoretical constructs, testing the assumptions of a quantitative theory is an integral part of the modeling approach.

## Overview of the Two-Stage Model of Memory

Two-stage (three-state) Markov models have been used with considerable success to address a number of problems in psychology (for review, see Greeno, 1974). Although different versions exist within this general class of models, varying both in terms of their complexity (as measured by the number of free parameters) and in terms of their domain of applicability (from animal conditioning studies [e.g., Theios, 1963] to learning to search in infancy [Heth & Cornell, 1983], to children's learning of logical concepts [Brainerd, 1982]), the use of two-stage models to measure storage and retrieval began nearly two decades ago with the work of Greeno and colleagues (Greeno, 1968, 1974; Humphreys & Greeno, 1970). The most recent implementation of this model (an 11-parameter version developed in Brainerd et al., 1982) has been used to partition storage and retrieval processes in episodic list-learning tasks involving children (both normally achieving [Brainerd, Howe, Kingma, & Brainerd, 1984a; Brainerd, Kingma, & Howe, 1986a; Howe, Brainerd, & Kingma, 1985a] and learning-disabled elementary schoolers [Brainerd, Kingma, & Howe, 1986b; Howe, Brainerd, & Kingma,

1985b]), college students (Brainerd et al., 1982; Brainerd, Howe, Kingma, & Brainerd, 1984b; Howe, 1987), and young and old adults (Howe & Hunter, 1985, 1986). Indeed, when strict criterion acquisition procedures are in place, it turns out that performance on most, if not all, long-term memory tasks (e.g., free and cued recall, paired-associate and serial learning, etc.) are well described by this two-stage mathematical system. I present a description of this system in both the context of an abstract memorization system and in terms of its storage and retrieval interpretation.[2]

In the two-stage model performance on episodic memory tasks in which subjects are required to reach a memory criterion of perfect recall is partitioned into three levels or states: (1) an "unmemorized" state U in which the probability of a correct response is 0; (2) a "partially memorized" state P in which both errors and successes occur and a correct response occurs with some average probability $0 < p < 1$; and (3) a "memorized" state M in which the probability of a correct response is 1. Improvement in performance (i.e., memorization) is described in terms of a discrete forward progression through these states until the list has been mastered.

This process of memorization is captured by 11 parameters whose theoretical definitions are summarized in Table 2.1. Seven of these parameters are *memorization* or *learning* parameters that measure the difficulty of escaping state U ($a'$, $a$, and $1$-$f$) and state P ($b'$, $b$, $c$, and $d$), and 4 are *performance* parameters that measure steady-state recall in state P ($1-r$, $1-e$, $g$, and $h$). At both a theoretical and an empirical level, these parameters have been mapped onto current cognitive models that factor memorization stages into a storage component and a retrieval component (Brainerd, 1985b; Greeno, James, DaPolito, & Polson, 1978; Halff, 1977; Howe, 1985). At a formal level, it is clear that memorization (arrival in state M) consists of two events or stages, namely, escape from states U and P. The first stage of memorization (escape from state U) is said to consist of storing a trace in long-term memory and the second stage (escape from state P) is said to consist of learning how to retrieve it in a reliable manner.

Consider storage first. As in other memory models (Estes, 1986; Flexser & Tulving, 1978; Greeno et al., 1978), it is assumed that information about concepts on a list is stored in a long-term memory trace (e.g., an array or matrix) that consists of feature or attribute values. Because most episodic memory tasks contain controls that ensure that a correct response cannot be made on the basis of output from short-term memory (e.g., inserting buffer activity between study and test trials, using supraspan lists, random presentation of materials), a correct response must be based on a representation of that item

---

[2]Note: The algebraic mechanics of this model, as well as the corresponding proofs, are tedious and space consuming to report, are readily available in a number of previous publications, and are not necessary to understand the basic operation of this model; therefore, specific mathematical details are not presented. Readers interested in the underlying mathematical details should consult Brainerd et al. (1982).

TABLE 2.1. Theoretical Definitions of Two-Stage Model Parameters

| Process and Parameter | Theoretical Definition |
|---|---|
| Storage | |
| $a'$ | Probability of storing an item on the first trial |
| $a$ | Probability of storing an item on any trial after the first trial |
| $1-f$ | Probability that a stored item remains in storage between the first and second test trials |
| Algorithmic Retrieval | |
| $b'$ | Probability of simultaneously acquiring a retrieval algorithm for an item that was stored on the first trial |
| $b$ | Probability of simultaneously acquiring a retrieval algorithm for items stored on any trial after the first one |
| $c$ | For any item where a retrieval algorithm was not available at the time of storage, the probability that a retrieval algorithm is acquired following a correct response |
| $d$ | For any item where a retrieval algorithm was not available at the time of storage, the probability that a retrieval algorithm is acquired following an incorrect response |
| Heuristic Retrieval | |
| $1-r$ | For any item stored on the first trial where recall is mediated by heuristic not algorithmic retrieval processes, the probability of a correct response |
| $1-e$ | For any item stored on any trial after the first trial where recall is mediated by heuristic not algorithmic retrieval processes, the probability of a correct response |
| $g$ | For any two consecutive test trials mediated by heuristic retrieval, the probability the an error is followed by a success |
| $h$ | For any two consecutive test trials mediated by heuristic retrieval, the probability that a success is followed by another success |

that has been stored in long-term memory. Therefore, it can be assumed that a change in performance from no correct responding to at least some correct responding (i.e., escape from state U) is mediated by storage processes. It follows that the parameters $a'$ and $a$, which give the probability of escaping state U on the first and subsequent study trials, respectively, reflect the difficulty of storing a trace in long-term memory in the early (Trial 1) and later phases of memorization. A third parameter, $1 - f$, measures the difficulty of retaining a stored trace early in the memorization process (i.e., between the first and second test trials).

Simply storing a trace in long-term memory does not guarantee that the information contained in that representation can be retrieved reliably on subsequent recall attempts. The remaining stage in the memorization process (escape from state P), therefore, is identified with processes involved in retrieval of information. Here, recall can occur with one of two probabilities—either with probability 1 (arrival in state M), in which case memorization is complete, or with some probability that while greater than zero is less than one (state P). In this latter case, further work must be done in order to memorize that item (Halff, 1977; Howe, 1985). These two types of retrieval have been referred to as *algorithmic* and *heuristic*, respectively (Halff, 1977; Howe, 1985). This distinction is primarily structural, not theoretical. Simply put, algorithmic retrieval consists of any operation that produces errorless recall, and heuristic retrieval consists of any operation that produces both recall successes and failures. If memorization is not complete, and recall is mediated by heuristic retrieval operations, the result is steady-state recall in the "partially memorized" state P, in which the probability of a correct response is measured by the parameters $1 - e$ and $1 - r$ on the first trial and by $g$ and $h$ for subsequent trials following an error or a success, respectively. Alternatively, the parameters $b'$ and $b$ give the probability that a retrieval algorithm is available at the time a trace was stored, on the first test trial and subsequent test trials, respectively. The parameters $c$ and $d$ give the probability that a retrieval algorithm is acquired sometime after storage is complete, following a successful or an unsuccessful heuristic retrieval attempt, respectively.

To summarize, memorization is partitioned into two events or stages, namely storage and retrieval. These events are mapped onto three levels of performance that are commonly observed in long-term memory tasks: state U, an item is not in storage and correct responding occurs with probability 0; state P, an item has been stored but because an algorithmic retrieval operation is not available, recall is mediated by heuristic retrieval in which the average probability of a correct response is $0 < p < 1$; and state M, an item is both stored and a retrieval algorithm that produces recall with probability 1 is available. Finally, in addition to providing independent measures of storage (the parameters $a'$, $a$, and $1 - f$), heuristic retrieval (the parameters $1 - r$, $1 - e$, $g$, and $h$), and algorithmic retrieval (the parameters $b'$, $b$, $c$, and $d$), three of these parameters (one from each of these groupings, namely, $a'$, $1 - r$, and $b'$) provide a measure of the difficulty of storage and retrieval early in the memorization process (Trial 1), whereas the remaining eight parameters measure the difficulty of storage and retrieval processes later in the memorization process (i.e., all subsequent trials to criterion).

# Current Research

In this section, the two-stage model is used to identify the storage and retrieval loci of developmental differences in young and elderly adult long-term memory. Eight episodic memory experiments were conducted, each of which was concerned with a somewhat different aspect of age-related declines in verbal long-term memory. Specifically, Experiments 1 through 4 were concerned with developmental differences in memory for concrete material that was either easy or hard (as measured by high and low meaningfulness ratings; Experiments 1 and 2, respectively) and abstract material that was either easy or hard (again, as reflected in high and low meaningfulness ratings; Experiments 3 and 4, respectively). Experiments 5 through 8 were concerned with developmental differences in free recall of organized material that varied in the number (two or four) of categories (Experiments 5 and 6, respectively) and cued recall of organized material that also varied in the number (two or four) of categories (Experiments 7 and 8). In order to avoid repetition, details concerning subjects, lists, and procedures that are common to all of the experiments are presented before the individual experiments themselves. Following this, each group of experiments will be described separately, including any methodological points that are unique to a given study.

## General Methodology

### Subjects

The subjects in Experiments 1 through 4 were 100 (43 males, 57 females) undergraduate students (age: M = 22 years, 2 months; SD = 3 years, 11 months) and 80 (24 males, 56 females) senior citizens (age: M = 69 years, 5 months; SD = 6 years, 11 months). The subjects in Experiments 5 through 8 were 120 (50 males, 70 females) undergraduate students (age: M = 21 years, 9 months; SD = 3 years, 8 months) and 80 (33 males, 47 females) senior citizens (age: M = 70 years, 2 months; SD = 6 years, 4 months). All subjects participated on a voluntary basis; the younger subjects were drawn from a university subject pool, and the elderly subjects from a pool of volunteers from the surrounding community. All of the older subjects were healthy, self-sufficient, and living in their own homes. Like the university sample, many of the elderly adults were not native residents of the city (i.e., they had moved there for retirement purposes from many other Canadian cities). All subjects were tested individually, with the younger subjects being tested in a university laboratory and the elderly subjects being tested in a quiet room in their homes.

## Lists and Procedure

In all experiments, subjects were required to memorize a 16-item word list. The words for Experiments 1 through 4 were drawn from the Toglia and Battig (1978) semantic word norms, and the words for Experiments 5 through 8 were drawn from the Battig and Montague (1969) production frequency norms (see Howard [1980] for the applicability of these norms in aging research).

Regardless of whether a free (Experiments 1 through 6) or cued (Experiments 7 through 8) recall procedure was employed, all subjects were tested using a standard episodic memorization paradigm that consisted of an alternating sequence of study-distractor-test cycles.[3] On each study trial, words were presented visually, one at a time in random order, at a 5-second rate. After the 16 items had been presented, subjects engaged in 30 seconds of distractor activity (circling pairs of letters as quickly as possible on a sheet of paper), to avoid possible short-term memory effects. Following completion of this buffer activity, subjects in the free recall experiments were required to orally recall as many of the items from the list as possible. A test trial was terminated, and a new cycle begun, when 20 seconds had elapsed without an item being recalled. Subjects in the cued recall experiments were given the category labels (in a random sequential order that varied across test trials) and asked to recall all the items that belonged to that category. For each category, recall continued until 20 seconds had elapsed without the production of a word, at which time either another category label was presented or a new cycle begun. This study-distractor-test procedure was continued until the subject was able to reach a criterion of perfect recall on two consecutive test trials.

## Experiments 1 Through 4

The primary purpose of the first four experiments was to determine the extent to which developmental differences in verbal memory are the result of age-related declines in storage mechanisms, retrieval mechanisms, or both, and whether these declines in storage and retrieval are differentially accelerated. In addition, these experiments were concerned with the generality of any pattern of storage–retrieval development that might emerge across concrete and abstract material that also differed in level of difficulty (as measured in terms of high and low values for rated meaningfulness).

---

[3]There is one exception to the general study-distractor-test cycle that occurs only on the first trial; that is, subjects are administered the sequence study-distractor-test-distractor-test. The reasons for inserting two distractor-test trials after the first study trial are technical in nature, having to do with providing sufficient degrees of freedom for parameter estimation (see Brainerd et al., 1982).

Concreteness and meaningfulness were selected for use in these experiments because of their well-known effects. In published reports, both concreteness and meaningfulness have been shown to influence the recall patterns of both young and old adults, although it is not always clear whether the magnitude of these effects is developmentally invariant (Craik, 1977; Craik & Masani, 1967; Hartley, Harker, & Walsh, 1980; Howe & Hunter, 1985, 1986; Kausler, 1982; Keitz & Gounard, 1976; Mason & Smith, 1977; Schaie & Gribbin, 1975; Winograd, Smith, & Simon, 1982). In terms of concreteness effects in verbal memory, performance measures typically indicate that: (1) concrete words are easier than abstract words; (2) the magnitude of this effect is not always developmentally invariant; and (3) young adults outperform old adults on both concrete and abstract materials (Howe & Hunter, 1985; Mason & Smith, 1977: Rowe & Schnore, 1971).

A similar pattern has been reported for meaningfulness effects in verbal memory. Specifically, regardless of whether the scale of meaningfulness is defined in a personal/generational sense or in the more classical verbal learning sense (anchored at one end by nonwords that have few, if any, associates and at the other end by words that have a rich network of associations [Toglia & Battig, 1978]), performance measures usually indicate that: (1) high meaningful terms are easier than low meaningful terms; (2) the magnitude of this effect is not always developmentally invariant; and (3) young adults outperform old adults on both high and low meaningful material (Craik & Masani, 1967; Salthouse, 1982; Schaie & Gribbin, 1975; Wittels, 1972). Because these effects are reasonably well established, and because the primary focus of this chapter is on the nature of age differences and similarities in storage and retrieval processes, both at a qualitative and quantitative level, discussion will center strictly on general developmental trends that might emerge across these factors rather than on direct contrasts between concrete and abstract or high and low meaningful materials.

As mentioned, the word for the lists in the first four experiments were drawn from the Toglia and Battig (1978) semantic word norms. In the first two experiments, subjects learned concrete word lists (as indicated by high concreteness ratings: Experiment 1: $M = 5.81$, $SD = .38$; Experiment 2: $M = 5.78$, $SD = .21$) that were rated high in meaningfulness (Experiment 1: $M = 5.19$, $SD = .18$) or rated low in meaningfulness (Experiment 2: $M = 3.82$, $SD = .17$). In the second two experiments, subjects learned abstract word lists (as indicated by low concreteness ratings: Experiment 3: $M = 3.52$, $SD = .30$; Experiment 4: $M = 3.58$, $SD = .34$) that were rated high in meaningfulness (Experiment 3: $M = 5.23$, $SD = .28$) or rated low in meaningfulness (Experiment 4: $M = 3.58$, $SD = .34$). All words were also rated as being highly familiar ($M = 6.17$, $SD = .20$; $M = 6.11$, $SD = .14$; $M = 6.28$, $SD = .34$; and $M = 6.04$, $SD = .19$; across the four experiments, respectively). A separate sample of 25 young adults and 20 old adults served as subjects in each of the four experiments.

Insofar as the results were concerned, global trends in the data were assessed by examining two performance statistics (trial of last error; total errors per item). Because the results of these analyses were the same, only the total errors per item are reported. The means and standard deviations of this statistic are shown in the first four rows of Table 2.2. Using a simple *t* test, significant differences between the age groups were obtained in all four experiments ($p < .05$). Although it is no surprise, these findings indicate that younger adults made fewer errors than older adults when memorizing verbal material.

The question to which principal interest attaches, however, is what accounts for these age differences? In order to answer this question, the parameters of the two-stage model must be estimated. Before using the two-stage model to interpret these developmental differences in terms of storage and retrieval processes, it must be shown that the model provides a statistically acceptable account of the data from these experiments. (Again, the specific mathematical details of these tests will not be presented here. Readers interested in the statistical machinery underlying these goodness-of-fit tests are referred to Brainerd [1985b] and Brainerd et al. [1982]). Because the results of these goodness-of-fit tests are tedious and space-consuming to report, and because there is ample prior evidence that this model provides a comprehensive account of both young and old adults' recall data (Howe & Hunter, 1985, 1986), detailed numerical analyses have been omitted. Instead, the rationale underlying these tests, as well as the specific results for these experiments, are simply reported in summary form.

The first step in the goodness-of-fit procedure consists of determining whether the two-stage model is necessary or whether the data are simpler than the two-stage model assumes. Using familiar likelihood-ratio tech-

TABLE 2.2. Means and Standard Deviations for Total Errors per Item by Experiment and Age

| | Young Adults | Old Adults |
|---|---|---|
| Free Recall of Concrete Words | | |
| Experiment 1 | 0.84 (.56)[a] | 1.51 (.65) |
| Experiment 2 | 1.02 (.83) | 2.43 (.96) |
| Free Recall of Abstract Words | | |
| Experiment 3 | 1.45 (.63) | 2.17 (1.44) |
| Experiment 4 | 1.59 (.80) | 3.31 (1.07) |
| Free Recall of Categorized Words | | |
| Experiment 5 | 0.60 (.41) | 1.18 (1.57) |
| Experiment 6 | 0.58 (.48) | 1.19 (1.20) |
| Cued Recall of Categorized Words | | |
| Experiment 7 | 0.56 (.37) | 0.97 (.60) |
| Experiment 8 | 0.65 (.44) | 1.06 (.63) |

[a]Standard deviations are given in parentheses.

niques, this *necessity test* examines the null hypothesis that a simpler model (with fewer parameters) provides as adequate an account of the data as the two-stage model. When these tests were conducted, the null hypothesis was soundly rejected for both the young and old adults in each of the four experiments ($p < .001$).

Having established that the data were at least as complex as supposed in the two-stage model, the second step in the goodness-of-fit procedure consists of determining whether the two-stage model is sufficiently complex to capture the data structure. Again, using standard likelihood-ratio techniques, this *sufficiency test* examines the null hypothesis that the two-stage model provides as adequate an account of the data as a more complex model (with more parameters) does. When these tests were conducted, the null hypothesis could not be rejected for the young or old adults in any of the four experiments ($p > .20$). Taken together, these results leave little doubt that the two-stage model provides a statistically adequate account of the free recall data of both young and old adults.

Because the two-stage model provides an accurate account of the free recall data, its parameters can be used to localize developmental differences in memory in terms of storage and retrieval processes. The numerical estimates of the storage, heuristic retrieval, and algorithmic retrieval parameters appear in the first eight rows of Table 2.3 for Experiments 1 through 4. To evaluate parameter differences as a function of age, it is necessary to use a series of *conditionwise* and *parameterwise* likelihood-ratio tests (readers interested in the mathematical details of the statistical machinery underlying these tests should consult Brainerd et al., 1982, Equations 53–55). Using a chi-square statistic with 11 degrees of freedom, the conditionwise test evaluates the null hypothesis that the values of the parameters as a whole do not differ across the pair of conditions that constitute each of the experiments. For the first four experiments, the null hypothesis was rejected in each case ($p < .001$), indicating that the numerical values of the parameters that measure storage and retrieval differed as a function of age. The parameterwise test, which is also a chi-square statistic but has only 1 degree of freedom, evaluates whether specific target parameters differ between the conditions of a particular experiment. Detailed presentation of these statistics has been omitted. A summary of the reliable ($p < .01$) parameter differences is given below.

Overall, the results of the parameterwise tests provided clear evidence that, regardless of the nature of the material being memorized (concrete or abstract, high or low in meaningfulness), young adults were generally better learners than old adults. More importantly, these analyses showed that age differences in adult memorization were (1) localized in specific subcomponents of both storage and retrieval processes, and (2) that these differences tended to be similar in magnitude, both in terms of the number of parameters affected and the average numerical magnitude of these effects.

Consider age differences that emerged at storage first. An examination of

TABLE 2.3. Estimates of the Theoretical Parameters by Experiment, Age, and List

| Experiment, Age, and List | Parameter | | | | | | | | | | |
|---|---|---|---|---|---|---|---|---|---|---|---|
| | Storage | | | Algorithmic Retrieval | | | | Heuristic Retrieval | | | |
| | $a'$ | $1-f$ | $a$ | $b'$ | $b$ | $c$ | $d$ | $1-r$ | $1-e$ | $g$ | $h$ |
| Free Recall of Concrete Words | | | | | | | | | | | |
| *Experiment 1* | | | | | | | | | | | |
| Young adults | .68 | 1.0 | .80 | .31 | .36 | .48 | .66 | .85 | .99 | .87 | .90 |
| Old adults | .61 | 1.0 | .68 | .31 | .31 | .37 | .38 | .82 | .96 | .50 | .78 |
| *Experiment 2* | | | | | | | | | | | |
| Young adults | .67 | 1.0 | .71 | .27 | 0.0 | .44 | .58 | .90 | 1.0 | .90 | .90 |
| Old adults | .45 | 1.0 | .60 | .22 | 0.0 | .30 | .35 | .81 | .86 | .53 | .71 |
| Free Recall of Abstract Words | | | | | | | | | | | |
| *Experiment 3* | | | | | | | | | | | |
| Young adults | .61 | 1.0 | .75 | .30 | 0.0 | .44 | .46 | .88 | .86 | .65 | .76 |
| Old adults | .55 | 1.0 | .51 | .19 | 0.0 | .34 | .39 | .91 | 1.0 | .59 | .74 |
| *Experiment 4* | | | | | | | | | | | |
| Young adults | .58 | 1.0 | .67 | .28 | 0.0 | .44 | .41 | .93 | 1.0 | .67 | .81 |
| Old adults | .36 | 1.0 | .40 | .23 | 0.0 | .21 | .40 | .90 | .86 | .57 | .72 |
| Free Recall of Categorized Words | | | | | | | | | | | |
| *Experiment 5* | | | | | | | | | | | |
| Young adults | .80 | 1.0 | .84 | .40 | .55 | .54 | .89 | .82 | 1.0 | .36 | .89 |
| Old adults | .81 | .94 | .90 | .53 | .72 | .36 | .11 | .68 | .88 | .59 | .81 |
| *Experiment 6* | | | | | | | | | | | |
| Young adults | .77 | 1.0 | .90 | .69 | .68 | .66 | .93 | .85 | .85 | .91 | .87 |
| Old adults | .73 | 1.0 | .53 | .64 | .39 | .31 | .35 | .74 | 1.0 | .63 | .79 |
| Cued Recall of Categorized Words | | | | | | | | | | | |
| *Experiment 7* | | | | | | | | | | | |
| Young adults | .82 | 1.0 | .90 | .53 | .79 | .58 | .92 | .81 | 1.0 | .64 | .86 |
| Old adults | .76 | 1.0 | .65 | .48 | .28 | .52 | .15 | .83 | 1.0 | .75 | .84 |
| *Experiment 8* | | | | | | | | | | | |
| Young adults | .77 | 1.0 | .89 | .65 | .69 | .61 | .91 | .77 | 1.0 | .80 | .89 |
| Old adults | .67 | .99 | .68 | .36 | .14 | .51 | .13 | .91 | .95 | .84 | .88 |

the first eight rows of Table 2.3 shows that in all four experiments younger adults were better than older adults at establishing a stable trace in long-term memory (as measured by $a$ in Experiments 1–4 and as well by $a'$ in Experiments 2 and 4). Importantly, however, these differences did not generalize to processes that mediate maintenance of traces stored early in the memorization sequence (as reflected in the invariance of the parameter $1-f$; bearing in mind, of course, the usual caveat concerning possible ceiling effects).

Next, consider age differences that emerged at retrieval. Recall that two forms of retrieval are differentiated in the two-stage model: algorithmic and heuristic. In terms of algorithmic retrieval, parameterwise tests showed that regardless of the material being memorized, younger adults were better than older adults at learning to access information in a reliable fashion (as measured by $b'$ in Experiment 3, $c$ in Experiments 1–4, and $d$ in Experiments 1 and 2). Similar to the findings at storage, age differences at retrieval did not generalize to all forms of retrieval. Specifically, with only a minor exception (the parameter $g$ in Experiments 1 and 2), differences in heuristic retrieval did not serve to discriminate between young and old adults.

Finally, to understand memory development in adulthood, it is as important to examine developmental invariances as it is to examine developmental differences. There are two basic forms of invariance: *qualitative* and *quantitative.* Quantitative invariances refer to parameters whose values remain constant across age, whereas qualitative invariances refer to relationships between parameters that remain constant across age. Examination of the first eight rows of Table 2.3 reveals one quantitative invariance: $1 - f = 1.0$. This finding, as already pointed out, places an important limitation on the generalizability of storage differences in adulthood.

Two qualitative invariances are also present in Table 2.3, $\{a', a\} \geqslant \{b', b, c, d\}$ and $g \leqslant h$ (see Brainerd et al., 1982, Equation 56, for the relevant likelihoodhood procedures involved in testing these parameter invariances). Both these invariances have been observed in previous free recall studies (Howe & Hunter, 1985). The first invariance indicates that regardless of the particular material being learned (concrete or abstract, high or low meaningful) both young and old adults find storing a trace easier than learning an algorithm with which to retrieve that trace reliably. The second qualitative invariance indicates that regardless of age and material, heuristic retrieval is easier following a previously successful application of that heuristic than following an unsuccessful application. This result is fairly common and has been interpreted in terms of a priming effect in the partially memorized state (Howe & Hunter, 1985).

To summarize, the results of the first four experiments indicate that regardless of age the overriding difficulty in memorizing verbal information in a free recall task is making reliable contact with that information in long-term memory. These results also tell us that although age differences in adult memorization are localized both at storage and retrieval, and these differences are reasonably similar in overall magnitude, generalizing to all of the components that comprise the processes of storage and retrieval is clearly unwarranted. That is, age differences at storage were confined to processes involved in establishing a trace in long-term memory and did not extend to processes involved in maintaining a stored trace early in memorization. Similarly, age differences at retrieval were confined primarily to algorithmic retrieval with few or no differences being observed at heuristic retrieval. These patterns are consistent with previous free recall research involving the two-stage model (Howe & Hunter, 1985), and suggest that a number of important memorization functions involved in the storage and retrieval of information tend to decline with age. Equally important, these results signal that caution should be exercised when generalizing these declines to all aspects of storage and retrieval processing.

## Experiments 5 Through 8

These last four experiments sought to test the generality of the above pattern of developmental differences and invariances in organized memory, both in a free (Experiments 5 and 6) and a cued recall (Experiments 7 and 8) paradigm. Like concreteness and meaningfulness, it is not clear whether age differences in organized recall are primarily the result of a decline in storage, retrieval, or both, and if both, whether these declines in storage and retrieval are differentially accelerated. What is clear from the previous literature on organizational processes in aging memory is that elderly adults tend to engage in spontaneous organizational restructuring of information less frequently and less effectively than younger adults (see reviews in Burke & Light, 1981; Guttentag, 1985; Kausler, 1982; Poon, 1985; Salthouse, 1982). As pointed out by Burke and Light (1981), these performance deficits are probably not the result of a simple production deficiency. For example, if production deficiencies do exist, then performance on recall tasks should improve more dramatically for elderly subjects than younger subjects when the basis of the organization is emphasized in some manner. This, in turn, should reduce or eliminate age differences in organized recall.

As it turns out, however, age differences do not disappear under enhanced conditions, whether these conditions involve manipulations at encoding such as varying instructions to organize (Hultsch, 1969), use of a sorting technique (Hultsch, 1971; Worden & Meggison, 1984), or use of a semantic orienting task (Craik, 1977; Craik & Simon, 1980). Similarly, age differences are reduced, but not eliminated, when category cues are provided at the time of study, test, or both (Hultsch & Craig, 1976; Smith, 1977). Given these results, it would appear that age-related declines in organized memory, like those seen more generally in long-term memory, are most likely rooted in qualitative and quantitative changes in the basic processes of storage and retrieval that are the essential determinants of recall performance (see discussions in Burke & Light, 1981; Craik & Rabinowitz, 1984).

In order to specify the locus of these age differences in terms of the basic processes that mediate organized memory, two 16-item lists were constructed from the Battig and Montague (1969) production frequency norms. In the two-category list (Experiments 5 and 7), 8 items were drawn from the "four-footed animal" category and the remaining 8 items were drawn from the "parts of the building" category. In the four-category list (Experiments 6 and 8), 4 items were drawn from the "four-footed animal" category, 4 from the "parts of a building" category, 4 from the "parts of the body" category, and 4 from the "clothing" category. All items were considered typical category members as they were drawn from the first 10 rank-order positions in the norms for that category. A standard free recall procedure was used in Experiments 5 and 6, whereas a standard cued recall procedure was used in Experiments 7 and 8 in which subjects were given the category labels as recall aids on test trials. A separate sample of 30 young adults and 20 old adults served as subjects in each of these four experiments.

As before, the results begin with a general assessment of the trends in the data using two performance statistics (trial of last error, total errors per item). Again, because the results were the same, only the total error per item statistic is reported. The means and standard deviations of this statistic are shown in the last four rows of Table 2.2. Using a simple $t$ test, significant differences between the age groups were obtained in all four experiments ($p < .05$). Like the previous experiments, then, younger adults made fewer errors than older adults when memorizing verbal material.

In order to determine the locus of these age differences in organized free and cued recall, goodness-of-fit tests were conducted on the two-stage model. Inasmuch as the two-stage model was again found to provide both a necessary ($p < .001$) and sufficient ($p > .20$) account of the data, it was concluded that young and old adults' free and cued recall of organized lists was a two-stage process to a very close approximation. The numerical estimates of the storage, algorithmic retrieval, and heuristic retrieval parameters appear in the last eight rows of Table 2.3.

Conditionwise tests again revealed that, at a global level, the numerical values of the storage and retrieval parameters differed as a function of age in each of these experiments ($p < .001$). Subsequent parameterwise tests ($p < .01$) provided clear evidence that for both free and cued recall of organized verbal material young adults were generally better than old adults. Like the first four experiments, these analyses showed that age differences in adult memorization were localized in specific subcomponents of both storage and retrieval processes. However, unlike the earlier experiments, developmental differences were *not* the same in magnitude at storage and retrieval. Specifically, age differences at retrieval, algorithmic retrieval in particular, tended to be larger than those at storage, both in terms of the number of parameters affected and in terms of the average numerical magnitude of these differencees. As well, consistent with previous research (Worden & Meggison, 1984), these differences tended to be larger for the four- than the two-category lists.

Consider age differences that emerged at storage first. An examination of the last eight rows of Table 2.3 shows that, in three of these four experiments, younger adults were better than older adults at establishing a stable trace in long-term memory (as measured by $a$ in Experiments 6–8 and as well by $a'$ in Experiment 8). Once again, however, these differences did not generalize to processes that mediate maintenance of traces stored early in the memorization sequence (as reflected in the invariance of the parameter $1 - f$).

Next, consider age differences that emerged at retrieval. In terms of algorithmic retrieval, parameterwise tests showed that with only a single exception (the parameters $b'$ and $b$ in Experiment 5 favoring the older adults), younger adults were better than older adults at learning to access information in a reliable fashion (as measured by $b'$ in Experiment 8, $b$ in Experiments 6–8, $c$ in Experiments 5, 6, and 8, and $d$ in Experiments 5–8). Once again, age differences at algorithmic retrieval did not generalize to heuristic retrieval. Specifically, with only a minor exception (the parameter $g$ in Experiments 5 [favoring the older adults] and 6 [favoring the younger adults]), differences in heuristic retrieval did not serve to discriminate between young and old adults.

In terms of parameter invariance, an examination of the last eight rows of Table 2.3 once again reveals the same quantitative invariance ($1 - f$ not significantly different from 1.0) and both qualitative invariances ($\{a', a\} \geqslant \{b', b, c, d\}$ and $\{g \leqslant h\}$). These latter results provide strong converging evidence that, regardless of the particular material being learned, both young and old adults find storing a trace easier than learning an algorithm with which to retrieve that trace reliably and that heuristic retrieval is easier following a previously successful application of that heuristic than following an unsuccessful application.

To summarize, these results again illustrate that (1) for both young and old adults, learning to retrieve is more difficult than storage, regardless of whether recall is free or cued; (2) developmental differences in long-term memory in adulthood exist both at storage and retrieval; and (3) age differences at storage do not extend to processes involved in trace maintenance early in memorization, nor do age differences at algorithmic retrieval extend to heuristic retrieval. The replication of these patterns both here and elsewhere (Howe & Hunter, 1985) provides strong converging evidence that while a number of important aspects of storage–retrieval functions decline with age, a number of them do not.

## General Discussion

A long-standing question about the development of memory in adulthood is whether changes at storage or at retrieval represent the more important source of decline in aging memory. Unfortunately, having relied primarily on a design-based approach, previous research has met with considerable difficulty when attempting to isolate developmental differences in storage and retrieval factors in long-term memory. Motivated by a need to clarify the role of these processes in aging memory, the present chapter provided an overview of the general two-stage model approach to factoring storage and retrieval in long-term memory and illustrated its use in eight experiments that examined the development of verbal memory in adulthood. The results of these experiments bear directly on this question, and reveal a number of important trends in long-term memory development in adulthood. In the discussion that follows, these findings will be examined in terms of the specific issues concerning the relative contributions of storage and retrieval to long-term memory development in adulthood, as well as the more general issues that confront theories of cognitive and memory development in adulthood.

## Relative Contributions of Storage and Retrieval to Memory Development in Adulthood

One developmentally invariant finding that emerged in all eight experiments was that, regardless of the type of material being memorized and regardless of whether recall was free or cued, both young and old adults found it easier to store a trace in long-term memory than to learn to retrieve it. Regardless of age, then, the overriding difficulty encountered by adults in episodic memory tasks of this sort is how to make reliable contact with the contents of long-term memory.

These invariances notwithstanding, advancing age in adulthood was associated with marked declines in memorization ability in all eight experiments. The question still remains, therefore, "Is memory development in adulthood primarily a consequence of variation in trace storage, trace retrieval, or some combination of the two?" Moreover, if it is the result of changes in both, are these changes differentially accelerated? The answer provided by this current research is that (1) memory development in adulthood is the consequence of decrements in both storage and retrieval processes, (2) these decrements are differentially accelerated, on average (as seen in Experiments 6–8), and (3) these decrements, rather than being generalizable to all aspects of storage and retrieval, tend to be confined to specific subcomponents of these processes.

These findings are valuable for a number of reasons. First, age differences favoring younger adults at trace storage emerged in seven of eight experiments reported in this chapter (Experiment 5 being the single exception), illustrating the importance of reconsidering storage as a central locus of developmental differences in episodic memory. Perhaps because there were a number of early failures to find developmental differences in interference effects during retention intervals, investigators tended to not consider storage as a potential source of age differences in long-term memory (for review, see Kausler, 1982). Indeed, in most contemporary writings the emphasis has been placed squarely on retrieval processes as the primary source of developmental differences in memory (see reviews in Burke & Light, 1981; Poon, 1985). Although clear developmental differences do exist at retrieval (see following discussion as well as Howe & Hunter, 1985, 1986), the findings reported in this chapter clearly indicate the pervasive nature of developmental differences in storing information in long-term memory.

Second, age differences primarily favoring young adults (the single exception occurring in Experiment 5) were observed at retrieval in all eight experiments, specifically in algorithmic retrieval. In fact, age differences at algorithmic retrieval tended to be larger, overall, than those observed at storage (primarily in terms of the number of parameters affected in at least three of eight experiments). Consistent with previous research (Howe & Hunter, 1985, 1986), it appears that while both storage and retrieval are important sources of age differences in long-term memory in adulthood, the magnitude of developmental differences at retrieval tends to be larger, on average, than those at storage.

Third, developmental differences in the processes that mediate long-term memory, while pervasive, tend not to generalize to all aspects of storage and retrieval. Specifically, whereas establishing a trace in long-term memory was easier for younger than older subjects, age differences were absent when it came to maintaining a previously stored trace, at least early in the memorization process. Similarly, developmental differences at retrieval tended to be confined to algorithmic retrieval processes for the most part and did not spread to heuristic retrieval processes. It is clear, therefore, that although a number of important developmental differences exist at storage and retrieval, there also exist a number of limitations that restrict the generalizability of these differences in long-term episodic memory. These results, as well as those reported elsewhere (Howe & Hunter, 1985, 1986), provide reasonable documentation that a comprehensive theory of memory development in adulthood must include consideration of memory components that vary with age as well as those that remain invariant.

## General Implications and Conclusions

It now appears that one answer to the question of what declines in adult memory is the ability to input information into memory and, to a somewhat greater extent, to reliably retrieve that information from memory. Moreover, what does not seem to differ is the ability to maintain a stored trace early in the memorization process (although large differences do exist over more protracted periods of time) (Howe & Hunter, 1986), or the ability to access that information using a general retrieval heuristic.

It is tempting to speculate on the nature of the relationship between the developments in verbal memory that were observed here and corresponding developments in that occur in other cognitive domains (e.g, thinking, problem solving, decision making, etc.). Unfortunately, however, such speculation, including any attempt to map changes in general cognitive functioning in adulthood onto problems encountered in establishing stable trace information in memory (storage) or in making reliable contact with that information (retrieval), would be premature given the absence of a comprehensive theory of memory development in adulthood. Although I do not formulate such a theory here, I conclude this chapter by commenting on some of the more salient issues that were raised by the modeling approach to studying memory development.

First, it is obvious from this research that an adequate theory of memory development must incorporate both qualitative and quantitative aspects of age differences and invariances. Clearly, it is not sufficient to make broad statements about some generalized age-related deficit in memory processes in adulthood. Rather, we need to specify as precisely as possible exactly what it is that does develop, the direction and extent of that development, and what remains developmentally invariant. A critical feature of the present approach is that it utilizes a framework (the two-stage model) within which the relative contributions of age differences in storage and retrieval processes to memory development in adulthood can be measured with a high degree of precision.

Second, an overriding conclusion from the use of this modeling approach, and one that is clearly illustrated in the pattern of findings in this chapter, is that whatever memory development is in adulthood, it probably is not the result of a uniform decline in a single factor. The global trends observed here, as well as elsewhere (Howe & Hunter, 1985, 1986; Wilkinson & Koestler, 1983), are considerably more complex than single-process theories anticipate. Indeed, the data are fundamentally inconsistent with any theory of memory development that seeks to explain age differences in recall by positing some mechanism whose decline exerts a unitary effect on long-term memory processes.

To illustrate, consider the recent debate concerning possible age-related declines in processing resources. Here, the processing of information in most tasks (including episodic memory tasks) is said to operate in a limited (cognitive) resource environment. In general, cognitive processes are viewed as lying on a continuum ranging from *predominantly automatic* to *predominantly controlled* or effortful. To the extent that processing demands of a task are automatic, age invariances should be observed. To the extent that processing demands of a task are controlled or effortful, age differences should be observed (cf. Hasher & Zacks, 1979). The extremes of these dimensions are viewed as being mutually exclusive with respect to a given process in a specific task. That is, a process or processing variable is typically considered to be either relatively automatic or relatively effortful in a given task, but not both. Thus, on the one hand, if the execution of a process is deemed relatively automatic, only age invariances should appear. On the other hand, if the execution of a process is deemed relatively effortful, only age differences should be observed. For example, encoding of organized material may require access (attention) to associative or semantic features of that information, which may, in turn, involve the use of controlled processes. If so, and if the elderly have limited attentional resources (Craik & Byrd, 1982; Rabinowitz, Craik, & Ackerman, 1982), then age differences in the effects of this variable on recall could emerge *across the board* simply because older adults' encodings contain less of the necessary associative and/or semantic information.

As it turns out, however, unless one is willing to either drop the condition of mutual exclusivity or make additional, post hoc assumptions concerning differences in the resource demands made by trace storage versus trace maintenance processes and heuristic versus algorithmic retrieval processes, these predictions are incompatible with the observation that age differences and invariances exist both at storage and at retrieval. In addition, there is a growing body of evidence which indicates that whether elderly subjects perform poorly on tasks is independent of where those tasks fall on the automatic–effortful continuum (Kausler, Lichty, & Hakami, 1984; Lehman & Mellinger, 1984). Therefore, although it may be useful at a general level to conceive cognitive and memory processes as lying on a continuum ranging from few to many resource demands, this concept is not consistent with a number of developmental findings. Moreover, even this general assumption has been challenged in a number of recent papers that have questioned the adequacy of the underlying structural assumption that cognitive processes operate in a limited resource environment (cf. Cheng, 1985; Navon, 1984; Salthouse, this volume).

Although it may be some time before a complete theory of memory development is articulated, the current chapter provides at least one starting point for this development. First, it illustrates the importance of using precise techniques, with known measurement properties, to partition the (memory) processes under study (in this case, storage and retrieval). Second, using one such technique, the results of a series of experiments provide converging evidence concerning the relative rates of decline and stability of storage-retrieval development in adulthood. Finally, the current chapter serves to underscore the essential idea that memory development, like the development of other cognitive functions (cf. Baltes & Willis, 1982; Denney, 1984; Labouvie-Vief, 1985; Reese & Rodeheaver, 1985), does not consist in adulthood of a simple, uniform decline in processing ability. Through the development and implementation of models that provide a comprehensive measurement technology, thereby increasing the tractability of (memory) processes that develop, the mechanism(s) responsible for (memory) development will become more apparent. When these processes are better understood, a more comprehensive theory will emerge that makes contact with, and specifies the relationship between, memory development on one hand and more general cognitive development in adulthood on the other.

*Acknowledgments.* Preparation of this chapter and the research reported herein were supported by Grant (No. A3334) from the Natural Sciences and Engineering Research Council of Canada. I thank Julia O'Sullivan for providing a number of important suggestions in her review of an earlier version of this chapter.

# References

Baltes, P.B., & Willis, S.L. (1982). Plasticity and enhancement of intellectual functioning in old age: Penn State's adult development and enrichment project (ADEPT). In F.I.M. Craik & S. Trehub (Eds.), *Aging and cognitive processes* (pp. 353–389). New York: Plenum Press.

Botwinick, J. (1977). Intellectual abilities. In J.E. Birren & K.W. Schaie (Eds.), *Handbook of the psychology of aging* (1st ed., pp. 580–605). New York: Van Nostrand Reinhold.

Battig, W. F., & Montague, W.E. (1969). Category norms for verbal items in 56 categories: A replication and extension of the Connecticut category norms. *Journal of Experimental Psychology: Monograph, 80* (No. 3, Pt. 2).

Brainerd, C.J. (1982). Children's concept learning as rule-sampling systems with Markovian properties. In C.J. Brainerd (Ed.), *Children's logical and mathematical cognition: Progress in cognitive development research* (pp. 177–212). New York: Springer-Verlag.

Brainerd, C.J. (1985a). Model-based approaches to storage and retrieval development. In C.J. Brainerd & M. Pressley (Eds.), *Basic processes in memory development: Progress in cognitive development research* (pp. 143–208). New York: Springer-Verlag.

Brainerd, C.J. (1985b). Three-state models of memory development: A review of advances in statistical methodology. *Journal of Experimental Child Psychology, 40,* 375–394.

Brainerd, C.J., Howe, M.L., & Kingma, J. (1982). An identifiable model of two-stage learning. *Journal of Mathematical Psychology, 26,* 263–293.

Brainerd, C.J., Howe, M.L., Kingma, J., & Brainerd, S.H. (1984a). On the measurement of storage and retrieval contributions to memory development. *Journal of Experimental Child Psychology, 37,* 478–499.

Brainerd, C.J., Howe, M.L., Kingma, J., & Brainerd, S.H. (1984b). Explaining category interference effects in associative memory. *Canadian Journal of Psychology, 38,* 454–477.

Brainerd, C.J., Kingma, J., & Howe, M. L. (1985). On the development of forgetting. *Child Development, 56,* 1103–1119.

Brainerd, C.J., Kingma, J., & Howe, M.L. (1986a). Spread of encoding and the development of organization in memory. *Canadian Journal of Psychology, 40,* 203–223.

Brainerd, C.J., Kingma, J., & Howe, M.L. (1986b). Long-term memory development and learning disability: Storage and retrieval loci of disabled/nondisabled differences. In S.J. Ceci (Ed.), *Handbook of cognitive, social, and neuropsychological aspects of learning disabilities* (pp. 161–184). Hillsdale, NJ: Erlbaum.

Burke, D.M., & Light, L.L. (1981). Memory and aging: The role of retrieval processes. *Psychological Bulletin, 90,* 513–546.

Cerella, J. (1985). Information processing rates in the elderly. *Psychological Bulletin, 98,* 67–83.

Chechile, R.A., & Meyer, D.L. (1976). A Bayesian procedure for separately estimating storage and retieval components of forgetting. *Journal of Mathematical Psychology, 13,* 269–295.

Chehile, R.A., & Richman, C.L. (1982). The interaction of semantic memory with storage and retrieval processes. *Developmental Review, 2,* 237–250.

Chechile, R.A., Richman, C.L., Topinka, C., & Ehrensbeck, K. (1981). A developmental study of the storage and retrieval of information. *Child Development, 52,* 251–259.
Cheng, P.W. (1985). Restructuring versus automaticity: Alternative accounts of skill acquisition. *Psychological Review, 92,* 414–423.
Craik, F.I.M. (1977). Age differences in human memory. In J.E. Birren & K.W. Schaie (Eds.), *Handbook of the psychology of aging* (1st ed., pp. 384–420). New York: Van Nostrand Reinhold.
Craik, F.I.M., & Byrd, M. (1982). Aging and cognitive deficits: The role of attentional processes. In F.I.M. Craik & S. Trehub (Eds.), *Aging and cognitive processes* (pp. 191–211). New York: Plenum Press.
Craik, F.I.M., & Masani, P.A. (1967). Age differences in the temporal integration of language. *British Journal of Psychology, 58,* 291–299.
Craik, F.I.M., & Rabinowitz, J.C. (1984). Age differences in the acquisition and use of verbal information: A tutorial review. In H. Bouma & D.G. Bouwhuis (Eds.), *Attention and performance X* (pp. 471–499). Hillsdale, NJ: Erlbaum.
Craik, F.I.M., & Simon, E. (1980). Age differences in memory: The roles of attention and depth of processing. In L.W. Poon, J.L. Fozard, L.S. Cermak, D. Arenberg, & L.W. Thompson (Eds.), *New directions in memory and aging* (pp. 95–112). Hillsdale, NJ: Erlbaum.
Denney, N.W. (1984). A model of cognitive development across the life span. *Developmental Review, 4,* 171–191.
Duchek, J.M. (1984). Encoding and retrieval differences between young and old: The impact of attentional capacity usage. *Developmental Psychology, 20,* 1173–1180.
Estes, W.K. (1986). Memory storage and retrieval processes in category learning. *Journal of Experimental Psychology: General, 115,* 155–174.
Flexser, A. J., & Tulving, E. (1978). Retrieval independence in recognition and recall. *Psychological Review, 85,* 153–171.
Greeno, J.G. (1968). Identifiability and statistical properties of two-stage learning with no success in the initial stage. *Psychometrika, 33,* 173–215.
Greeno, J.G. (1974). Representation of learning as discrete transition in a finite state space. In D.H. Krantz, R.C. Atkinson, R.D. Luce, & P. Suppes (Eds.), *Contemporary developments in mathematical psychology* (pp. 1–43). San Francisco, CA: Freeman.
Greeno, J.G., James, C.T., DaPolito, F.J., & Polson, P.G. (1978). *Associative learning: A cognitive analysis.* Englewood Cliffs, NJ: Prentice-Hall.
Guttentag, R.E. (1985). Memory and aging: Implications for theories of memory development during childhood. *Development Review, 5,* 56–82.
Halff, H.M. (1977). The role of opportunities for recall in learning to retrieve. *American Journal of Psychology, 90,* 383–406.
Hartley, J.T., Harker, J.O., & Walsh, D.A. (1980). Contemporary issues and new directions in adult development of learning and memory. In L.W. Poon (Ed.), *Aging in the 1980s: Psychological issues* (pp. 239–252). Washington, DC: American Psychological Association.
Hasher, L., & Zacks, R.T. (1979). Automatic and effortful processes in memory. *Journal of Experimental Psychology: General, 108,* 356–388.
Heth, C.D., & Cornell, E.H. (1983). A learning analysis of spatial concept development in infancy. In J. Bisanz, G. Bisanz, & R.V. Kail, Jr. (Eds.), *Learning in children: Progress in cognitive development research* (pp. 61–84). New York: Springer-Verlag.
Horn, J.L. (1982). The theory of fluid and crystallized intelligence in relation to con-

cepts of cognitive psychology and aging in adulthood. In F.I.M. Craik & S. Trehub (Eds.), *Aging and cognitive processes* (pp. 237-278). New York: Plenum Press.

Howard, D.V. (1980). Category norms: A comparison of the Battig and Montague (1969) norms with the responses of adults between the ages of 20 and 80. *Journal of Gerontology, 35,* 225-231.

Howe, M.L. (1985). Storage and retrieval of associative clusters: A stages-of-learning analysis of associative memory traces. *Canadian Journal of Psychology, 39,* 34-53.

Howe, M.L. (1987). *Associative symmetry in the acquisition and retention of long-term memory traces.* Manuscript submitted for publication.

Howe, M.L., Brainerd, C.J., & Kingma, J. (1985a). Development of organization in recall: A stages-of-learning analysis. *Journal of Experimental Child Psychology, 39,* 230-251.

Howe, M.L. Brainerd, C.J., & Kingma, J. (1985b). Storage-retrieval processes of normal and learning-disabled children: A stages-of-learning analysis of picture-word effects. *Child Development,* 56, 1120-1133.

Howe, M.L., & Hunter, M.A. (1985). Adult age differences in storage-retrieval processes: A stages-of-learning analysis of developmental interactions in concreteness effects. *Canadian Journal of Psychology, 39,* 130-150.

Howe, M.L., & Hunter, M.A. (1986). Long-term memory in adulthood: An examination of the development of storage and retrieval processes at acquisition and retention. *Developmental Review, 6,* 334-364.

Hultsch, D.F. (1969). Adult age differences in the organization of free recall. *Developmental Psychology, 1,* 673-678.

Hultsch, D.F. (1971). Adult age differences in free classification and free recall. *Developmental Psychology, 4,* 338-342.

Hultsch, D.F., & Craig, E.R. (1976). Adult age differences in the inhibition of recall as a function of retrieval cues. *Developmental Psychology, 12,* 83-84.

Humphreys, M.S., & Greeno, J.G. (1970). Interpretation of the two-stage analysis of paired-associate memorizing. *Journal of Mathematical Psychology,* 7, 275-292.

Kausler, D.H. (1982). *Experimental psychology and human aging.* New York: Wiley.

Kausler, D.H. (1985). Episodic memory: Memorizing performance. In N. Charness (Ed.), *Aging and human performance* (pp. 101-141) New York: Wiley.

Kausler, D.H., Lichty, W., & Hakami, M.K. (1984). Frequency judgements for distractor items in a short-term memory task: Instructional variation and adult age differences. *Journal of Verbal Learning and Verbal Behavior, 23,* 660-668.

Keitz, S.M., & Gounard, B.R. (1976). Age differences in adults' free recall of pictorial and word stimuli. *Educational Gerontology, 1,* 209-210.

Labouvie-Vief, G. (1985). Intelligence and cognition. In J.E. Birren & K.W. Schaie (Eds.), *Handbook of the psychology of aging* (2nd ed., pp. 500-530). New York: Van Nostrand Reinhold.

Lehman, E.B., & Mellinger, J.C. (1984). Effects of aging on memory for presentation modality. *Developmental Psychology, 20,* 1210-1217.

Mason, S.E., & Smith, A.D. (1977). Imagery in the aged. *Experimental Aging Research, 3,* 17-32.

Navon, D. (1984). Resources—A theoretical soup stone? *Psychological Review, 91,* 216-234.

Perlmutter, M., & Mitchell, D.B. (1982). The appearance and disappearance of age differences in adult memory. In F.I.M. Craik & S. Trehub (Eds.), *Aging and cognitive processes* (pp. 127-144). New York: Plenum Press.

Poon, L.W. (1985). Differences in human memory with aging: Nature, causes, and clinical implications. In J.E. Birren & K.W. Schaie (Eds.), *Handbook of the psychology of aging* (2nd ed., pp. 427–462). New York: Van Nostrand Reinhold.

Rabinowitz, J.C., Craik, F.I.M., & Ackerman, B.P. (1982). A processing resource account of age differences in recall. *Canadian Journal of Psychology, 36,* 325–344.

Reese, H.W., & Rodeheaver, D. (1985). Problem solving and complex decision making. In J.E. Birren & K.W. Schaie (Eds.), *Handbook of the psychology of aging* (2nd ed., pp. 474–499). New York: Van Nostrand Reinhold.

Rowe, E.J., & Schnore, M.M. (1971). Item concreteness and reported strategies in paired associate learning as a function of age. *Journal of Gerontology, 26,* 470–475.

Salthouse, T.A. (1982). *Adult cognition: An experimental psychology of human aging.* New York: Springer-Verlag.

Schaie, K.W., & Gribbin, K. (1975). Adult development and aging. *Annual Review of Psychology, 26,* 65–96.

Smith, A.D. (1977). Adult age differences in cued recall. *Developmental Psychology, 13,* 326–331.

Smith, A.D. (1980). Age differences in encoding, storage, and retrieval. In L.W. Poon, J.L. Fozard, L.S. Cermak, D. Arenberg, & L.W. Thompson (Eds.), *New directions in memory and aging* (pp. 23–45). Hillsdale, NJ: Erlbaum.

Theios, J. (1963). Simple conditioning as two-stage all-or-none learning. *Psychological Review, 70,* 403–417.

Toglia, M.P., & Battig, W.F. (1978). *Handbook of semantic word norms.* Hillsdale, NJ: Erlbaum.

Wilkinson, A.C., & Koestler, R. (1983). Repeated recall: A new model and tests of its generality from childhood to old age. *Journal of Experimental Psychology: General, 112,* 423–451.

Wilkinson, A.C., & Koestler, R. (1984). Generality of a Markov model for repeated recall. *Journal of Mathematical Psychology, 28,* 43–72.

Winograd, E., Smith, A.D., & Simon, E.W. (1982). Aging and the picture superiority effect in recall. *Journal of Gerontology, 37,* 70–75.

Wittels, I. (1972). Age and stimulus meaningfulness in paired-associate learning. *Journal of Gerontology, 27,* 372–375.

Worden, P.E., & Meggison, D.L. (1984). Aging and the category-recall relationship. *Journal of Gerontology, 39,* 322–324.

# 3. Memory Self-Knowledge and Self-Efficacy in the Aged

*David F. Hultsch, Christopher Hertzog, Roger A. Dixon, and Heather Davidson*

While following trends in cognitive psychology, gerontologists have become increasingly interested in the ways social and personality processes may contribute to cognitive functioning. In the domain of memory, this interest has led to suggestions that age-related changes in basic memory processes may be only one contributing factor in the typically observed decline in performance in later life. In particular, individuals' performance may be shaped not only by their actual skills, but also by their knowledge of the cognitive demand characteristics of the situation and their perceptions of the likely outcomes of their behaviors in such a situation. Such self-knowledge and self-perceptions have been labeled *metamemory*. As originally proposed by Flavell and his colleagues (Flavell, 1971; Flavell & Wellman, 1977), emphasis was placed on knowledge about memory. In particular, they suggested that memory performance may be affected by (a) knowledge of the memory demand characteristics of particular tasks or situations, and (b) knowledge of potentially employable strategies relevant to a given task or situation. More recently, the concept has been expanded to include the individual's sense of self-efficacy with respect to memory, either generally or in relation to a given task or situation. Several writers have suggested that perceived self-efficacy may be a particularly important determinant of memory-related behavior in older adults (Hultsch, Dixon, & Hertzog, 1985; Lachman, Steinberg, & Trotter, 1987; West & Berry, 1987).

Two broad methodologies have been used to examine adults' memory self-knowledge and perceived memory self-efficacy. The most prevalent has relied on self-report questionnaires. In recent years, a number of these instruments have been developed for use with adults, including the Short Inventory of Memory Experiences (SIME; Herrmann & Neisser, 1978), the Memory Functioning Questionnaire (MFQ; Gilewski, Zelinski, Schaie, & Thompson, 1983), and the Metamemory in Adulthood instrument (MIA; Dixon & Hultsch, 1983b, 1984) (see Dixon, in press; Gilewski & Zelinski, 1986 for reviews of available questionnaires). In general, these questionnaires have assessed a variety of knowledge and self-efficacy dimensions in relation to a variety of "everyday" memory-demanding situations. The Dixon and Hultsch (1983b) instrument also examines several affective and motivational dimensions that may be associated with such memory-demanding situations.

The second methodology has indexed metamemory through the application of a number of experimental paradigms (see Cavanaugh, in press, for a review). One widely used approach requires subjects to monitor their memory before, during, or following performance of a specific memory-demanding task. The focus may be on assessments of the memorability of particular items as well as the task as a whole. Experimentally based measures of metamemory have generally indexed memory self-knowledge and perceived self-efficacy in relation to "standard" laboratory tasks.

In this chapter, we focus on research that has used the questionnaire approach to index metamemory. Initial work with these questionnaires has produced promising results. There is evidence for their reliability and factorial validity (Dixon, in press; Gilewski & Zelinski, 1986). In addition, previous work has provided some indiction of the presence of age-related differences on some dimensions of metamemory, as well as evidence of a number of linkages between individuals' self-knowledge and self-efficacy about memory and their actual performance on memory tasks (Chaffin & Herrmann, 1983; Dixon & Hultsch, 1983a; Dixon, Hertzog, & Hultsch, 1986; Zelinski, Gilewski, & Thompson, 1980). However, it is equally clear that several fundamental issues remain unresolved despite these preliminary positive results. One set of issues relates to the definition and measurement of the metamemory construct itself. A second set of issues revolves around inconsistencies in the pattern of age-related differences on various dimensions of metamemory. Finally, a third set of issues is associated with the question of whether measures of metamemory are (or should be) veridical indicators of actual memory ability. In the following sections, we examine these three sets of issues in turn.

## The Definition and Measurement of Metamemory

### Dimensions of Metamemory

Metamemory involves an essential central distinction between remembering and thinking about remembering. However, as Wellman (1983) noted, the construct rapidly becomes fuzzy once we move away from this central distinction. It seems clear that there may be several dimensions of metamemory, but the question of how many dimensions are required to adequately define the domain remains unresolved. Four broad dimensions that may be relevant are suggested in Table 3.1. The first dimension reflects factual knowledge about memory tasks and memory processes. Examples of this dimension include knowing that short lists of items are easier to remember than long ones, and that organizing the elements of a list of items is likely to improve recall. The remaining three dimensions reflect self-knowledge or perceptions about memory rather than factual knowledge. Memory monitoring involves self-knowledge about how one typically uses one's memory as well as the current state of one's memory; for example, reports of strategy use, feeling-of-knowing judgments (e.g, "I know that I know that"), and assessments of the accuracy of one's responses (e.g., "I got that right"). Memory self-efficacy refers one's sense of mastery within the memory domain. Examples of this dimension include beliefs about memory capacity, short- and long-term changes in memory functioning, and the degree to which memory functioning is amenable to self-control. Finally, memory-related affect encompasses a variety of states that may be related to, or generated by, memory-demanding situations including anxiety, depression, fatigue, etc.

The dimensions outlined in Table 3.1 fit Wellman's (1983) broad definition of metamemory in that they all reflect cognitions about memory. However, they have received varying degrees of research attention. In particular, the bulk of work has focused on the first two dimensions. Indeed, developmental differences in memory knowledge were largely the basis for the original definition of metamemory proposed by Flavell (1971). Memory monitoring indices have been widely used in many experimental paradigms designed to examine metamemory. A focus on memory self-efficacy has been emphasized particularly by researchers interested in memory and aging. Attention to affective states generated by memory-demanding situations has received the least attention.

TABLE 3.1. Hypothetical Dimensions of Metamemory

| Dimension | Content |
|---|---|
| Memory knowledge | Factual knowledge about memory tasks, processes, strategies, etc. |
| Memory monitoring | Self-knowledge about current memory use, contents, states, etc. |
| Memory self-efficacy | Beliefs about memory abilities, strengths, weaknesses, etc. |
| Memory-related affect | Affective states generated by or associated with memory-demanding situations |

This diversity is reflected in the numerous questionnaires that have been developed to measure the metamemory. For example, some questionnaires such as the Memory Complaints Questionnaire make no distinction among different dimensions of metamemory, yielding only a total score (e.g., Zarit, 1982; Zarit, Cole, & Guilder, 1981; Zarit, Gallagher, & Kramer, 1981). Inspection of the items from this and other "single score" measures suggests that multiple dimensions have been combined. Other questionnaires appear to examine a single dimension or facet of a dimension in some depth. For example, several questionnaires such as the SIME (Herrmann & Neisser, 1978) assess individuals' perceptions of the difficulty they have remembering within particular content domains (e.g., names, errands, conversations). Such questionnaires may be thought of as in-depth assessments of perceived memory capacity, which can be considered to be one facet of memory self-efficacy. Finally, other questionnaires appear to explicitly tap several of the dimensions outlined in Table 3.1. For example, the MFQ (Gilewski et al., 1983) contains subscales that index aspects of memory monitoring and memory -self efficacy. Our own measure, the MIA (Dixon & Hultsch, 1983b, 1984), incorporates elements from all four dimensions noted above. Since the MFQ and MIA have been widely used in aging work, we briefly describe these two questionnaires.

The 64 items of the MFQ are distributed into eight a priori scales as shown in Table 3.2. The instrument is a shortened version of a 92-item instrument originally developed by Zelinski et al. (1980). In the original sample, Cronbach's alpha for the various subscales ranged from .82 to .93, and 3-year test-retest reliabilities ranged from .22 to .64 (Zelinski et al., 1980). Factor analysis of the a priori scales revealed three common factors including Frequency of Forgetting, Seriousness, and Mnemonics/Retrospective Functioning. This factor structure replicated in young (29–39 years) and old-old (71+ years) age groups, but not a young-old (55–70 years) age group. In this latter group, the three factors were Frequency of Forgetting, General Rating, and Mnemonics.

The 120-item MIA is composed of eight factor-analytically-defined dimensions, seven of which are summarized in Table 3.3. (In our recent work we have dropped the original Activity subscale for conceptual and measurement reasons.) As summarized in Table 3.4, Cronbach's alpha for the various subscales ranged from .71 to .92 across multiple samples. The demonstrated reliability of the MIA (and the MFQ) is reassuring. Several writers (e.g., Dixon & Hertzog, in press; Gilewski & Zelinski, 1986) have noted that many of the metamemory instruments now available have unknown or low levels of reliability. Further, there are important consequences of low reliability for determining convergent and discriminant validity, and for estimating metamemory/memory performance relationships (e.g., Dixon & Hertzog, in press; Rushton, Brainerd, & Pressley, 1983). We will return to this issue later.

Prior work with multiple samples also indicated that the subscales of the MIA are factorially valid (Dixon & Hultsch, 1983b). More recently, Hertzog,

TABLE 3.2. A Priori Subscales of the Memory Functioning Questionnaire (MFQ)[a]

| Subscale | Sample Item |
|---|---|
| 1. General rating | 1. How would you rate your memory in terms of the kinds of problems you have? (+ = no problems) |
| 2. Retrospective functioning | 2. How is your memory compared to what it was . . . (a) 1 year ago? (+ = much better) |
| 3. Frequency of forgetting | 3. How often do these present a memory problem for you . . . (a) names? (+ = never) |
| 4. Frequency of forgetting when reading novels | 4. As you are reading a novel, how often do you have trouble remembering what you have read . . . (a) in opening chapters, once you have finished the book? (+ = never) |
| 5. Frequency of forgetting when reading newspapers and magazines | 5. When you are reading a newspaper or magazine article, how often do you have trouble remembering what you have read . . . (a) in the opening paragraphs, once you have finished the article? (+ = never) |
| 6. Remembering past events | 6. How well do you remember things that occurred . . . (a) last month? (+ = very good) |
| 7. Seriousness | 7. When you actually forget in these situations, how serious a problem do you consider the memory failure to be . . . (a) names. (+ = not serious) |
| 8. Mnemonics | 8. How often do you use these techniques to remind yourself about things . . . (a) keep an appointment book. (+ = never) |

[a]Based on Gilewski et al. (1983).

Dixon, Schulenberg, and Hultsch (1987) tested the hypothesis that the eight subscales of the MIA tap higher order metamemory factors reflective of memory knowledge, memory self-efficacy, and memory-related affect dimensions. Data from the six separate studies involving a total of 750 subjects were combined to yield two half-samples for cross-validation purposes. Each of the samples were partitioned into young, middle-aged, and old groups to examine the consistency of factor structure at different ages. A multiple groups confirmatory factor analysis was conducted on the data, using the first half-sample to develop a model and the second half-sample to validate it.

Although the models did not fully cross-validate, both analyses indicated that there are at least two higher order factors in the MIA. The first, labeled

TABLE 3.3. Seven Dimensions of the Metamemory in Adulthood (MIA) Instrument[a]

| Dimension | Description | Sample Item |
|---|---|---|
| 1. Strategy | Knowledge and use of information about one's remembering abilities such that performance in given instances is potentially improved (+ = high use) | Do you write appointments on a calendar to help you remember them? |
| 2. Task | Knowledge of basic memory processes, especially as evidenced by how most people perform (+ = high knowledge) | For most people, facts that are interesting are easier to remember than facts that are not. |
| 3. Capacity | Perception of memory capacities as evidenced by predictive report of performance on given tasks (+ = high capacity) | I am good at remembering names. |
| 4. Change | Perception of memory abilities as generally stable or subject to long-term decline (+ = stability) | The older I get the harder it is to remember things clearly. |
| 5. Anxiety | Feelings of stress related to memory performance (+ = high anxiety) | I do not get flustered when I am put on the spot to remember new things. |
| 6. Achievement | Perceived importance of having a good memory and performing well on memory tasks (+ = high achievement) | It is important that I am very accurate when remembering names of people. |
| 7. Locus | Perceived personal control over remembering abilities (+ = internality) | Even if I work on it my memory ability will go downhill. |

[a]Based on Dixon & Hultsch (1983b).

Memory Self-Efficacy, involves beliefs about competence associated with memory-demanding situations. The second, tentatively labeled Memory Knowledge, combined knowledge about memory and affect related to memory. Factor loadings for Memory Knowledge were invariant across the three age groups; Strategy, Task, Achievement, and Anxiety consistently loaded on this factor. In contrast, there were significant age differences in the weights associated with the Memory Self-Efficacy factor. It was generally

TABLE 3.4. Internal Consistency (Cronbach's Alpha) for Seven MIA Subscales for Multiple Samples

| | Sample | | | | |
|---|---|---|---|---|---|
| Subscale | Dixon & Hultsch (1983b) $N = 120$ | Dixon & Hultsch (1983b) $N = 108$ | Dixon & Hultsch (1983b) $N = 150$ | Hultsch et al. (1987) $N = 388$ | Hultsch et al. (1987) $N = 342$ |
| Strategy | .86 | .86 | .85 | .84 | .82 |
| Task | .83 | .81 | .83 | .78 | .78 |
| Capacity | .86 | .82 | .86 | .85 | .81 |
| Change | .93 | .90 | .91 | .91 | .92 |
| Anxiety | .83 | .84 | .83 | .87 | .86 |
| Achievement | .76 | .78 | .79 | .78 | .76 |
| Locus | .71 | .78 | .77 | .78 | .71 |

defined by Capacity, Change, Anxiety, and Locus, but loadings for the Change and Locus subscales were substantially higher in the old than in the young.

In sum, metamemory seems to be most productively considered as a multidimensional construct. At minimum, it is possible to differentiate memory knowledge from memory self-efficacy dimensions. Multiple facets may exist within these broad dimensions. In addition, there may be age differences in the structure of these dimensions. In particular, the composition of memory self-efficacy dimensions may be different for older as compared to younger adults. Specifically, perceptions of change in memory and perceptions of reduced control over memory are more salient for the elderly.

## Convergent and Discriminant Validity

Until now, psychologists interested in constructing metamemory questionnaires have focused on developing and validating their own instruments, paying relatively little attention to the similarity of their instrument to others. As discussed by several reviewers (Dixon, in press; Gilewski & Zelinski, 1986; Herrmann, 1982), further work investigating the validity of metamemory questionnaires for adult populations is critically needed. In particular, traditional issues associated with construct validity of psychological measures (e.g., Cronbach & Meehl, 1955; Messick, 1981) have yet to be addressed with respect to metamemory questionnaires (Dixon, in press; Dixon & Hertzog, in press). One issue is the degree of convergent validity between different metamemory questionnaires. As outlined above, different questionnaires emphasize different domains of metamemory. For example, the MIA measures affect about memory not explicitly assessed by other questionnaires. There is, however, reason to wonder whether memory self-efficacy, as measured by the MIA Capacity scale, is the same construct as measured by the MFQ or the SIME. The principal scales from the MFQ and the SIME are relatively similar to one another. Both query the respondent about frequency of forgetting problems in specific domains of memory, such as forgetting names. An overall frequency-of-forgetting score is then calculated by summing frequency-of-forgetting ratings across the domain of forgetting instances. Although there are some differences between the SIME and the MFQ in terms of the selection of forgetting instances and the specificity of question wording (see Gilewski & Zelinski, 1986), it is reasonable to expect a high degree of convergent validity between the two scales.

If the MFQ and SIME also measure memory self-efficacy with their frequency-of-forgetting scales, then they should display convergent validity with some MIA scales (particularly Capacity). There is, however, a greater opportunity for divergence between the MIA and the other two scales, given differences in the way self-efficacy questions are phrased in the MIA (see Table 3.3). There is at this time some limited evidence that the MIA and the SIME are significantly correlated. Cavanaugh and Poon (1985) found evidence of a substantial correlation between the MIA Capacity scale and the total score on the SIME, but with a very small sample of older adults. There has been, before the work described in this chapter, no information relating the MFQ to the MIA or the SIME.

A second issue regarding the validity of metamemory questionnaires is their discriminant validity from other, theoretically related constructs. Can memory self-perceptions be differentiated from well-established constructs such as locus of control, self-esteem, and personality? Surprisingly, little effort has been made to this point to demonstrate that cognitive psychologists have not merely rediscovered such well-known constructs and given them a different label! This is an obvious concern for the MIA, in which it seems quite plausible that measures of perceived locus of control or anxiety regarding memory might measure nothing more than general locus of control and trait anxiety. In addition, it is plausible that such measures are highly influenced by the emotional state of the respondent at the time of the self-rating. Zarit (1982) has suggested that older adults' complaints about their memory may reflect their degree of depression as much, if not more, than their actual memory capacity. Indeed, some studies have found higher correlations between memory complaints and depression than between memory complaints and actual memory performance (e.g., Kahn, Zarit, Hilbert, & Niederehe, 1975; West, Boatwright, & Schleser, 1984). Although such findings do not necessarily indicate that perceived memory self-efficacy is determined by depression, they do indicate that close examination of the issue is required.

In order to address the validity of the MIA and MFQ, we have recently conducted a major study that used confirmatory factor analysis to explicitly evaluate the convergent validity of the two questionnaires and their discriminant validity from related constructs. Several methodologists have noted that confirmatory factor analysis is an ideal tool for assessing validity (e.g., Bentler, 1978; Hertzog, 1985; Joreskog, 1974). Like its counterpart, structural equation models, confirmatory factor analysis estimates relations among latent variables (factors) that are disattenuated for measurement error. This means, for example, that it is meaningful to test whether a factor correlation is 1.0 in a population (because 1.0 is a true upper bound of the latent variable correlation; see Joreskog, 1974). A meaningful operational definition of convergent validity, then, is that two latent variables have a disattenuated correlation of 1.0. Similarly, confirmatory factor analysis is helpful in assessing discriminant validity. With this approach, low correlations among factors imply a low degree of shared variance in the latent construct (and not any artifact of poor reliability). Thus, showing low correlations among factors implies discriminant validity of the constructs reflected in those factors.

The validation study included two samples drawn from rather different populations. One sample was drawn from a medium-sized western Canadian city (Victoria, British Columbia). The second sample was drawn from a semirural area in the eastern United States (Annville, Pennsylvania). The Victoria sample consisted of 378 individuals (100 university students, 278 adults aged 55–78 years), whereas the Annville sample included 447 adults (age range, 20–78 years). Additional details regarding the samples may be found in Hultsch, Hertzog, and Dixon (1987).

## Convergent Validity of the MIA and MFQ

Do the MIA and the MFQ measure the same dimensions of metamemory? Clearly, the MFQ does not measure the same aspects of memory-related affect, but there appears to be substantial overlap in other domains. The critical dimension, given our previous discussion, is memory self-efficacy. The Hertzog, Dixon, Schulenberg, and Hultsch (1987) analysis suggested that the MIA scales of Capacity, Change, Anxiety, and Locus all loaded on a dimension we interpreted as Memory Self-Efficacy. A content analysis of the MFQ suggested that its Global Rating Scale, Memory Problems, and Remote Memory scales do indeed measure interrelated aspects of Memory Self-Efficacy. The MFQ also measures in great depth self-reported memory problems for reading materials. This also seemed to be an aspect of Memory Self-Efficacy, although it seemed plausible that its specificity would cause a less-than-perfect correlation of it with a more general Memory Self-Efficacy factor.

Our content analysis of the MFQ is consistent with an unpublished study of the factor structure of the MFQ reported by Gilewski et al. (1983). Their confirmatory factor analysis of the MFQ found one strong factor that seems to be Memory Self-Efficacy (including high loading on the Memory Problems and Memory Rating indicators). Two weaker factors were also reported, which in essence appeared to be dominated by single measures: Strategy Use and Perceived Seriousness. The Gilewski et al. (1983) analysis thus appears to identify a strong Memory Self-Efficacy factor in the MFQ that in theory should converge with the Memory Self-Efficacy factor in the MIA found by Hertzog, Dixon, Schulenberg, and Hultsch (1987).

Aside from Memory Self-Efficacy, there are other overlapping scales between the two questionnaires. Both contain a self-reported strategy use scale. Both contain a scale asking individuals to assess perceived change in memory capacity (MIA Change, MFQ Retrospective). Although these may be primary markers of a Memory Self-Efficacy factor, it is plausible that indicators of perceived change would form a factor independent of Memory Self-Efficacy.

Hertzog, Hultsch, and Dixon (1987) conducted an extensive series of confirmatory factor analyses designed to evaluate the degree of convergence between the MIA and MFQ scales. Analyses were conducted in three phases. First, an exploratory model was developed using the data from the Annville sample. Second, this model was replicated (cross-validated) in the Victoria adult sample. Finally, a multiple groups factor analysis was run to determine age-related invariance in the joint factor structure of the two scales. We shall only summarize the salient results of the analyses here.

The exploratory analysis of the Annville sample forced immediate reassessment of some of our hypotheses about the factor structure of the metamemory scales. First, the zero-order correlations among the MIA Task, Strategy, Locus, and Achievement scales were lower than in the original Dixon and Hultsch (1983b) samples. These correlations, generally below .3, indicated that we would not be able to replicate the second factor (labeled Memory Knowledge) found by Hertzog, Dixon, Schulenberg, and Hultsch (1987). In fact, the low correlation of the MIA Task with either the MIA or the MFQ Strategy scales was a surprising finding, for it indicated that simply stripping the more affect-related MIA scales such as Achievement from the factor would not suffice in defining a memory knowledge factor. On the other hand, the high correlation of the two strategy use scales suggested that a convergent Strategy factor could be modeled. Second, the Seriousness scale of the MFQ had virtually zero correlation with other scales and was hence eliminated from the analysis.

After a series of model-building exercises, we arrived at a basic specification that appeared to account for the structure of the two questionnaires. The model specified two Memory Self-Efficacy factors (one for each questionnaire), a MFQ Reading Self-Efficacy factor (marked by problems in remembering materials from novels and problems remembering newpapers and magazines), a strategy use factor, a memory-related affect factor (marked chiefly by MIA Achievement), a Change factor (marked by MIA Change, MFQ Retrospective, and Locus), and an MIA Task factor (treated as a single indicator).

The model fit well in both samples. The LISREL Adjusted Goodness-of-Fit index was .945 for the Annville sample and .943 for the Victoria sample.

This index has a maximum of 1.0 when a model fits a set of data perfectly, and fits greater than .9 are usually considered excellent for this index.

Table 3.5 reports the factor loadings for this model for both the Annville sample and the Victoria sample. We estimated standardized solutions in both samples that can act to accentuate sample differences in the model's parameter estimates. Moreover, the two samples differed widely in age range, so differences might be expected both because of sample differences in variances and age differences in the factor structure of metamemory. The similarity, then, of the standardized factor loadings reported in Table 3.5 is impressive. Indeed, when *t* tests of the differences between sample estimates were computed, none of the estimates differed significantly from each other. The largest difference, that for the loading of Anxiety on the Memory-Related Affect factor, yielded a *t* test of 1.79, which is not significant at the 5% level of confidence.

We did conduct a more direct test of age differences in factor loading (see Hertzog, Hultsch, & Dixon 1987 for more details). The two samples were split into two age groups. The old sample approximated the age range of the Victoria sample, and a middle-aged group was then constructed from the 20-to 55-year-olds.[1] In the Victoria sample, the student group defined a young age group to supplement the old group already analyzed. We then ran a series of simultaneous multiple group factor analyses (Joreskog, 1971) designed to test group differences in factor loading. None of the groups differed significantly in factor loading. The result was somewhat surprising, for it disagreed with the findings of Hertzog, Dixon, Schulenberg, and Hultsch (1987), who found significant age group differences in the loading of the MIA scales on a Memory Self-Efficacy factor. The explanation of the discrepant results is happily straightforward. There were significant age group differences in the correlation of the Change factor with the Memory Self-Efficacy factor. As might be expected, perceived change was more highly correlated with self-efficacy in the old groups. In the Hertzog, Dixon, Schulenberg, and Hultsch (1987) analysis of the MIA, it was not possible to separately estimate the Change factor. Thus, the different relationship of change to self-efficacy was absorbed, as it were, into the loading of MIA Change and MIA Locus on the Memory Self-Efficacy factor. In sum, it appears that the factor solutions were replicable across multiple groups, and that the different age groups had equivalent factor loadings, but differed in factor correlations.

Table 3.6 reports the factor correlations for the four different age groups.[2] Table 3.6 includes crucial information regarding the question of convergent validity: the correlation between the MIA and MFQ Memory Self-Efficacy factors. We can now see the beneficial effect of using confirmatory factor analysis to assess convergent validity. As discussed above, if it were the case

---

[1]Most of these subjects were aged 33 or older.

[2]The models computed factor covariance matrices, but these have been standardized for ease of interpretation and discussion.

TABLE 3.5. Factor Loadings of Metamemory Scales for Annville (A) and Victoria (V) Samples

| | Factors[a] | | | | | | | | | | | |
|---|---|---|---|---|---|---|---|---|---|---|---|---|
| | $MSE_{MIA}$ | | $MSE_{MFQ}$ | | RD | | STRAT | | AFF | | CHANGE | |
| Scale | A | V | A | V | A | V | A | V | A | V | A | V |
| STRAT[a] | 0[b] | 0 | 0 | 0 | 0 | 0 | 1.0[c] | 1.0[c] | 0 | 0 | 0 | 0 |
| TASK | 0 | 0 | 0 | 0 | 0 | 0 | 0 | 0 | 0 | 0 | 0 | 0 |
| CAP | .844 | .843 | 0 | 0 | 0 | 0 | 0 | 0 | .235 | .314 | 0 | 0 |
| CHA | .514 | .612 | 0 | 0 | 0 | 0 | 0 | 0 | 0 | 0 | .500 | .505 |
| ANX | −.633 | −.702 | 0 | 0 | 0 | 0 | 0 | 0 | .332 | .165 | 0 | 0 |
| ACH | 0 | 0 | 0 | 0 | 0 | 0 | 0 | 0 | .847 | .944 | 0 | 0 |
| LOC | .250 | .279 | 0 | 0 | 0 | 0 | 0 | 0 | .343 | .300 | .336 | .335 |
| G.RATING | 0 | 0 | .448 | .544 | 0 | 0 | 0 | 0 | 0 | 0 | 0 | 0 |
| RETRO | 0 | 0 | .151 | .220 | 0 | 0 | 0 | 0 | 0 | 0 | .334 | .345 |
| FORGET | 0 | 0 | .853 | .850 | 0 | 0 | 0 | 0 | 0 | 0 | 0 | 0 |
| READ1 | 0 | 0 | 0 | 0 | .856 | .882 | 0 | 0 | 0 | 0 | 0 | 0 |
| READ2 | 0 | 0 | 0 | 0 | .849 | .822 | 0 | 0 | 0 | 0 | 0 | 0 |
| PAST | 0 | 0 | .650 | .741 | 0 | 0 | 0 | 0 | 0 | 0 | 0 | 0 |
| MFQSTRAT | 0 | 0 | 0 | 0 | 0 | 0 | −.719 | −.695 | 0 | 0 | 0 | 0 |

[a]Abbreviations: *Factors:* $MSE_{MIA}$—Memory Self-Efficacy, MIA scale; $MSE_{MFQ}$—Memory Self-Efficacy, MFQ Scale; RD—Memory Self-Efficacy, Reading; STRAT—Memory Strategy Use: AFF—Memory-Related Affect.
*Scales:* STRAT—MIA Strategy Use: CAP—MIA Capacity; CHA—MIA Change; ANX—MIA Anxiety; ACH—MIA Achievement; LOC—MIA Locus of Control; G.RATING—MFQ Global Memory Rating; RETRO—MFQ Retrospective; FORGET—MFQ Problems; READ1—MFQ Problems Remembering Novels; READ2—MFQ Problems Remembering Magazines; PAST—MFQ Remote Memory; MFQSTRAT—MFQ Strategy Use.
[b]All 0 entries were fixed by hypothesis.
[c]Denotes fixed parameter.

TABLE 3.6. Metamemory Factor Correlations in Four Groups

| | Groups | | | |
|---|---|---|---|---|
| Factors[a] | Victoria (old) | Annville (old) | Annville (middle-aged) | Victoria (young) |
| $MSE_{MIA}$, $MSE_{MFQ}$ | .879 | .963 | 1.004[b] | .836 |
| $MSE_{MIA}$, RD | .667 | .730 | .736 | .567 |
| $MSE_{MFQ}$, RD | .742 | .749 | .806 | .576 |
| $MSE_{MIA}$, STRAT | −.194 | −.368 | −.258 | −.177 |
| $MSE_{MFQ}$, STRAT | −.117 | −.205 | −.227 | −.152 |
| RD, STRAT | −.113 | −.074 | −.124 | −.139 |
| $MSE_{MIA}$, AFF | −.096 | −.210 | −.131 | −.166 |
| $MSE_{MFQ}$, AFF | .087 | −.148 | −.005 | .105 |
| RD, AFF | −.057 | −.157 | .005 | −.029 |
| STRAT, AFF | .320 | .293 | .267 | .376 |
| $MSE_{MIA}$, TASK | .089 | .095 | −.004 | .103 |
| $MSE_{MFQ}$, TASK | .049 | .195 | .057 | .188 |
| RD, TASK | .006 | .225 | .144 | .238 |
| STRAT, TASK | .082 | .087 | .274 | .124 |
| AFF, TASK | .320 | .178 | .180 | .269 |
| $MSE_{MIA}$, CHANGE | .367 | .637 | .336 | .127 |
| $MSE_{MFQ}$, CHANGE | .324 | .488 | .172 | .105 |

[a]Abbreviations: *Factors:* $MSE_{MIA}$—Memory Self-Efficacy, MIA scale; $MSE_{MFQ}$—Memory Self-Efficacy, MFQ Scale; RD—Memory Self-Efficacy, reading; STRAT—Memory Strategy Use; AFF—Memory-Related Affect.

[b]The maximum likelihood estimate for the factor covariance did, when rescaled, convert to a correlation greater than 1.0. This can happen in latent variable models of this kind, especially when factor loadings are constrained equal over groups.

that the two scales measure the same Memory Self-Efficacy construct, then the correlation between the two Memory Self-Efficacy factors should be 1. The first row of correlations in Table 3.6 shows that these correlations were uniformly large, albeit larger in the Annville than in the Victoria groups. Correlations of this magnitude justify the conclusion that the two scales are, indeed, measuring the same construct. It should be noted, however, that formal tests of this hypothesis, achieved by constraining the factor correlation to equal 1 (see Joreskog, 1974), are statistically significant for the Victoria samples.

Practically speaking, the divergence from 1 is relatively trivial, but some patterns in the estimated factor correlations indicate differences between the MIA and MFQ Memory Self-Efficacy factors in their relations to other factors. For example, the Reading Self-Efficacy factor (taken from the MFQ) correlates more highly with the MFQ Memory Self-Efficacy factor than with the MIA Memory Self-Efficacy factor. It seems likely that the minor differences are a function of method variance associated with the different types of questions and Likert response formats; indeed, Hertzog, Hultsch, and Dixon (1987) reported results from a model consistent with this hypothesis. Thus, with respect to the major metamemory factor, Memory Self-Efficacy, the MIA and MFQ converge to measure the same construct. The viability of the Strategy Use factor also indicates convergence of the MIA and MFQ in measuring self-reported use of memory strategies (especially, external aids).

The correlations reported in Table 3.6 also support the conclusion that there are multiple dimensions of metamemory. In all four samples there is a small, negative relationship between Memory Self-Efficacy and Strategy Use, with individuals low in self-efficacy more likely to report more strategy use. All four samples also show virtually zero correlations between Memory Self-Efficacy, whether measured by the MIA or by the MFQ, and the MIA Task scale. This finding buttresses the contention that knowledge about how memory functions is independent of memory self-efficacy beliefs.

## Discriminant Validity

We are now conducting a series of multivariate analyses exploring the discriminant validity of the metamemory factors from related constructs. At this point we can draw some preliminary conclusions from patterns of simple correlations of the metamemory scales with scales measuring personality, locus of control, and affective states.

Table 3.7 presents correlations of the MIA scales with measures of personality taken from the Jackson Personality Inventory and the Jackson Personality Research Form for the Annville sample. The highest correlations involve the MIA Anxiety scale with the personality scales Anxiety, Self-Esteem, and Conformity. This finding supports the hypothesis that part of the variance in MIA Anxiety is associated with the personality dimension of Neuroticism (and of course, more specifically, trait Anxiety). With respect to the first three scales listed in Table 3.7, Locus, Capacity, and Change, the correlations are relatively low. There therefore appears to be little cause for concern that Memory Self-Efficacy, as measured by these scales, is a reexpression of basic personality dimensions.

It is also interesting to note the low correlations of MIA Locus with the three scales taken from the Levenson Internal/External Locus of Control scale (Internal, Powerful Others, and Chance). Levenson (1974) argued that internal control orientations (as assessed by her Internal scale) are distinct from two aspects of an external control orientation (as measured by Powerful Others and Chance). One would expect a high correlation of MIA Locus with Levenson Internal if, in fact, the MIA Locus scale was just a reexpression of a general internal control orientation. The small correlations reported in Table 3.7 provide no basis, then, for arguing that Locus is just another measure of generalized locus of control. This result agrees well with work by Lachman (1983, 1986), who has shown that control beliefs are both general and domain-specific. Lachman also demonstrated that control

TABLE 3.7. Correlations of MIA Subscales With Personality and Locus of Control Measures

| | MIA Subscales | | | | | | |
|---|---|---|---|---|---|---|---|
| Measure | LOC | CAP | CHA | ANX | ACH | STRAT | TASK |
| JPI Anxiety[a] | −.050 | −.082 | −.073 | .438 | .216 | .177 | −.045 |
| JPI Affect | .073 | .045 | −.076 | .238 | .244 | .193 | .045 |
| JPI Energy | .173 | .248 | .219 | −.281 | .011 | −.087 | .029 |
| JPI Self-esteem | .082 | .315 | .255 | −.423 | −.035 | −.094 | .017 |
| JPI Conformity | −.048 | −.169 | −.145 | .388 | .226 | .234 | .060 |
| PRF Endurance | .194 | .209 | .182 | −.218 | .109 | −.110 | −.003 |
| Internal | .160 | .170 | .156 | −.140 | .091 | −.012 | .170 |
| Others | −.037 | −.054 | −.076 | .253 | .175 | .143 | .086 |
| Chance | −.014 | −.041 | −.048 | .169 | .063 | .028 | −.063 |
| VW DEP | .050 | .124 | .092 | −.361 | −.187 | −.054 | .002 |
| CES-D DEP | −.004 | −.122 | −.107 | .289 | .175 | −.013 | −.057 |
| CES-D WB | −.040 | −.166 | −.133 | .234 | .133 | −.018 | −.035 |
| VW WB | .067 | .138 | .145 | −.309 | −.144 | .003 | .011 |

[a]Abbreviations: JPI—Jackson Personality Inventory; PRF—Jackson Personality Research Form; VW Dep—Veit/Ware Depression; CES-D DEP—CES-D Depression scale; CES-D WB—CES-D Well-Being scale; VW WB—Veit/Ware Well-Being scale; LOC—MIA Locus of Control; CAP—MIA Capacity; CHA—MIA Change; ANX—MIA Anxiety; ACH—MIA Achievement; STRAT—MIA Strategy; TASK—MIA Task.

beliefs about intellectual functioning predicted performance on intelligence tests, whereas the Levenson scales did not. It does appear from Table 3.7 that there are modest correlations of Levenson Internal Locus of Control with all three indicators of Memory Self-Efficacy, and that Memory Self-Efficacy correlates more with internal than external locus of control.

The remaining correlations in Table 3.7 are from two measures of psychological well-being and depression. The Veit/Ware scales refer to revisions by Veit and Ware (1983) of a questionnaire measuring aspects of well-being and distress that was originally administered as part of a federal government study of health and well-being in the United States. Similar measures of well-being and distress were taken from the Center for Epidemiological Studies Depression scale (CES-D; see Radloff, 1977). The Veit/Ware and CES-D scales are scored in opposite directions of the relationships. Examination of these correlations shows that the MIA scales generally correlate at low levels with the measures of perceived well-being and depression. The major exception, again, is the MIA Anxiety scale. There is little cause for concern, however, that perceived memory self-efficacy is indistinguishable from depression.

As indicated, a second set of issues involves the degree to which responses on the MIA are influenced by concurrent affective state—particularly when

TABLE 3.8. Correlations of MIA Subscales With Mood State Variables

| Mood State Variable | | MIA Subscales | | | | | | |
|---|---|---|---|---|---|---|---|---|
| | | LOC[a] | CAP | CHA | ANX | ACH | STRAT | TASK |
| Cattell | Anxiety | −.075 | −.128 | −.112 | .358 | .100 | .065 | −.073 |
| Cattell | Fatigue | −.116 | −.194 | −.211 | .270 | .039 | .079 | −.019 |
| Cattell | Depression | −.129 | −.260 | −.265 | .416 | .105 | .035 | −.093 |
| Cattell | Well-Being | .119 | .142 | .090 | −.187 | −.019 | −.029 | −.010 |
| MA[a] | Anxiety | −.090 | −.200 | −.152 | .361 | .101 | .048 | −.038 |
| MA | Fatigue | −.080 | −.130 | −.105 | .203 | .032 | .053 | −.022 |
| MA | Depression | −.059 | −.144 | −.088 | .192 | .116 | −.021 | −.042 |
| MA | Well-Being | .124 | .023 | .094 | −.240 | −.023 | −.022 | .023 |
| MA | Vigor | .170 | .233 | .192 | −.252 | .030 | −.080 | −.005 |

[a]Abbreviations: MA—Mood Adjective Rating Scale; LOC—MIA Locus of Control; CAP—MIA Capacity; CHA—MIA Change; ANX—MIA Anxiety; ACH—MIA Achievement; STRAT—MIA Strategy; TASK—MIA Task.

responding to questions about control, anxiety, and achievement motivation. Table 3.8 presents the correlations of the MIA with two sets of mood state measures: (a) scales from Cattell's Eight State Questionnaire, and (b) mood adjective rating scales, with adjectives used from the Profile of Mood States and from Lebo and Nesselroade (1978). These correlations were consistent with those already reported for personality, control, and depression. MIA Anxiety showed salient correlations with mood states of anxiety and depression. None of the other MIA scales showed much relationship to the mood rating variables.

In sum, our preliminary analyses of the discriminant validity data suggest that (a) MIA Anxiety has substantial relationships to trait anxiety and related affective states; (b) none of the other MIA scales shows strong relationships to these variables; (c) the Memory Self-Efficacy factor identified in the MIA is not merely generalized locus of control, although there appears to be a modest relationship between internal locus of control and Memory Self-Efficacy; and (d) the small correlations seem to rule out the hypothesis that Memory Self-Efficacy ratings are highly related to depression or concurrent depressive affect.

## Age and Sex Differences in Metamemory

Researchers interested in metamemory and aging have, of course, examined the basic question of the existence of age and other group (e.g., gender) differences in metamemory. The answer to this basic question has not been particularly straightforward. Specifically, the consistency and robustness of such group differences are somewhat unclear. This lack of clarity may result, in part, from some of the measurement issues noted. Studies have varied widely in the definition of the construct and the particular instrument used to operationalize it. However, inconsistencies have also appeared in work administering the same questionnaire to different samples. Nevertheless, examination of multiple data sets has begun to paint a reasonably consistent picture that permits us to unravel some of the confusion present in the literature.

## Age Differences

As noted, the literature presents a plethora of conclusions regarding adult age differences in metamemory. For example, although several studies have failed to find age differences in reported use of memory strategies (Dixon & Hultsch, 1983b; Gilewski et al., 1983; Perlmutter, 1978), others have reported that older adults use fewer strategies than younger adults (Weinstein, Duffy, Underwood, MacDonald, & Gott, 1981). There has also been disagreement about whether older adults report more memory failures in everyday activities than younger adults. Some studies (e.g., Gilewski et al., 1983: Perlmutter, 1978) report negative age differences, but others (e.g., Sunderland, Harris, & Baddeley, 1983) have found that younger adults actually reported more such incidents than older adults. Similarly, a mixed pattern of results appears for indicators of perceived memory abilities or capacities. Although Dixon and Hultsch (1983b), Gilewski et al. (1983), and Zelinski et al. (1980) found older adults had a poorer perception of their memory for various content domains than younger adults, Chaffin and Herrmann (1983) found a mixed pattern of results (including positive, equivalent, and negative age differences) across domains, and Bennett-Levy and Powell (1980) reported a positive age effect on their measure.

Given the diversity of measurement approaches used in the work summarized above, it is extremely difficult to distinguish age effects from measurement effects. However, data on multiple samples are available for at least two multidimensional metamemory instruments: the MIA and the MFQ. In the case of the MIA, data are available for seven samples varying in size and nationality (Cavanaugh & Poon, 1985; Dixon & Hultsch, 1983b; Gutman, 1987; Hultsch et al., 1987). The nature of the samples and the pattern of age differences emerging on the various subscales of the MIA in the different samples are shown in Table 3.9. Although there are inconsistencies across the samples, the pattern of results suggests that there may be reliable age differences on the Capacity, Change, and Locus subscales. Significant age differences on these indicators are observed in most of the samples. Further, in most instances, the age effects associated with these subscales are accounting for substantial portions of variance (Capacity: range = 3–10%; Change: range = 13–37%; Locus: range = 3–19%). Across multiple samples, then, there is evidence to suggest that, compared to younger adults, older

TABLE 3.9. Summary of Significant Age-Related Differences for Subscales of the MIA Over Multiple Samples

| Sample Characteristics/ Sources | MIA Subscales[a] | | | | | | |
|---|---|---|---|---|---|---|---|
| | STRAT | TASK | CAP | CHA | ANX | ACH | LOC |
| 1. N = 120; 2 age groups (18–37, 50–81) Dixon & Hultsch (1983b) | | –[b] | – | – | | | – |
| 2. N = 108; 3 age groups (21–30, 40–58, 60–84) (Dixon & Hultsch, 1983b) | | | – | – | | | – |
| 3. N = 150; 3 age groups (21–39; 40–58; 60–74) (Dixon & Hultsch, 1983b) | | – | – | | | | – |
| 4. N = 46; 2 age groups (M = 19.0, M = 76.9) (Cavanaugh & Poon, 1985) | | | – | – | | | |
| 5. N = 360; 4 age groups (20–26, 55–61, 62–68, 69–78) (Hultsch et al., 1987) | +[b] | | – | – | | | – |
| 6. N = 415; continuous age sample 20–78 (Hultsch et al., 1987) | | | – | – | | | –(t)[b] |
| 7. N = 376; 4 age groups (54–61, 62–68, 60–75, 76–93) (Gutman, 1987) | | | | – | | + | |

[a]Abbreviations: STRAT—MIA Strategy; TASK—MIA Task; CAP—MIA Capacity; CHA—MIA Change; ANX—MIA Anxiety; ACH—MIA Achievement; LOC—MIA Locus of Control.
[b]+, older adults score significantly higher ($p < .01$) than younger adults;
–, older adults score significantly lower ($p < .01$) than younger adults;
(t), trend toward significance at $p < .05$.

adults see themselves as having less memory capacity, report that their memory has declined over the years, and believe that there is little that they can do to enhance their memory or prevent its deterioration.

It should be noted that the age differences observed appear to be most pronounced when a contrast is drawn between a young university student sample and middle-aged and older community residents. For example, Hultsch et al. (1987) tested two large samples that differed in their demographic characteristics. One sample was designed to represent the entire adult age range, and consisted of younger, middle-aged, and older adults, none of whom was enrolled full-time in university at the time of testing. Hierarchical regression analyses of the data from this sample indicated significant linear effects related to age on the Capacity and Change subscales, and a marginally significant trend on the Locus subscale.

The other sample was designed to be comparable to the "traditional" cross-sectional sample typically used in cognitive aging research. In this case, the younger adults were university students and the middle-aged and older adults were healthy, community-dwelling volunteers. In this sample, the significant age effects, which included the Capacity, Change, and Locus subscales, generally resulted from differences between the youngest group and the remaining groups. Differences among the various older groups were generally not significant. Similarly, a hierarchical regression analysis conducted on the data from the middle-aged and older age groups from this sample did not show any significant linear trends. This suggests that age differences at the mean level within the middle to older age ranges may be relatively fragile. Thus, some of the discrepant findings in the literature may result partially from the characteristics of the subjects sampled from these portions of the life span.

In the case of the MFQ, results from four separate samples are available. The sample characteristics and pattern of age effects across them are shown in Table 3.10. The pattern of results suggests consistent age differences are present on the Retrospective Functioning subscale. There are less consistent indications of differences on the Global Rating and memory problems associated with reading. In general, it appears that the MIA and MFQ are differentially sensitive to detecting mean age differences. Such differences are more likely to be found with the MIA than with the MFQ. The strongest evidence for this conclusion comes from the Hultsch et al. (1987) study, in which both questionnaires were administered to two large samples. As indicated in Tables 3.9 and 3.10, age differences were found on both measures in the traditional sample contrasting young university students and older community residents. However, even in this case, the magnitude of the effects were generally smaller in the case of the MFQ than in the case of the MIA. In the other sample that sampled community residents (nonstudents) from the entire age range, several significant age differences emerged on the MIA, but only trends were observed in the case of the MFQ.

The differential sensitivity of various questionnaires to age differences

TABLE 3.10. Summary of Significant Age-Related Differences for Subscales of the MFQ Over Multiple Samples

| Sample Characteristics/ Source | MFQ Subscales[a] | | | | | | | |
|---|---|---|---|---|---|---|---|---|
| | G.RATING | RETRO | FORGET | READ1 | READ2 | PAST | SERIOUS | MFQSTRAT |
| 1. N = 639; 3 age groups (16–54, 55–70, 71–89) (Gilewski et al., 1983) | –[b] | – | – | – | – | – | – | |
| 2. N = 264; 3 age groups (16–54, 55–70, 71–89) (Gilewski et al., 1983) | – | – | – | – | – | – | | |
| 3. N = 360; 4 age groups (20–26, 55–61, 62–68, 69–78) (Hultsch et al., 1987) | – | – | | – | – | | | |
| 4. N = 415; continuous age sample (20–78) (Hultsch et al., 1987) | | –(t) | | | –(t) | | | +(t)[b] |

[a]Abbreviations: G.RATING—MFQ Global Memory Rating; RETRO—MFQ Retrospective; FORGET—MFQ Problems; READ1—Problems Remembering Novels; READ2—Problems Remembering Magazines; PAST—MFQ Remote Memory; SERIOUSNESS—MFQ Seriousness; MFQSTRAT—MFQ Strategy Use.

[b]+, older adults score significantly higher ($p < .01$) than younger adults;
–, older adults score significantly lower ($p < .01$) than younger adults;
(t), trend toward significance at $p < .05$.

may be related to the phrasing of the questions. For example, Hultsch et al. (1987) found no age differences on subscales consisting of questions that ask people to report the extent to which they experience episodes of forgetting in particular domains (e.g., MFQ Frequency of Forgetting). In contrast, age differences were observed on subscales consisting of questions that ask people to rate their memory relative to some unspecified anchor (e.g., MIA Capacity). Age differences are particularly apparent on subscales consisting of questions that ask people to rate their memory relative to the anchor of their own past performance (e.g., MIA Change; MFQ Retrospective Functioning). One possible explanation of this pattern is that, although older adults perceive that their memory has declined from previously higher levels of functioning, they do not view this loss as a "problem," either because their current level of functioning conforms to what they expect or because the incidents of forgetting do not seriously interfere with achieving everyday goals. Sunderland, Watts, Baddeley, & Harris (1986) have presented data that are consistent with this latter notion.

### Sex Differences

The question of whether there are gender differences in memory knowledge and perceptions is unresolved. In some instances, samples have been composed of individuals of predominately one gender (Dixon & Hultsch, 1983b). In other instances, although both genders have been represented in the sample, differences between them have not been explicitly examined. In our recent analysis (Hultsch et al., 1987), we found some evidence for gender differences on the MIA and MFQ that are consistent across samples, although they do not account for large amounts of variance. Specifically, women appear to report more strategy use and greater anxiety associated with memory-demanding situations than men. Significant differences were observed on the MIA Strategy subscale in both samples and on the MFQ Mnemonics subscale in one sample. Differences were also observed on the MIA Anxiety subscale in both samples. In all instances, however, the effects accounted for 3% or less of the variance.

## Metamemory/Memory Relationships

One of the thorniest questions facing researchers interested in metamemory concerns the relationship between thinking about remembering and actually remembering. The most straightforward view assumes there should be close linkages between these two activities. For example, work in which metamemory is conceptualized largely as factual knowledge about memory tasks and strategies quickly leads to the hypothesis that actual performance in memory-demanding situations may be wholly or partially dependent on such metamemorial knowledge (Flavell & Wellman, 1977). Experimental work, particularly with children, has provided some support for the notion that performance differences among different age groups may be related to differences in knowledge of task demands and strategy use (Cavanaugh & Perlmutter, 1982).

It is becoming increasingly clear, however, that the relationship between metamemory and actual memory performance is not straightforward. For example, as Herrmann (1982, 1984) and others have pointed out, the evidence supporting the predictive validity of the various metamemory questionnaires is relatively limited. The general pattern of results suggests that correlations in the .20–.30 range are typical. Such findings have led some writers to question the validity of self-report measures of metamemory and to reject their use as substitutes for performance measures in clinical settings (Sunderland et al., 1986).

As we noted earlier, some questionnaires have been developed without attention to the usual steps associated with instrument development. Thus, it is possible that some of the difficulty may be related to measurement problems. For example, zero-order correlations of metamemory scales with memory performance may be attenuated by measurement errors. It is well known that the maximum population correlation between two variables is the square root of the product of their reliabilities (Nunnally, 1978). Given low reliability in the metamemory scale, we could get low correlations because the scale is a poor measure, not because metamemory and memory are unrelated. As Rushton et al. (1983) point out, scales that aggregate multiple items should have better reliability than other metamemory measures and thus correlate higher with performance measures. The MIA scales fulfill this criterion.

Of course, aggregate scales are still, to a lesser degree, unreliable. Hence they are also subject to attenuation from measurement error. One of the features of our work is the use of structural equation models to estimate correlations among latent variables such as the metamemory dimensions discussed above. The principal advantage of such approaches is that they *completely* disattenuate correlations between variables for measurement error (Schaie & Hertzog, 1985). In other words, when one estimates a latent variable for metamemory and a latent variable for memory performance, the maximum possible correlation between these latent variables is not bounded by reliability: The latent variable correlation ranges between $-1$ and 1. This disattenuation is accomplished by using multiple measures of each latent variable in the structural equation model (Joreskog, 1974; Long, 1983). The structural equation approach also has the advantage of maximizing the validity of the latent variable (e.g., Embretson, 1983).

We have also argued that metamemory is a multidimensional construct (Dixon & Hertzog, in press), and studies that have used unidimensional measures have almost unanimously failed to find significant relationships with performance (Kahn et al., 1975). Similarly, it is clear that memory performance is itself a multidimensional construct. As a result of the multidimensional nature of the domains, then, the obtained pattern of metamemory–memory correlations will be a function of which indicators were selected from which domain.

Evidence for the importance of domain specificity is convincing, although the exact patterns remain to be clarified. Dixon and Hultsch (1983a), for example, found that several metamemory subscales predicted memory for text performance in several samples. In addition, there was evidence to suggest age-related differences in the pattern of the correlations. It appeared that two indicator of memory knowledge (Task and Strategy) were the best overall predictors of performance for all adults in all samples. Certain age differences were evident, however. Younger adults' performance was predicted by what they knew about retrieval strategies and physical reminders (Strategy), what they believed about their capacity to perform on given tasks (Capacity), and what they knew about memory tasks and processes in general (Task). In contrast, older adults' performance was predicted by what they knew about memory tasks and precesses is general (Task), their level of motivation to achieve in memory-demanding situations (Achievement), and their belief in the degree of control they exercise over their memory functioning (Locus). These results suggest the possibility that the performance of older adults is more related to their beliefs about their memory self-efficacy than is the case for younger adults. However, this may not be the case for all performance measures. In another analysis, Dixon et al. (1986) examined the relationship of the MIA to performance on a battery of psychometric measures. In this instance, moderate correlations (range: .25 to .53) were observed mostly between the Strategy and Task subscales and several memory and verbal comprehension tests. The subscales reflecting memory self-efficacy showed little relationship to these traditional cognitive performance measures.

These results suggest that certain metamemory–memory performance relationships may be more likely to appear with performance tasks that are high in ecological validity. Such a finding is not surprising considering the fact that most metamemory questionnaires solicit self-evaluations of memory capacity in relation to everyday memory situations. Direct support for this notion comes from studies that have reported significant correlations of various components of metamemory with story recall but not with word recall (Sunderland et al., 1983; Zelinski et al., 1980). Similarly, Berry, West, and Scogin (1983) found that self-reports about memory predicted performance on a set of everyday memory tasks better than performance on a set of traditional laboratory tasks. Such results suggest the need for more careful consideration of the domains of metamemory and memory performance being examined. Indeed, it may be suggested that metamemory may be most relevant for memory-related behaviors typically not considered at all. For example, the decision to enter a memory-demanding situation in the first place may be determined in part by individuals' perceptions of their self-efficacy in such situations.

Despite some consistencies, it is clear that the relationship between individuals' self-knowledge and self-efficacy about their memory and memory performance is complex. There is sufficient evidence to reject a straightforward interpretation of individuals' self-reports about their memory as veridical reports of their experience. For example, Sunderland et al. (1983), examining the relationship between reports of memory problems and performance for patients suffering from closed head injuries, showed that patients' self-reports showed only weak correlations with their actual performance, whereas relatives reports of the patients' problems showed stronger relationships with the same measures. Similarly, some other studies using community-dwelling adults have found instances of negative correlations between subjective ratings of memory and memory performance (Cavanaugh & Poon, 1985; Dixon et al., 1986). Thus, individuals with poor memories may be poor at recalling instances of memory failure resulting in an overestimate of memory abilities. The absence of evidence for veridical self-reports of memory suggests that metamemory questionnaires are of limited usefulness for clinical purposes.

However, it is becoming increasingly clear that cognitive processes do not operate in isolation from personality and social processes. If one accepts the possibility of interfaces among such processes, we should not necessarily expect self-reports about memory to be veridical indicators of actual memory ability. Assessments of components such as memory self-efficacy will vary considerably across individuals, and perhaps within individuals across even relatively brief intervals of time. The question is whether these individual differences in accuracy are systematic, and whether they relate to other behaviors in memory-demanding situations. If older persons' perceptions of their memory prove to be one link in a process relating the social and cognitive domains, then the metamemory construct is of interest even if it is not a substitute for performance measures.

## Summary and Conclusions

Several multidimensional metamemory questionnaires with demonstrated reliability and factorial validity (including the MIA and MFQ) have been developed. Our recent work, summarized here, has shown that the MIA and MFQ converge to measure memory self-efficacy and strategy use. In addition, the MIA measures aspects of memory-related affect and knowledge about memory-demanding situations. We have also demonstrated the discriminant validity of the MIA with respect to various personality traits and states. Recent research also suggests that there are consistent and reliable age differences in metamemory, mostly related to a sense of self-efficacy. Older adults perceive less capacity, greater change, and less control than younger adults. These differences appear to be relatively substantial when the comparison is between young university students and older adults. Differences within the middle to older ages ranges are less robust. In addition, the MIA appears to be somewhat more sensitive to age-related differences than the MFQ.

The issue of metamemory/memory performance relations remains somewhat unclear. Generally, predictive relationships are relatively modest. Latent variable analysis may help clarify the ambiguities associated with measurement error problems. We are currently pursuing this strategy with our data set. In addition, a focus on additional measures of memory-related behaviors such as the decision to enter memory-demanding situations may be required. In sum, we have made considerable progress in the domains of measurement and descriptive research related to metamemory. Attention must now be turned toward the development of an explanatory process model that will permit understanding of the ways in which cognitive and personality/social domains interact to produce the behaviors we have labeled metamemory.

*Acknowledgments.* The research conducted in our laboratories, and the preparation of this chapter, was supported by Research Grant 492-84-002 from the Social Sciences and Humanities Research Council of Canada to David Hultsch, and Research Grant AG06162 from the National Institute on Aging to Christopher Hertzog. Dr. Hertzog's work is also supported by a Research Career Development Award from the National Institute on Aging. Ms. Davidson is supported by a predoctoral fellowship from the Natural Sciences and Engineering Research Council of Canada. The cooperation of Robert K. Nielsen, M.D., the other physicians, and the members of the Annville Family Practice, Annville, Pennsylvania is deeply appreciated.

## References

Bennett-Levy, J., & Powell, G.E. (1980). The subjective memory questionnaire (SMQ). An investigation into the self-reporting of 'real life' memory skills. *British Journal of Social and Clinical Psychology, 19,* 177–188.

Bentler, P.M. (1978). The interdependence of theory, methodology, and empirical data: Causal modeling as an approach to construct validation. In D.B. Kandel (Ed.), *Longitudinal research on drug abuse: Empirical and methodological issues* (pp. 267–302). Washington, DC: Hemisphere.

Berry, J.M., West, R.L., & Scogin, F., (1983, November). *Predicting everyday and laboratory memory skill.* Paper presented at the meeting of the Gerontological Society of America, San Francisco, CA.

Cavanaugh, J.C. (in press). The importance of awareness in memory aging. In L.W. Poon, D.C. Rubin, & B.A. Wilson (Eds.), *Everyday cognition in adulthood and old age.* Cambridge: Cambridge University Press.

Cavanaugh, J.C., & Perlmutter, M. (1982). Metamemory: A critical examination. *Child Development, 53,* 11–28.

Cavanaugh, J.C., & Poon, L.W. (1985, August). *Patterns of individual differences in secondary and tertiary memory performance.* Paper presented at the meeting of the American Psychological Association, Los Angeles, CA.

Chaffin, R., & Herrmann, D.J. (1983). Self-reports of memory ability by old and young adults. *Human Learning, 2,* 17–28.
Cronbach, L.J., & Meehl, P.E. (1955). Construct validity in psychological tests. *Psychological Bulletin, 52,* 281–302.
Dixon, R.A. (in press). Questionnaire research on metamemory and aging: Issues of structure and function. In L.W. Poon, D.C. Rubin, & B.A. Wilson (Eds.), *Everyday cognition in adulthood and old age.* Cambridge; Cambridge University Press.
Dixon, R.A., & Hertzog, C. (in press). A functional approach to memory and metamemory development in adulthood. In F.E. Weinert & M. Perlmutter (Eds.), *Memory development across the life-span: Universal changes and individual differences.* Hillsdale, NJ: Erlbaum.
Dixon, R.A., Hertzog, C., & Hultsch, D.F. (1986). The multiple relationships among Metamemory in Adulthood (MIA) scales and cognitive abilities in adulthood. *Human Learning, 5,* 165–177.
Dixon, R.A., & Hultsch, D.F. (1983a). Metamemory and memory for text relationships in adulthood: A cross-validation study. *Journal of Gerontology, 38,* 689–694.
Dixon, R.A., & Hultsch, D.F. (1983b). Structure and development of metamemory in in adulthood. *Journal of Gerontology, 38,* 682–688.
Dixon, R.A., & Hultsch, D.F. (1984). The Metamemory in Adulthood (MIA) instrument. *Psychological Documents, 14,* 3.
Embretson (Whitley), S. (1983). Construct validity: Construct representation versus nomothetic span. *Psychological Bulletin, 93,* 179–197.
Flavell, J.H. (1971). First discussant's comments: What is memory development the development of? *Human Development, 14,* 272–278.
Flavell, J.H., & Wellman, H.M. (1977). Metamemory. In R.V. Kail, Jr., & J.W. Hagen (Eds.), *Perspectives on the development of memory and cognition* (pp. 3–34). Hillsdale, NJ: Erlbaum.
Gilewski, M.J., & Zelinski, E. (1986). Questionnaire assessment of memory complaints. In L.W. Poon (Ed.), *Handbook for clinical memory assessment of older adults* (pp. 93–107). Washington, DC: American Psychological Association.
Gilewski, M.J., Zelinski, E.M., Schaie, K.W., & Thompson, L.W. (1983, August). *Abbreviating the metamemory questionnaire: Factor structure and norms for adults.* Paper presented at the meeting of the American Psychological Association, Anaheim, CA.
Gutman, M.P. (1987). *Memory perceptions and memory performance in older adults.* Unpublished Master's thesis, Department of Psychology, University of Victoria, Victoria, British Columbia.
Herrmann, D.J. (1982). Know thy memory: The use of questionnaires to assess and study memory. *Psychological Bulletin, 92,* 434–452.
Herrmann, D.J. (1984). Questionnaires about memory. In J.E. Harris & P.E. Morris (Eds.), *Everyday memory, actions and absent-mindedness* (pp. 133–152). Academic Press: London.
Herrmann, D.J., & Neisser, U. (1978). An inventory of everyday memory experiences. In M.M. Gruneberg, P.E. Morris, & R.N. Sykes (Eds.), *Practical aspects of memory* (pp. 35–51). London: Academic Press.
Hertzog, C. (1985). Applications of confirmatory factor analysis to the study of intelligence. In D.K. Detterman (Ed.), *Current topics in human intelligence* (pp. 59–97). Norwood, NJ: Ablex.
Hertzog, C., Dixon, R.A., Schulenberg, J., & Hultsch, D.F. (1987). On the differentia-

tion of memory beliefs from memory knowledge: The factor structure of Metamemory in Adulthood scale. *Experimental Aging Research, 13,* 101–107.

Hertzog, C., Hultsch, D.F., & Dixon, R.A. (1987). *Evidence for the convergent validity of two self-report metamemory questionnaires.* Unpublished manuscript, School of Psychology, Georgia Institute of Technology, Atlanta, GA.

Hultsch, D.F., Dixon, R.A., & Hertzog, C. (1985). Memory perceptions and memory performance in adulthood and aging. *Canadian Journal on Aging, 4,* 179–187.

Hultsch, D.F., Hertzog, C., & Dixon, R.A. (1987). Age differences in metamemory: Resolving the inconsistencies. *Canadian Journal of Psychology, 41,* 193–208.

Joreskog, K.G. (1971). Simultaneous factor analysis in several populations. *Psychometrika, 36,* 409–426.

Joreskog, K.G. (1974). Analyzing psychological data by analysis of covariance matrices. In D.H. Krantz, R.C. Atkinson, R.D. Luce, & P. Suppes (Eds.), *Contemporary developments in mathematical psychology* (Vol. 2, pp. 1–56). San Francisco: W.H. Freeman.

Kahn, R.L., Zarit, S.H., Hilbert, N.M., & Neiderehe, G. (1975). Memory complaint and impairment in the aged: The effects of depression and altered brain function. *Archives of General Psychiatry, 32,* 1569–1573.

Lachman, M.E. (1983). Perceptions of intellectual aging: Antecedent or consequence of intellectual functioning. *Developmental Psychology, 19,* 482–498.

Lachman, M.E. (1986). Locus of control in aging research: A case for multidimensional and domain-specific assessment. *Journal of Psychology and Aging, 1,* 34–40.

Lachman, M.E., Steinberg, E.S., & Trotter, S.D. (1987). The effects of control beliefs and attributions on memory self-assessments and performance. *Psychology and Aging, 2,* 266–271.

Lebo, M.A., & Nesselroade, J.R. (1978). Intraindividual differences of mood change during pregnancy identified in five P-technique factor analyses. *Journal of Research in Personality, 12,* 205–224.

Levenson, H. (1974). Activism and powerful others: Distinctions within the concept of internal-external locus of control. *Journal of Personality Assessment, 38,* 377–383.

Long, J.S. (1983). *Covariance structure models: An introduction to LISREL.* Beverly Hills, CA: Sage.

Messick, S. (1981). Constructs and their vicissitudes in educational and psychological measurement. *Psychological Bulletin, 89,* 575–588.

Nunnally, J.C. (1978). *Psychometric theory* (2nd ed.). New York: McGraw-Hill.

Perlmutter, M. (1978). What is memory aging the aging of? *Developmental Psychology, 14,* 330–345.

Radloff, L. (1977). The CES-D scale: A self-report depression scale for research in the general population. *Journal of Applied Psychological Measurement, 1,* 385–401.

Rushton, J.P., Brainerd, C.J., & Pressley, M. (1983). Behavioral development and construct validity: The principle of aggregation. *Psychological Bulletin, 94,* 18–38.

Schaie, K.W., & Hertzog, C. (1985). Measurement in the psychology of adulthood and aging. In J.E. Birren & K.W. Schaie (Eds.), *Handbook of the psychology of aging* (2nd ed., pp. 61–92). New York: Van Nostrand Reinhold.

Sunderland, A., Harris, J.E., & Baddeley, A.D. (1983). Do laboratory tests predict everyday memory? A neuropsychological study. *Journal of Verbal Learning and Verbal Behavior, 22,* 341–357.

Sunderland, A., Watts, K., Baddeley, A.D. & Harris, J.E. (1986). Subjective memory assessment and test performance in elderly adults. *Journal of Gerontology, 41,* 376–384.

Veit, C., & Ware, J.E., Jr. (1983). The structure of psychological distress and well-being in general populations. *Journal of Consulting and Clinical Psychology, 51,* 730–742.

Weinstein, C.E., Duffy, M., Underwood, V.L., MacDonald, J., & Gott, S.P. (1981). Memory strategies reported by older adults for experimental and everyday learning tasks. *Educational Gerontology, 7,* 205–213.

Wellman, H.M. (1983). Metamemory revisited. In M.T.H. Chi (Ed.), *Trends in memory development research* (pp. 31–51). Basel: Karger.

West, R.L., & Berry, J.M. (1987, August). Self-efficacy and memory performance: Measurement issues. In J.M. Berry & J.C. Cavanaugh (Chairs), *Cognitive and memory self-efficacy in adults.* Symposium conducted at the meeting of the American Psychological Association, New York.

West, R.L., Boatwright, L.K., & Schleser, R. (1984). The link between memory performance, self-assessment, and affective status. *Experimental Aging Research, 10,* 197–200.

Zarit, S.H. (1982). Affective correlates of self-report about memory of older adults. *International Journal of Behavioral Geriatrics, 1,* 25–34.

Zarit, S.H., Cole, K.D., & Guider, R.L. (1981). Memory training strategies and subjective complaints of memory in the aged. *The Gerontologist, 21,* 158–164.

Zarit, S.H., Gallagher, D., & Kramer, N. (1981). Memory training in the community aged. Effects on depression, memory complaint, and memory performance. *Educational Gerontology, 6,* 11–27.

Zelinski, E.M., Gilewski, M.J., & Thompson, L.W. (1980). Do laboratory tests relate to self-assessments of memory ability in the young and old? In L.W. Poon, J.L. Fozard, L.S. Cermak, D. Arenberg, & L.W. Thompson (Eds.), *New directions in memory and aging. Proceedings of the George A. Talland Memory Conference* (pp. 519–544). Hillsdale, NJ: Erlbaum.

# 4. Memory for Activities: Rehearsal-Independence and Aging

*Donald H. Kausler and Wemara Lichty*

Our primary objectives in this chapter are to give an overview of what we have discovered to date about adult age differences in activity memory proficiency, and to present a model for conceptualizing activity memory in general and adult age differences in activity memory proficiency in particular. In our studies, activities consist of continuous performances on each of a series of tasks, such as solving anagrams, tracing mazes, and searching for words within a matrix of letters. Completion of the series is followed by a memory test, either for the content of the individual activities or for a non-content attribute of the activities, such as the temporal order in which they were performed.

At the time we began our research program, we expected to find little, if any, in the way of adult age differences in the proficiency of memory for activities. The expected null effect for age variation followed from our conceptualization of activity memory as a form of rehearsal-independent episodic memory. However, we have consistently found substantial age deficits in various components of activity memory. Of interest therefore is the extent to which adult age differences in these components are affected by variations in procedural and task conditions. The variable of greatest concern has been that of incidental versus intentional memory instructions. Given the presumed rehearsal-independent nature of activity memory, little if any advantage of intentional over incidental memory was expected, regardless of the age of our subjects. The expected null effect for instructional variation has been confirmed repeatedly in our studies. Before describing our research program, however, some discussion of the relevance of activity memory to both basic memory theory and gerontological memory theory is in order.

## Basic Concepts and Issues

### Rehearsal-Independent Versus Rehearsal-Dependent Memory

In the everyday world, we perform many activities—working on a crossword puzzle, repairing a broken appliance, writing a letter, balancing a checkbook, and so on. Memory of an activity usually persists even though there was no apparent attempt to commit it to memory and therefore little likelihood of rehearsing it either during or after its performance. Many of our other everyday memories seem to be characterized similarly by such rehearsal-independency. That is, as with activity memory, memory occurs incidentally, and therefore in the absence of deliberate rehearsal. For example, we have memories, at least partial, of the contents of our conversations with other people and of the television programs we have watched. It seems highly unlikely that participating in a conversational exchange or watching a television program is accompanied by rehearsal of the content of the conversation or the content of the program. To the extent that the processes of activity memory are representative of the processes of rehearsal-independent forms of episodic memory in general, our knowledge of adult age differences in activity memory should have important implications for adult age differences in other forms of rehearsal-independent episodic memory.

Despite the relevance of rehearsal-independent forms of episodic memory to the everyday functioning of elderly people, these forms have been largely ignored by both basic and gerontological memory researchers. Instead the primary focus of episodic memory research has been on rehearsal-dependent forms of memory. By rehearsal-dependency we mean that the extent of memory for episodic events is contingent on the success of rehearsing those events—the greater the success (defined in terms of either the amount or the quality of rehearsal), the greater the subsequent memorability. Rehearsal-dependent forms of memory are tested in the laboratory by the use of traditional paired-associate, serial, free recall, and prose learning tasks. In general, elderly adults perform at a level well below that of young adults on these tasks (see Craik, 1977; Kausler, 1982; Salthouse, 1982). Age deficits in rehearsal-dependent memory are commonly explained in terms of the diminished capacity of elderly adults' working memory, relative to the capacity of young adults (e.g., Light & Anderson, 1985), resulting in less proficient rehearsal of the list-based episodic events by elderly than by young adults. Various hypotheses have been offered to describe the age-related change in rehearsal proficiency. For example, it has been postulated both that elderly adults rehearse to-be-remembered episodes less elaboratively than do young adults and that elderly adults are less likely than young adults to incorporate contextual information as they rehearse to-be-remembered episodes (see Burke & Light, 1981).

The focus of aging research on rehearsal-dependent memory is understandable, given the fact that most aging research studies simply extend earlier basic memory studies by including age variation as an additional independent variable. Rehearsal-dependent memory is of major concern to basic memory theorists and researchers, as it should be. It enters prominently into the everyday academic performances of college students, the standard subject population for basic memory research. Although rehearsal-dependent forms of memory (e.g., learning new face–name associations) continue as part of the everyday performances of people long removed from academic settings, they probably do so less often than in the everyday performances of college students.

## Automaticity of Memory

There is an obvious relatedness between what we are referring to as rehearsal-independent memory and the currently popular concept of automatic memory (Hasher & Zacks, 1979, 1984). Rehearsal-independency, in the sense of a "rehearsal bypass," is a core concept of automaticity. As noted by Hasher and Zacks, "Automatic processes function at optimal levels, continuously and independently of intention . . . and these processes require only that the event be attended to. . . . The information encoded in this way is no different than it is when intention is activated." (1984, p. 1373). Thus, incidental memory for activities must be equivalent to intentional memory if this form of memory is to be considered automatic. Hasher and Zacks (1979) have reasoned that automaticity of encoding occurs for information that is essential for maintaining continuity with the everyday world. Automaticity is hypothesized to be ensured either by being innately programmed in the human organism or by being the consequence of years of frequent practice during childhood. It has been most commonly associated with the encoding of certain noncontent attributes of to-be-remembered words, in particular their frequency of occurrence and their temporal ordering. Surely, memory for one's own activities is at least as essential for maintaining continuity with the everyday world as is memory for noncontent attributes of words.

According to Hasher and Zacks (1979, 1984), rehearsal-independency (i.e., equivalence of incidental and intentional memory) is only one of a number of criteria that must be satisfied in order for a particular form of memory to be considered automatic. One of these other criteria, the absence of age differences in memory proficiency, is of particular interest to us. This criterion follows from a basic assumption of automaticity, namely that the proficiency of encoding rehearsal-independent episodic events is unaffected by working memory capacity. Consequently, the proficiency of encoding rehearsal-independent events is expected to be unaffected by the presumed decrement in working memory's capacity from early to late adulthood, in contrast to the pronounced adverse effect of the decrement on the proficiency of rehearsal-dependent forms of memory (Figure 4.1). The concept of capacity, of course, remains a nebulous one (see Salthouse, this volume), with various references to capacity in terms of "cognitive resources," "cognitive energy," "space" for maintaining information briefly, and "space" for operating on briefly maintained information.

The apparent rehearsal-independent nature of activity memory in the everyday world qualifies it as a strong candidate for automaticity and therefore for immunity to age-related deficits. Thus, we began our studies on activity memory confident of finding negligible effects for both instructional variation (i.e., incidental versus intentional memory) and age variation (i.e., young versus old). The negligible effects were expected both for the memory of the content of activities and for the memory of certain noncontent attributes of those activities. The Hasher and Zacks (1979) concept of automaticity seemingly applies only to the encoding of noncontent attributes of episodic events, whether the events be words in a list or activities in a series. However, we believe that the content of certain events, such as activities, is also encoded automatically. The essential component of our conceptualiza-

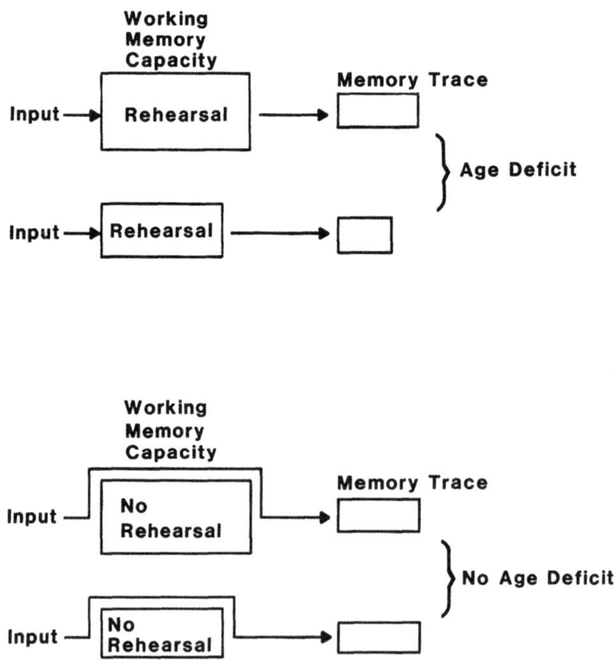


FIGURE 4.1. Top: Processes hypothesized to determine age deficits in encoding for rehearsal-dependent forms of episodic memory. Bottom: Processes hypothesized to determine the absence of age deficits for rehearsal-independent forms of episodic memory.

tion of automaticity is that the episodic event, whether it be content per se or an accompanying attribute of that content, is encoded without the involvement of active rehearsal. It is rehearsal that is a highly age-sensitive process. Consequently, the lack of the involvement of rehearsal in activity memory implies that there should be little decrement in encoding proficiency with normal aging.

Our confidence in the absence of age deficits, however, was tempered somewhat by our awareness of elderly adults' frequent complaints about memory problems, problems that seemingly include rehearsal-independent as well as rehearsal-dependent forms of memory (Lowenthal et al., 1967). To what extent self-reported memory problems reflect reality is questionable, however. True age-related problems with memory could be limited to only rehearsal-dependent forms of memory, but these problems could be generalized to all forms of memory when elderly people give self-reports of their memory proficiencies.

## Memory for Content

"I balanced my checkbook yesterday." Note that memory in this case is for both the content of an activity (i.e, balancing the checkbook) and a noncontent attribute of that activity (i.e., when it was performed). Our concern in this section is with age differences in memory for the content of tasks as they are affected by variations in both the nature of that content (e.g., motor versus cognitive) and the conditions under which the tasks are performed (e.g., incidental versus intentional memory instructions). Age differences in memory for noncontent attributes will be considered in the next section.

Our standard procedure consists of having subjects perform for several minutes on each of 12 or more laboratory tasks. After a delay of 2 minutes, filled with informal conversation, they receive either a free recall test or a recognition test of those activities. Recall of an activity is scored as being correct if a subject either names it correctly (e.g., "Anagram Solving") or describes it adequately (e.g., "unscrambling letters to make words"). In most cases, recall consists of the latter. Recognition is tested by presenting a series of task descriptions in random order, with half being activities performed previously and the other half new activities, and requesting an "old/new" decision for each activity in the series. Memory for content is then assessed for both young and elderly subjects who perform under various procedural and task conditions.

### Incidental Versus Intentional Memory

A major objective of our studies has been to demonstrate the rehearsal-independent nature of memory for activities. Our procedure is the standard one employed in earlier tests of automaticity, specifically for memory of such attributes as the frequency of occurrence for words in a study list (Attig & Hasher, 1980; Kausler & Puckett, 1980). The procedure calls for variation in instructions whereby half the subjects at each age level receive incidental memory instructions and half intentional memory instructions. In the incidental memory condition, our subjects are given no hint of an eventual memory test. They are simply asked to perform each task for the purpose of contributing normative information about performance scores on that task for people of different ages.

Our procedure is stronger in the sense of inducing a true incidental memory set than is that employed in most studies on memory for noncontent attributes (see Mandler, Seegmiller, & Day, 1977), in which subjects are told that they will receive a later memory test—they simply are not informed as to the nature of the attribute to be tested (Attig & Hasher, 1980, Kausler & Puckett, 1980). In our intentional memory condition, our subjects are informed of the normative value of their performance scores, but they are also told that they will be asked to recall their activities and that they should make the effort to remember as many activities as possible. This condition replicates closely the intentional memory condition employed in most studies on memory for noncontent attributes (Attig & Hasher, 1980).

The recall scores obtained under these instructional conditions in our initial study (Kausler & Hakami, 1983) are shown in the top panel of Figure 4.2. It may be seen that recall under incidental memory conditions was as proficient as recall under intentional memory conditions for both young adults (college students) and elderly adults (mean age, 65.7 years; range, 56 to 76 years). This pattern of a null effect for instructional variation regardless of age has been replicated a number of times in our laboratory. The results from one of these replications (Kausler, Lichty, Hakami, & Freund, 1986), employing a different set of tasks than in our initial study, are given in the bottom panel of Figure 4.2. In fact, in this study, and in several of our other studies as well, there was a nonsignificant trend for recall to be greater incidentally than intentionally.

The null effect for instructional variation seemingly confirms the rehearsal-independent nature of activity memory over the course of the adult lifespan. However, a caveat is in order. Greene (1986) recently demonstrated that accuracy of frequency-of-occurrence memory for words is significantly greater intentionally than incidentally when considerable stress is given to the importance of measuring frequency information. The frequency judgment task is commonly viewed as being the prototypal one for testing the characteristics of automatic memory (Hasher & Zacks, 1979, 1984). Greene's results appear to suggest that even this prototypal form of automatic memory may be affected by rehearsal when that rehearsal is sufficiently intense (see also Maki & Ostby, 1987).

Presumably, other forms of memory believed to be automatic in the sense of incidental memory/intentional memory equivalence may be similarly affected by efforts to induce intensive rehearsal. We have begun a study in our

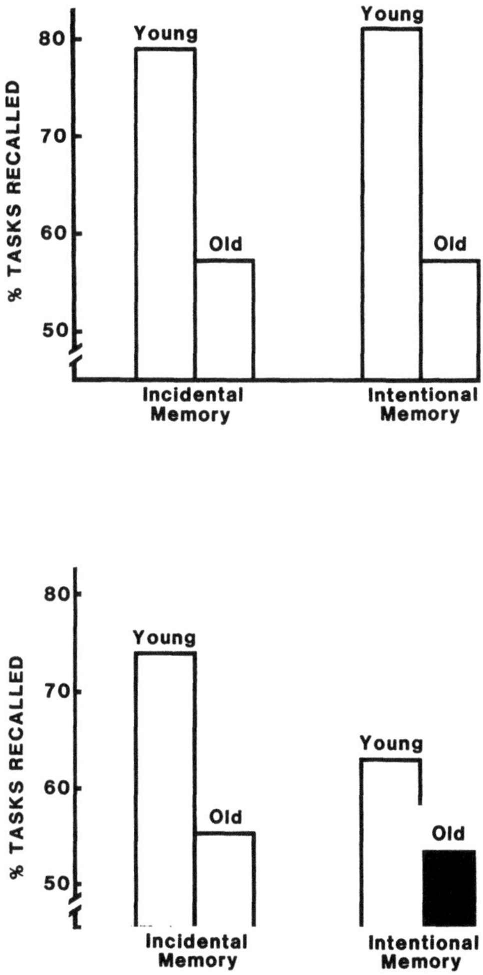


FIGURE 4.2. Age differences in recall of activities under incidental and intentional memory conditions. Top: Adapted from data in Kausler and Hakami (1983). Bottom: Adapted from data in Kausler, Lichty, Hakami, and Freund (1986).

laboratory that includes a "stress" intentional memory condition comparable to that of Greene. That is, the importance of remembering the performed activities is stressed heavily, and subjects are asked to maintain their rehearsal of each activity while performing it, even if it means lowering their task performance score. Significantly higher activity recall scores under this condition, relative to scores obtained under out standard incidental and intentional conditions, would undoubtedly have important theoretical implications. However, it should be noted that the "stress" condition is a somewhat unnatural one in the sense of having unlikely counterparts in everyday activity memory.

Further support for our belief that activity memory is not a rehearsal-dependent form of episodic memory comes from our analyses of serial position effects in the recall of activities. Of interest in these analyses is the probability of an activity's recall at each ordinal position in the series of tasks. (To avoid potential confounding of serial position by task content, our tasks are balanced over positions.) A representative outcome (Kausler & Hakami, 1983) is presented in the top panel of Figure 4.3. The probabilities shown here are for combined incidental and intentional memory conditions, given the negligible Instruction × Position interaction effect at each age level.

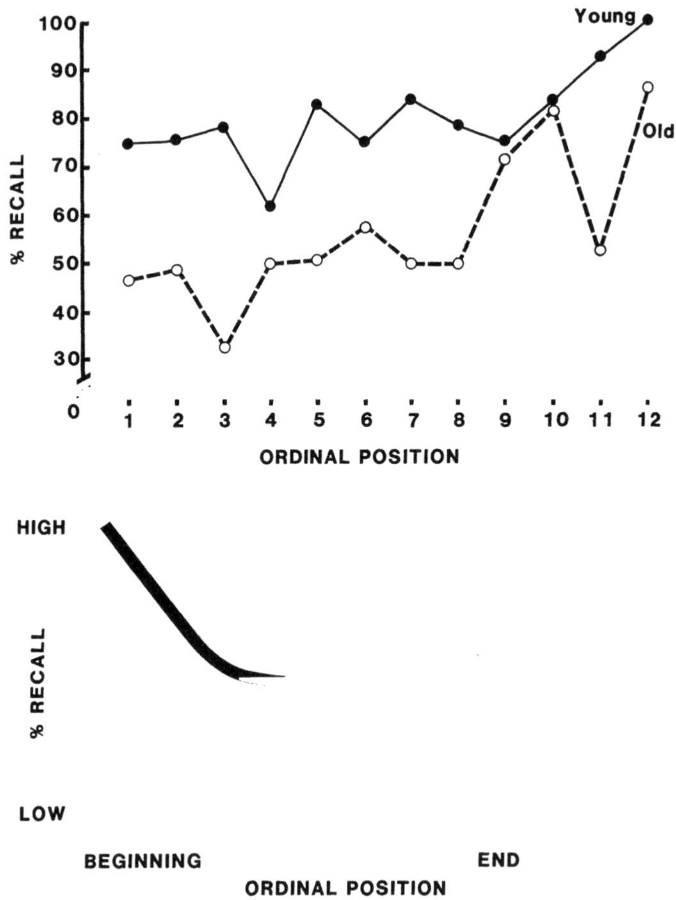


FIGURE 4.3. Top: Serial position effects for recall of a series of activities (adapted from data in Kausler & Hakami, 1983). Bottom: Serial position effects usually found for the free recall of a single word list.

Clearly apparent for both young and elderly subjects is a pronounced recency effect; that is, activities performed at the end of the series have a substantially higher probability of recall than activities performed in the middle of the series. The fact that 2 minutes of a rehearsal-preventing activity followed the last task in the series implies that the recency effect is unlikely to be the consequence of direct recall from a short-term store. Also apparent is the absence of a primacy effect defined in terms of enhanced probabilities of recalling activities performed early in the series, again relative to midseries probabilities. This pattern of a recency effect combined with the absence of a primary effect contrasts sharply with the pattern found for the free recall of a single list of words following a single study trial (Keppel & Mallory, 1969). As illustrated in the bottom panel of Figure 4.3, the free recall of a single word list yields a pronounced primacy effect and little, if any recency effect.

An inspection of Figures 4.2 and 4.3 reveals another important outcome of our studies—the age sensitivity of activity memory, at least as measured by recall. A significant age difference, favoring young adults, in the recall of activities has been found in four of our studies (Kausler & Hakami, 1983; Kausler, Lichty, & Davis, 1985; Kausler et al., 1986; Lichty, Kausler, & Martinez, 1986). Overall, our young subjects averaged recalling 75.6% of the activities, and our elderly subjects, 60.0%. The age deficit is especially alarming, given the generally superior nature of the elderly subjects employed in our studies. Their self-reported health is excellent or good, their vocabulary test scores are well above those of our young subjects, and their educational level is high (e.g, mean years of formal education = 16.21 in Kausler and Hakami's 1983 study).

The magnitude of the age deficit found in our studies is strikingly comparable to that found by Bromley (1958) in an early study that may be viewed as involving activity memory. Bromley administered the Wechsler intelligence test to groups of young and elderly adults. After completion of the test, the subjects were given an incidental memory test in which they were asked either to name the subtests of the Wechsler or to describe them. Recall averaged 75.1% and 61.8% of the subtests for young and elderly subjects, respectively.

The presence of an age deficit seemingly indicates that activity memory fails to satisfy a major criterion for automaticity established by Hasher and Zacks (1979, 1984), namely, a null effect for age variation. A plausible interpretation is that age deficits in the registration of memory traces in the long-term episodic store are highly generalizable. That is, an age-related decline in the transmission of traces to the store occurs for information encoded automatically as well as for information encoded effortfully via rehearsal. Interestingly, significant age defícts have also been found in recent studies of memory for word frequency information (Kausler, Lichty, & Hakami, 1984; Salthouse, Kausler, & Saults, 1988) and memory for word temporal information (Kausler, Salthouse, & Saults, in press). Thus, even these generally accepted forms of automatic memory, defined soley in terms of rehearsal-independence, appear to be age sensitive.

There is, however, an important alternative explanation of age deficits in the recall of activities. Recall of information in the long-term episodic store is likely to be effortful regardless of the means by which that information reached the store. Consequently, recall is likely to deline in proficiency during late adulthood as working memory's capacity declines. Activities may be encoded as effectively by elderly adults as by young adults—the former may simply be less capable of the subsequent retrieval of traces when asked to recall them. The inability to separate completely the effects of encoding and retrieval processes on memory proficiency remains a haunting problem in memory research, given the nature of the interaction between those processes (Smith, 1980).

Retrieval failure may occur when information that had been encoded adequately is inaccessible during a search of the store's content, for whatever reason. However, it may also occur simply because the to-be-retrieved information had not been encoded adequately in the first place. A familiar method for distinguishing between encoding and retrieval processes as the source of age deficits on a memory task is to contrast the magnitudes of the age differences found with recognition and recall tests. Recognition is presumably a less effortful form of retrieval than recall, and is therefore less susceptible to decrements attributable to age-related declines in working memory's capacity for exerting cognitive effort. Consequently, the absence of an age effect on a recognition test may be viewed as indicating age equivalence in encoding proficiency, with the age difference in recall being solely attributable to an age-related decrement in retrieval proficiency.

Recognition tests have been given in several of our studies, in each case following an initial recall test. Our typical finding is that a statistically significant age difference persists, even though our elderly subjects have very high hit rates and very low false-alarm rates. For example, Lichty et al. (1986) found the hit rate for recognizing prior old activities as old was .99 and .95 for young and elderly subjects, respectively, and the false-alarm rate for recognizing new activities as old was .01 and .07, respectively. Interpretation of these modest age differences is made difficult by the obvious possibility of a ceiling effect for hits and a floor effect for false alarms. In addition, there are other serious methodological problems encountered in attempting to distinguish between encoding and retrieval processes on the basis of comparisons between recall and recognition scores (Brainerd, 1985; Howe, this volume). Fortunately, alternative procedures for separating the contributions of encoding and retrieval processes to adult age differences in rehearsal-dependent memory have been introduced recently (e.g., Howe, this volume; Wilkinson & Koestler, 1983). Perhaps these procedures will eventually be extended to rehearsal-independent forms of memory as well.

Despite our reservations about recognition scores, it is interesting to note that the age difference in hit rate for activities is considerably less pronounced than the age difference in hit rate for rehearsal-dependent, word-list memory. For example, hit rates were .81 and .69, in a study by Erber (1974, and .94 and .76, in a study by Rankin and Kausler (1979), for young and elderly subjects, respectively. The implications of the absence of an age difference in recognition for our rehearsal-independent task will be considered later in this chapter.

## Type of Activity

Much of our research on activity memory has centered on determining the extent to which age differences in recall are affected by variations in conditions other than instructions. Our functional analysis began with variation in the type of activity performed in the laboratory. Conceivably, some activities yield more distinctive, and therefore more accessible, memory traces than other activities. In fact, some traces may be sufficiently distinctive that their recall should be as proficient for elderly as for young subjects thus eliminating the age deficit in recall. This hypothesis was tested initially by Kausler and Hakami (1983). The 12 tasks performed by their young and elderly subjects were grouped in four categories of three tasks each (with tasks randomly ordered in the series). The categories were: perceptual-motor (e.g., letter cancellation and card sorting), verbal learning (e.g., paired-associate learning and serial learning), generic memory (e.g., naming instances of taxonomic categories and word–picture matching), and problem solving (e.g., solving anagrams and solving arithmetic problems). As noted earlier, the main effect of age was significant in this study. However, the main effect needs to be viewed cautiously in light of the significant Age × Type of Activity interaction effect that was also found in this study.

The nature of this interaction may be seen from the percentages of subjects recalling each type of activity (Figure 4.4). Recall by young subjects significantly exceeded that of elderly subjects for the perceptual-motor, verbal learning, and generic memory tasks, but not for problem-solving tasks. Moreover, the null effect for age variation on problem-solving tasks cannot be attributed to a ceiling effect present for young subjects. Conceivably, tasks vary in the amount of mental, or cognitive, effort required to initiate and to maintain performance on them (Tyler, Hertel, McCallum, & Ellis, 1979). Problem solving tasks are likely to demand more mental effort than, say, simple perceptual-motor tasks. Greater effort, in turn, may enhance the distinctiveness of activity memory traces, but, apparently, only for elderly individuals. An inspection of Figure 4.4 reveals that problem-solving activities were recalled more proficiently than other kinds of activities by elderly subjects. By contrast, recall of activities by young subjects was relatively unaffected by variation in type of activity. The mental effort dimension in Kausler and Hakami's study (1983) is admittedly speculative and post hoc in nature. Unfortunately, further research on this important task attribute is hindered by the absence of a means of direct assessment of mental effort.

Another potentially important task dimension is one anchored by "cognitive" on one end and by "motor" on the other end. That is, some tasks, such as

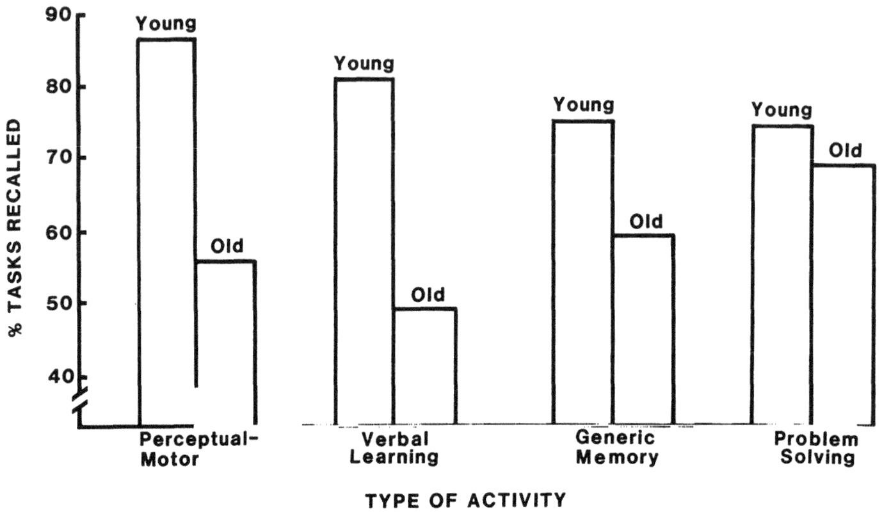


FIGURE 4.4. Age differences in recall of perceptual-motor, verbal learning, generic memory, and problem-solving activities (adapted from data in Kausler & Hakami, 1983).

anagram solving, are predominantly cognitive in nature, while other tasks, such as picking up objects and placing them in a specified location, are predominantly motor in nature. Bäckman (in press) has postulated that motor activity yields a multimodal memory trace that includes visual and tactile information as well as kinesthetic information. Multimodal traces are presumed to offer greater "contextual support" for older adults than do the unimodal traces yielded by cognitive activities. Greater contextual support, in turn, is expected to diminish the retrieval deficits commonly found in late adulthood. Thus, Bäckman's hypothesis predicts a pronounced reduction, if not elimination, of age differences in the recall of motor activities relative to cognitive activities.

This hypothesis has been tested twice in our laboratory. In the first study (Lichty et al., 1986), a mixed series of 12 tasks was performed (randomly ordered); half were primarily cognitive in nature (e.g., word searching and anagram solving) and half were primarily motor in nature (e.g., putting rubber bands on a tube and laying paper clips on the lines of a design). As in our earlier studies, separate groups of young and elderly subjects performed under incidental and intentional memory conditions. Here too the effects of instructional variation were not significant, either as a main effect or as an interaction effect with age. Accordingly, the recall percentages reported in Figure 4.5 are for the combined instructional groups. There was a trend ($p < .10$) for recall scores overall to be greater for motor tasks (74%) than for cognitive tasks (68%), in agreement with the hypothesized greater ease of retrieval for motor activity traces. However, contrary to our expectancy, the age

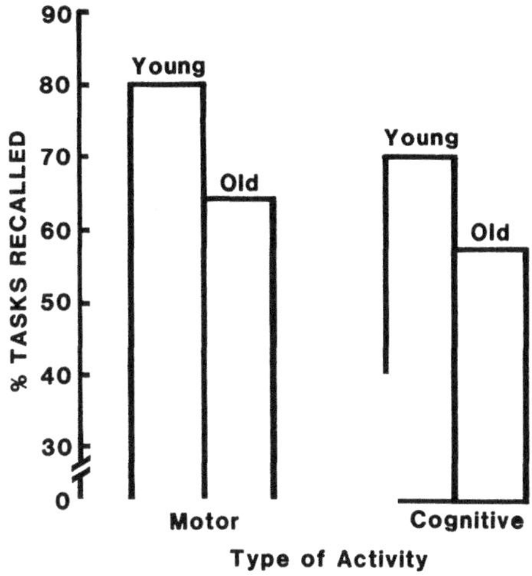


FIGURE 4.5. Age differences in recall of motor versus cognitive activities (adapted from data in Lichty, Kausler, & Martinez, 1986).

deficit was as pronounced for motor rasks as for cognitive tasks. That is, the age main effect was significant, but the Age × Type of Task interaction effect fell far short of significance.

There was an important modification in the procedure of the second study (Lichty, 1986): All 12 tasks performed in the laboratory were motor in nature, rather than a mixed series of cognitive and motor tasks. In addition, only an intentional memory condition was employed. This time the outcome provided apparent support for the multimodal hypothesis in the sense of a statistically nonsignificant age difference, with young adults recalling 67% of their activities and elderly adults 63%. This is the only one of our studies in which the age difference for recall scores failed to attain statistical significance. Interpretation of the reduced age deficit is complicated by the fact that recall scores for the elderly subjects were no greater than they were for the cognitive tasks employed by Lichty et al. (1986) (62%). The reduced age deficit found by Lichty clearly stems not from the enhanced recall of motor tasks by her elderly subjects, but rather from the unexplained low level of recall by her young subjects (67%) relative to the level of recall by young subjects of comparable activities in the study by Lichty et al. (1986) (81%). Again, the major difference between the two studies is in the use of mixed versus unmixed series of tasks. To what extent and why this variation may affect recall, especially for young adults, is a topic for future research.

Problems in identifying task dimension that are reliably related to the magnitude of age differences in recall should not hide the fact that there are considerable individual differences among tasks in their recallability for both young and elderly adults. This is true even though all the tasks performed share a common attribute, such as being either predominantly motor or predominately cognitive in nature. Moreover, the magnitude of the age differences varies greatly from task to task. Listed in Table 4.1 are the 12 motor tasks employed by Lichty et al. (1986) (6 were performed by half of the subjects at each age level, the remaining 6 by the other half), together with their recall scores and their age differences in recall. Comparable scores for the 12 cognitive tasks employed in this study are listed in Table 4.2. Note that some activities are clearly more memorable than other activities regardless of age. In addition, tasks that are more memorable for young adults also tend to be more memorable for elderly adults. The rank-order correlation coefficient between young and elderly recall scores was significant for the 12 motor tasks (.74, $p < .05$) and approached significance for the 12 cognitive tasks (.48, $p < .10$). Most important, for many activities, recall of elderly adults differs nonsignificantly from that of young adults. In fact, for only 4 of the 24 tasks entering into this study did the age difference favoring young adults attain statistical significance, and for 3 tasks the age difference actually favored elderly adults. Determining why some activities yield more distinctive memory traces than other activities and why some activities show less pronounced age deficits in recallability than other activities are important objectives of our future research on activity memory.

## Level of Task Performance

An intriguing issue concerns the relationship between performance level on a given task and the subsequent recallability of the underlying activity. Con-

TABLE 4.1. Recall Scores (% of Subjects Recalling a Task Performance) for Young and Elderly Subjects on 12 Different Motor Tasks[a]

| | Recall Score | | |
|---|---|---|---|
| Task | Young | Elderly | Age Difference |
| Clay modeling | 100 | 100 | 0 |
| Cutting shapes | 100 | 83 | 17 |
| Pegboard | 100 | 67 | 33[b] |
| Placement in vertical slots | 92 | 83 | 9 |
| Paper clips | 92 | 75 | 17 |
| Disk transfer | 83 | 75 | 8 |
| Movement on wires | 83 | 75 | 8 |
| Metallic designs | 83 | 42 | 41[b] |
| Rubber bands | 75 | 58 | 17 |
| Connecting rings | 50 | 25 | 25 |
| Drawing circles | 50 | 67 | −17 |
| Tweezers manipulation | 50 | 50 | 0 |

[a]From data in Lichty, Kausler, and Martinez (1986).
[b]$p < .05$, chi-square test.

TABLE 4.2. Recall Scores (% of Subjects Recalling a Task Performance) for Young and Elderly Subjects on 12 Different Cognitive Tasks[a]

| Task | Recall Score | | Age Difference |
|---|---|---|---|
| | Young | Elderly | |
| Identical pictures | 100 | 75 | 25 |
| Word search | 100 | 83 | 17 |
| Estimation of length | 83 | 75 | 8 |
| Hidden patterns | 83 | 50 | 33[b] |
| Anagrams | 83 | 75 | 8 |
| Instances of categories | 83 | 50 | 33[b] |
| Cube comparison | 75 | 50 | 25 |
| Incomplete words | 75 | 58 | 17 |
| Vocabulary | 75 | 83 | −8 |
| Nearer point | 67 | 58 | 9 |
| Calendar | 58 | 33 | 25 |
| Digit symbol | 33 | 58 | −25 |

[a]From data in Lichty, Kausler, and Martinez (1987).
[b]$p < .05$, chi-square test.

ceivably, tasks that are performed proficiently are more likely to be recalled later than are tasks performed less proficiently. This does not seem to be the case, however. We have consistently found little covariation between task performance level and subsequent recall versus failure of recall of that task (biserial *r*). For example, Kausler and Hakami (1983) reported *rs* for their 12 tasks that were all less than .20. In Lichty's study (1986), the correlation coefficients for her 12 tasks ranged from −.29 to .39 for young adults and from −.34 to .36 for elderly adults, with none of the coefficients attaining statistical significance. Competence on a given task appears to be a negligible factor determining later recall of that task's activity.

## Task Duration

The final procedural variable we have introduced in our studies to date is that of the duration of performing an activity. In the everyday world, our activities obviously vary considerably in the amount of time devoted to them, and the memorability of these activities may well be a function of that amount. Understanding the effect of activity duration on later recallability and on age differences in recallability has obvious practical implications. It also has important theoretical implications, as described by Kausler et al. (1986):

> On the one hand, it is conceivable that both the overall level of recall and the magnitude of age deficit in recall should increase as the duration of performing activities increases. Longer durations offer greater opportunity for encoding contextual information generated by performers' thoughts about the task at hand and

> about their competence on that task than do shorter durations. To the extent that the subsequent retrieval of contextual information enhances the retrievability of content information (Tulving, 1983), recall of activity content should increase for both young and elderly adults as the duration of activity participation increases. However, the magnitude of the age deficit in recall should also increase as duration increases, given the prevailing view that the proficiency of encoding contextual information declines from early to late adulthood (e.g., Burke & Light, 1981).
>
> On the other hand, variation in activity duration may have little, if any, effect on either the overall level of recall or the magnitude of the age deficit in recall. Performing an activity appears to be somewhat analogous to the maintenance rehearsal of verbal materials. Naveh-Benjamin and Jonides (1984) recently demonstrated that maintenance rehearsal is a two-stage activity. The first stage is an effortful one in which a program for rehearsing a verbal item is operationalized. The second stage is essentially an automatic one that involves repetitive execution of the activated program. Long-term memory traces of the rehearsal activity are largely the product of the first stage and are therefore independent of the duration of the second stage. Operationalizing a program to perform a laboratory activity is seemingly analogous to the second stage. This analogy implies an independence between activity duration and later recall of performing that activity. That is, both the duration main effect and the Age × Duration interaction effect are expected to be negligible. (p. 80)

Variation in duration of performance was introduced by Kausler et al. (1986) in a within-subjects design. Fifteen tasks were performed by each subject; all were component tests of the Reference Tests for Cognitive Factors (e.g., dot connecting, maze tracing; Ekstrom, French, Harman, & Derman, 1976). Five tasks were performed for 45 seconds each, five for 90 seconds each, and five for 180 seconds each (with each task appearing equally often in each duration condition). The recall results obtained for young and elderly subjects are shown in Figure 4.6 (combined for incidental and intentional memory conditions; p. 98 and Figure 4.2). The only statistically significant effect was the main effect for age. That is, neither the main effect for duration nor the Age × Duration interaction effect attained significance. Noteworthy is the negligible overall increment in recall scores from 45 seconds duration (60%) to 180 seconds (65.7%). The absence of an Age × Duration interaction effect implies that an age difference in encoding contextual information while continuing performance on a task is an unlikely reason for a difference in recall. However, these results do support the concept of a two-stage sequence in performing activities that is analogous to the two-stage sequence of maintenance rehearsal. The contextual information and stage-sequence concepts are discussed further later in this chapter.

## Memory for Noncontent Attributes

Memory for activities may consist not only of what activities were performed (i.e., content), but also when in a series they were performed and how often. Memories for these noncontent attributes correspond closely to what are called temporal and frequency-of-occurrence memory in the traditional

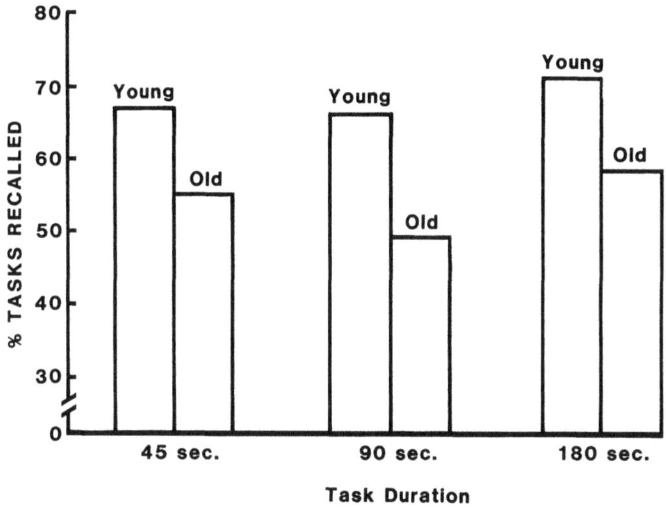


FIGURE 4.6. Age differences in recall of activities as a function of a task duration (adapted from data in Kausler, Lichty, Hakami, & Freund, 1986).

word-list memory literature. As noted earlier, temporal and frequency attributes of episodic events are commonly viewed as being encoded automatically. Accordingly, they are expected to be encoded as proficiently by elderly adults as by young adults. Tests of these hypotheses were the primary focus of our studies on the temporal and frequency attributes of activities as episodic events.

## Temporal Memory

Everyday activity memory often involves temporal decisions about previously performed activities. For example, we are often asked such questions as "When did we get together for bridge?" and "Was it Thursday you mowed the lawn?" Our frequent ability to respond correctly to such questions indicates that we do store, in whatever manner, temporal information about our own performances.

Until our studies on activity memory were initiated, the only research on temporal memory had been on memory for either words or pictures presented in a lengthy list. A temporal memory test consists either of presenting each item in the list and asking subjects the placement of that item in the list (e.g., first fourth, second fourth, and so on; see Toglia & Kimble, 1976) or giving the subjects all of the words from the list and asking them to reconstruct the order in which they appeared (Zacks, Hasher, Alba, Sanft, & Rose, 1984). For the former procedure, temporal memory proficiency is assessed by a subject's proportion of correct assignments of items to list segments; for the latter procedure, proficiency is assessed by the magnitude of the correlation coefficient between true word order and the subject's reconstructed order. The guiding conceptualization for research on word temporal memory is that temporal information is encoded automatically, thus making word temporal memory both rehearsal independent and age insensitive (Hasher & Zacks, 1979; Toglia & Kimble, 1976). In general, the available evidence does support the rehearsal-independent nature of word temporal memory in the sense that temporal memory scores are no greater when obtained under intentional memory than under incidental memory conditions (McCormack, 1981; Toglia & Kimble, 1976). The evidence regarding age insensitivity over the adult life span is more ambiguous. Some investigators (e.g., Perlmutter, Metzger, Nezworski, & Miller, 1981) have found a null effect when contrasting young and elderly subjects, while others (e.g., McCormack, 1982) have found a pronounced age deficit.

Our interest in temporal memory for activities has naturally centered on both its potential rehearsal-independency and its potential age insensitivity. Our first study (Kausler, Lichty, & Davis, 1985) required a modification of the procedure employed in our content memory studies. Young and elderly subjects performed on a series of 16 tasks (all component tests of the Reference Tests for Cognitive factors; Ekstrom et al., 1976) separated into four time blocks of four tasks each by the insertion of rest breaks between blocks. In addition to our standard incidental and intentional memory conditions (again, with intentional memory subjects being fully informed as to the temporal memory tests to follow the series of tasks), a third instructional condition was included. Subjects in this condition were informed that a recall test would be given, and that they should attempt to remember their activities (a free recall test was actually administered after the temporal memory tests were completed). Thus, this condition was incidental with respect to the forthcoming temporal memory tests. All subjects first received a temporal placement test in which they were given the instructions for each task in a random order and were asked to identify for each the time block (i.e., one through four) in which the task had been performed. They were then given a reconstruction test requiring them to order the tasks (via their instruction sheets) in the order in which they had been performed.

For the temporal placement test only the main effect for age was statistically significant, with young adults averaging 60% correct time block identifications and elderly adults 51%. The results for the three instructional conditions are illustrated in the top panel of Figure 4.7. It may be seen that identifications were as accurate incidentally as intentionally regardless of age. There was, however, a modest trend for elderly subjects to identify fewer tasks correctly when they were expecting a free recall test rather than a temporal memory test. A comparable outcome was obtained for correlations between true and reconstructed orders (see the bottom panel of Figure 4.7). Again, only the main effect for age was significant, with mean correlation coefficients *(r)* of .83 and .59 for young and elderly subjects, respectively. As

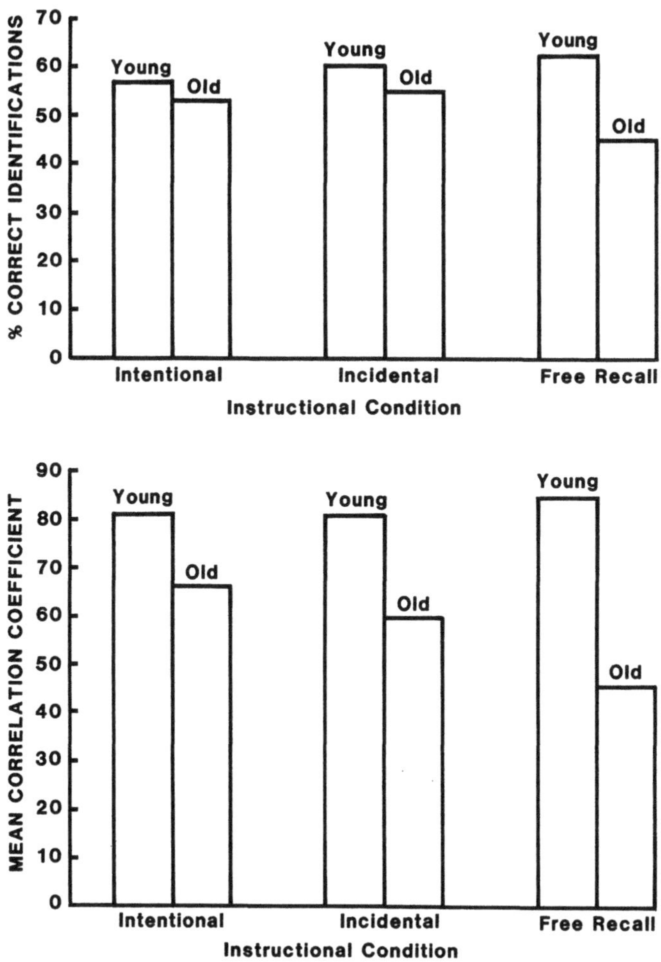


FIGURE 4.7. Top: Age differences in time block identification of activities under varying instructional conditions. Bottom: Age differences in correlation coefficients between true order and reconstructed order of activities under varying instructional conditions (adapted from data in Kausler, Lichty, & Davis, 1985).

with identification scores, there was a trend toward lower scores for elderly subjects under the free recall condition than under the other two conditions. Finally, the covariation between the two temporal memory scores was moderately high for both young ($r = .54$) and elderly subjects ($r = .59$).

The age sensitivity of temporal memory for activities has also been demonstrated in two large-scale normative studies (Kausler et al., in press; Salthouse et al., 1988). In each study, large samples of adults, noncollege students ranging in age from 20 to 70 years, were employed. There were 45 subjects in the 20- to 39-year-old range, 48 in the 40- to 59-year-old range, and 36 in the 60- to 79-year-old range for the first study; comparable sample sizes were 79, 77, and 77 for the second study. In both studies, subjects performed on a series of eight tasks (e.g., digit symbol test, number comparison test, and paired-associate learning test), each for several minutes. After the eighth task they received an unexpected activity temporal memory test requiring them to reconstruct the order in which the eight tasks had been performed.

The overall correlation between age and score on the temporal memory test (i.e., a subject's correlation between true and reconstructed order) was significant in each study; $r = -.25$ for the first study and $r = -.31$ for the second. For subjects in the 20–39, 40–59, and 60–79 age groups, the mean correlation coefficients for Study 1 and Study 2 were .70 and .74, .64 and .64, and .49 and .53, respectively. A separate group of college students was also included in each study. Their mean correlation coefficients were .91 in Study 1 and .86 in Study 2, both values being substantially higher than those found for noncollege-student young adults. Note that the difference between temporal memory scores for college students and elderly adults closely approximated that found by Kausler, Lichty, and Davis (1985) for a much longer series of activities. At this point, we are fairly well convinced that temporal memory for activities, like content memory for activities, is a rehearsal-independent form of memory, but one nevertheless that diminishes in proficiency over the course of the adult life span.

## Frequency-of-Occurrence Memory

The frequencies of performing specific tasks embedded within a series of tasks may vary, just as the frequencies of encountering specific words embedded within a lengthy list may vary. As noted earlier, memory for word frequency is commonly accepted as the prototype of automatic memory. However, the status of the automaticity of encoding word frequency information has been challenged by the results obtained in two recent studies. One of these challenges is the finding mentioned earlier that intensive intentional memory instructions serve to enhance the accuracy of frequency estimates by young adults (Greene, 1986). Another is the finding that dividing attention between studying list words and performing another task simultaneously had deleterious effects on the accuracy of frequency estimates (Naveh-Benjamin & Jonides, 1986). According to Hasher and Zacks (1979), memory for frequency information should be unaffected by division of attention. In addition, the evidence for age insensitivity, another criterion for automaticity of encoding frequency information, has been conflicting. Although some investigators (Attig & Hasher, 1980; Hasher & Zacks, 1979; Kausler & Puckett, 1980) have reported a null effect for adult age variation, others (Kausler, Hakami, & Wright, 1982; Kausler et al., 1984; Salthouse et al., 1988) have found a moderate but statistically significant age difference favoring young adults in accuracy of frequency judgments. The study by Kausler, Lichty, and Freund (1985) was intended, in part, to determine if two of the criteria of automaticity, rehearsal-independency and age insensitivity, apply to the encoding of frequency information for a series of activities performed in the laboratory.

Young (college students) and elderly (mean age, 71 years; range, 62.8 to 80.4 years) subjects received a series of tasks under either incidental or intentional memory conditions. Intentional subjects in this case were informed of the forthcoming frequency estimation test and were asked to keep track of the frequency they performed each task. Some of the tasks were planned and performed once (task duration = 90 seconds); others were performed two, three, or four times. At the end subjects were given a test series of task descriptions and were requested to estimate the number of times each task had been performed. The test series also included descriptions of tasks that had not been performed at all, thus having correct frequency estimates of zero.

The only variable to influence the magnitude of frequency estimates was the actual number of times each task had been performed (i.e., 0, 1, 2, 3, or 4). Both instructional variation and age variation had negligible effects on frequency estimates. As shown in Figure 4.8, young and elderly subjects (combined for instructional conditions) were both quite accurate in their frequency estimates. For each age group mean estimated frequencies approximated closely actual frequencies of task performances. In contrast to the encoding of activity temporal information, the encoding of activity frequency information appears to be largely unaffected by normal aging.

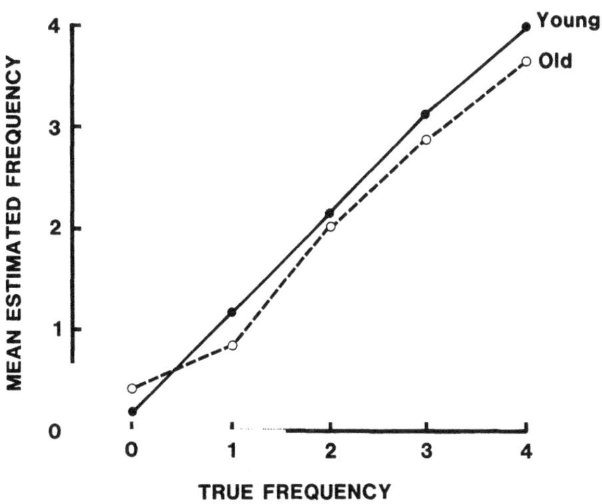


FIGURE 4.8. Covariation between true and estimated frequencies of activities for young and elderly subjects (adapted from data in Kausler, Lichty, & Freund, 1985).

## Comparison of Age Differences

Our normative studies (Kausler et al., 1988; Salthouse et al., 1988) offered a unique opportunity to compare age-related deficits for subjects performing on both rehearsal-dependent and rehearsal-independent memory tasks. Our objective in these studies was to obtain normative data on various cognitive tasks for subjects spanning a large segment of the adult life span. Among the tasks in our battery were a paired-associated learning task (two study-test trials on an eight-pair list), a word temporal memory task (reconstructing the order in which 16 words had been presented), and a frequency judgment task (words presented zero, two, three, or five times in a lengthy study list). The paired-associate task served to assess rehearsal-dependent memory proficiency; the other two tasks assessed rehearsal-independent memory proficiency. A third measure of rehearsal-independent memory proficiency was provided by the previously discussed activity temporal memory test that followed the last task in the series.

Shown in Figure 4.9 are age deficits for subjects in the 40- to 59- and 60- to 79-year-old range, expressed as percentage loss scores relative to the performance levels of noncollege subjects in the 20- to 39-year-old range. It may be seen that the magnitude of the age deficit for subjects in the 60–79 age range was approximately as large for the two temporal tasks as for the rehearsal-dependent paired-associate task. However, the rate of decline was

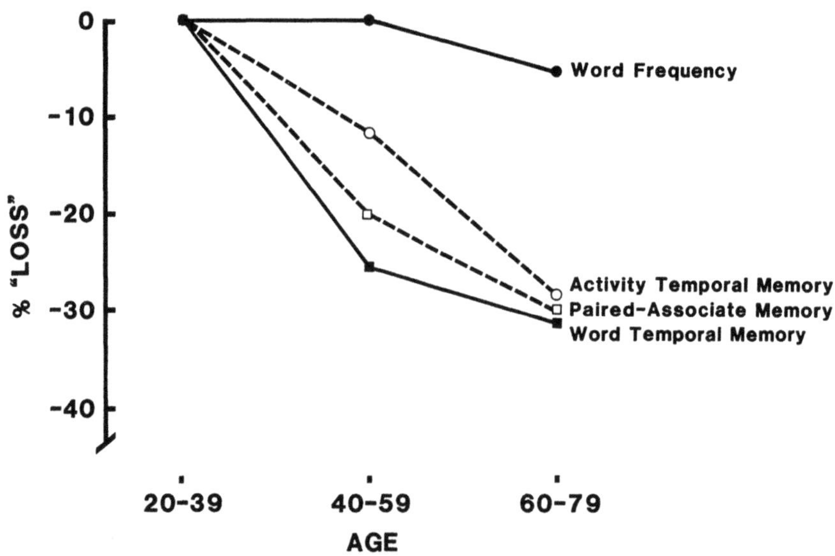


FIGURE 4.9. Age deficits on various memory tasks expressed relative to performance scores of young adults (adapted from data in Kausler, Salthouse, & Saults, in press; Salthouse, Kausler, & Saults, 1988).

considerably less pronounced for activity temporal memory than for either word temporal memory or paired-associate memory. By contrast, the age-related decline by age 60 to 79 years for word frequency memory was modest, although statistically significant. Encoding frequency information for words, as well as for activities, seems to be a process much less age-sensitive than encoding temporal information for either words or activities.

## Reality Monitoring

In the everyday world, some activities are planned to be performed but are interrupted before performance begins. An important issue concerns the extent of adult age differences in the ability to discriminate between the planning of activities and their actual executions. This discrimination seemingly corresponds closely to what Johnson (1977) has labeled "reality monitoring." Reality monitoring is commonly investigated by a modification of the word-frequency judgment task in which subjects must discriminate between externally generated frequencies (i.e., physical occurrences) versus internally generated frequencies (i.e., imaginal occurrences) (Johnson, Raye, Hasher, & Chromiak, 1979). Our use of the frequency judgment paradigm (Kausler, Lichty, & Freund, 1985) required a modification of the basic procedure described earlier to simulate reality monitoring of activities.

Specifically, an activity was planned by giving subjects task instructions in preparation for performance. For some tasks, the frequency of planning corresponded to the frequency of actual performance. That is, a task planned zero times was never performed, a task planned once was performed once, and so on. Our previously reported data for frequency estimates were for these tasks. For other tasks, there was a discrepancy between planning and actual performance. Thus, some tasks were planned once, but never performed; other tasks were planned twice but performed either once or not at all. Subsequently, subjects were asked to estimate the frequencies with which these tasks were actually performed. Both young and elderly adults were found to be quite capable of discriminating between planning and performing. That is, estimating performance frequencies was virtually unaffected, regardless of age, by additional plannings that were not followed by carrying out the expected activities. For example, frequency estimates for tasks planned twice but performed only once averaged 1.03 for young adults and 1.12 for elderly adults, values comparable to those found in the planned-once, performed-once condition (see Figure 4.8). These results imply that reality monitoring proficiency is unaffected by normal aging, at least as it involves discriminating between the planning of an activity and the actual initiation of that activity.

Another aspect of reality monitoring was also investigated by Kausler, Lichty, and Freund (1985). Their subjects were asked to estimate how often activities had been planned, as well as how often they had been performed. Reality monitoring in this case refers to the ability to resist distortion of planning frequency estimates by actual performances of the planned activities. For example, are activities planned and performed only once judged higher in frequency of planning than activities also planned only once, but never performed? Similarly, are activities planned and performed twice judged higher in frequency of planning than activities planned twice but performed only once or not at all? Our results indicate that there is an asymmetry in the proficiency of reality monitoring and that is equally true for young and elderly adults. That is, reality monitoring is less proficient, regardless of age, in judging planned performances than in judging true performances. For example, the mean frequency estimates of planning were 1.09 and .73 for young and elderly subjects, respectively, in the planned once-not performed condition and 1.34 and 1.27 in the planned once-performed once condition. The reason for the distortion of planning estimates by actual performances remains unknown.

## Action Memory

Unknown to us when we began our studies on activity memory, Cohen (1981) had initiated a program of research on what we will call action memory (it is also referred to as subject-performed-task memory, or SPT memory). In his studies, young adults are given a series of actions to perform and are subsequently asked to recall those actions. In contrast to our continuous activities, Cohen's episodic events consist of discrete actions, each lasting only several seconds, made in response to the experimenter's commands. Some actions require only motor responses (e.g., "Snap your fingers"), while others require interacting with an object present (e.g., "Pick up the pin"). The obvious similarity between activity memory and action memory makes it imperative that we examine the extent to which action memory conforms to rehearsal-independency and age insensitivity.

### Rehearsal-Independency

Cohen (1981, 1983) has provided several important tests of the nonstrategic nature of action memory—or its rehearsal-independency, in our terms. These tests have not included a comparison of the recall of actions under incidental and intentional memory conditions. However, a number of other procedural variations have yielded a convincing demonstration of action memory's rehearsal-independency. For example, recall of actions was found to be no greater following deep processing than following shallow processing (Cohen, 1981), in contrast to the usual superiority found for deep processing when rehearsal-dependent memory is involved (Craik & Tulving, 1975). In fact, Cohen discovered a recall advantage for deep processing only when the verbal commands had to be remembered (i.e., without performing the actions). Similarly, recall of actions stressed by the experimenter as being important to recall was essentially equivalent to the recall of actions downgraded in their importance (Cohen, 1983). On the other hand, recall of verbal commands, again in the absence of their execution, was markedly affected by the emphasis placed on their importance. Cohen and Bean (1983) also reported comparable levels of recall for educable mentally retarded subjects and their normal control subjects. If action memory is mediated by strategic rehearsal processes, then recall should be adversely affected by the diminished proficiency of those processes in retarded individuals. Finally, both Cohen (e.g., 1983) and Helstrup (1986) have repeatedly found a recency effect and the absence of a primacy effect in the recall of a series of actions, a finding that closely parallels the serial position effects characteristic of recalling a series of continuous activities.

Thus, action memory, like activity memory, seems to satisfy the rehearsal-independence criterion established by Hasher and Zacks (1979) for automaticity. However, Bäckman, Nilsson, and Chalom (1986) have demonstrated recently that action memory may not satisfy a related criterion of automaticity, namely the absence of an adverse effect for time-sharing with a simultaneously present task (i.e., divided attention). Their added task, performed by half their subjects, consisted of subtracting two consecutive digits from a number provided by the experimenter while performing the action ordered by the experimenter. Under nondivided and divided attention conditons, subjects recalled approximately 80% and 60%, respectively, of their actions. Bäckman et al. (1986) gave an interesting interpretation for the significant decrement in recall under the divided attention condition. They argued that the memory trace for a specific action consists of two kinds of information, information pertaining to the verbal command and information pertaining to the action per se. Under nondivided attention, the verbal component is established readily, and it enhances the subsequent retrievability of the total trace. Performance of the verbal secondary task (i.e., subtracting from a number), however, reduces the efficacy of encoding the verbal command, thereby reducing the amount of retrievable memory trace information.

Of particular interest to us is the possibility that the task names provided our subjects (e.g., "Anagram Solving") correspond to the verbal commands given to the Bäckman et al. subjects. Conceivably, task names may be encoded along with activities, yielding a compounded memory trace. However, as noted earlier, our subjects rarely recall task names, recalling instead descriptions of their activities (e.g., "unscrambling letters to make words"). Nevertheless, the potential role played by verbal labels in determining activity recall remains an important topic for future investigation.

## Age Variation

Adult age differences in the recall of discrete actions were investigated initially by Bäckman (Bäckman, 1985; Bäckman & Nilsson, 1984, 1985). The procedure in each study consisted of giving young and elderly subjects seven or eight series of actions, each series composed of 12 actions to perform. The end of each series was followed by an immediate recall test. In addition, the last series recall test was followed by a final, delayed recall test in which subjects attempted to recall all of the actions performed over the multiple series. In two of his studies, other groups of subjects were given only the verbal commands to recall without having performed the actions. The results of these studies are summarized in Table 4.3. Age diffferences in immediate recall of actions (averaged over all of the series) were slight and failed to attain statistical significance in any of the three studies. Nor did the age differences in the delayed recall of actions. By contrast, the age differences favoring young adults were pronounced for both the immediate and the delayed recall of verbal commands. Thus, Bäckman's results imply that the ability to recall discrete actions, in contrast to the ability to recall continuous activities, is immune to age-related deficits. If true, memory for discrete actions seemingly qualifies more completely for classification as an automatic form of memory than does memory for continuous activities.

Interestingly, there is another attribute of memory for discrete actions that appears to strengthen its classification as a form of automatic memory. This attribute, another identified by Hasher and Zacks (1979, 1984) as a criterion of automaticity, is the absence of nonspecific transfer or "learning-how-to-

TABLE 4.3. Summary of Studies on Adult Age Differences in Recall of Actions Versus Recall of Verbal Commands

| Study | Condition | Recall (%) Young | Elderly |
|---|---|---|---|
| Bäckman and Nilsson (1984) | Immediate action recall | 69 | 60 |
| | Immediate verbal recall | 59 | 32 |
| | Delayed action recall | 56 | 45 |
| | Delayed verbal recall | 42 | 15 |
| Bäckman and Nilsson (1985) | Immediate action recall | 65 | 62 |
| | Immediate verbal recall | 58 | 42 |
| | Delayed action recall | 53 | 47 |
| | Delayed verbal recall | 40 | 22 |
| | Delayed verbal recall | 40 | 22 |
| Bäckman (1985) | Immediate action recall | 61 | 57 |
| | Delayed action recall | 51 | 50 |
| Lichty (1986) | Action recall after brief delay | 63 | 48 |
| Cohen, Sandler, and Schroeder (1987) | Immediate action recall (14 actions) | 66 | 59 |
| Cohen, Sandler, and Schroeder (1987) | Immediate action recall (37 actions) | 45 | 34 |

learn." That is, no improvement in proficiency of performance is expected to occur with practice on the task. In Bäckman's studies, subjects receive multiple lists of actions to perform, but they show little improvement in the amount recalled from the first to last list (L. Bäckman, personal communication, 1985). This invariance in performance with practice contrasts sharply with the progressive increment in proficiency with practice found for rehearsal-dependent tasks, such as paired-associate learning (see Kausler, 1974). Noteworthy is the fact that other presumably automatic memory tasks, such as word temporal memory, have failed to satisfy the "absence of nonspecific transfer" criterion (Zacks et al., 1984). Unfortunately, successive lists of to-be-performed continuous activities have not been employed in our studies. Consequently, no evidence is available regarding practice effects for this form of memory.

There is good reason to dispute the "age-insensitive" classification for action memory implied by Bäckman's results. First, Bäckman did find a modest, albeit nonsignificant, age difference favoring young adults in each of his studies. Second, other investigators have recently contrasted young and elderly adults in memory for a single series of actions performed under intentional memory conditions (Cohen, Sandler, & Schroeder, 1987; Lichty, 1986) and have found a more pronounced age difference than that reported by Bäckman (see Table 4.3). Conceivably, an important difference between these studies and those of Bäckman is in the longer list of actions performed (e.g., 18 in Lichty's study) in the former studies. Of further importance is the fact that the subjects performing the discrete actions in Lichty's study were the same subjects who performed the continuous activities in the study discussed earlier (see p. 106). Thus, the significant age deficit for discrete action recall was obtained for the same subjects who manifested only a modest, nonsignificant age difference for continuous activity recall.

Our reference thus far has been to an age deficit in recall of discrete actions. A different picture emerges when a recognition test is employed. Such a test was included in Lichty's study (1986). Half her subjects performed one set of 18 actions (Set A), and the other half a different set of 18 actions (Set B). Following the recall test, all subjects received all 36 commands in a random order and identified each as being old (Set A for the first half, Set B for the second half) or new (reversal of the sets). Hit rates for identifying old actions were virtually perfect for both young (.99) and elderly subjects (.98), and false-alarm rates for incorrectly identifying new actions as old were essentially zero at each age level. Thus, the recall versus recognition comparison for action memory parallels closely that found for continuous activity memory. Interpretation of this comparison is, of course, again complicated by obvious ceiling and floor effects.

Lichty's study also revealed that individual differences among discrete actions in their recallability are as pronounced as individual differences among continuous activities in their recallability. This may be seen in Table 4.4 for a representative sample of 12 of 36 actions performed by Lichty's sub-

TABLE 4.4. Recall Scores (% of Subjects Recalling a Discrete Action) for Young and Elderly Subjects on a Representative Sample of Actions[a]

| Action | Recall Score | | Age Difference |
|---|---|---|---|
| | Young | Elderly | |
| Put on the hat | 100 | 58 | 42[b] |
| Bounce the ball | 92 | 42 | 50[b] |
| Unzip the zipper | 83 | 67 | 16 |
| Stir the tea in the cup | 75 | 58 | 17 |
| Pick up the chalk | 75 | 42 | 33[b] |
| Put the cap on the pen | 67 | 83 | −17 |
| Take the lid off the box | 67 | 50 | 17 |
| Fasten the safety pin | 58 | 58 | 0 |
| Close the purse | 58 | 17 | 41[b] |
| Open the penknife | 50 | 50 | 0 |
| Look through the magnifying glass | 42 | 33 | 9 |
| Put on the thimble | 33 | 42 | −9 |

[a]From data in Lichty (1986).
[b]$p < .05$, chi-square test.

jects. The overall pattern is much like that found for continuous activities; that is, a pronounced age difference favoring young adults was present for only some actions, attaining significance for only a few (5 out of 36, but approaching significance, $p < .10$, for another 8 actions). In addition, for 7 of 36 activities there was a reversal of the age difference. However, the correlation between young and elderly recall scores over all 36 actions was less pronounced ($r = .30$) than the comparable correlation found for continuous activities (see p. 106). Unfortunately, the reasons for variability both in overall recallability and in age differences in recallability remain as unidentified for discrete actions as they do for continuous activities (Cohen, Peterson, & Mantini-Atkinson, 1987).

Finally, performance of her subjects on both discrete actions and continuous activities permitted Lichty to examine the covariation between subjects' total recall scores for the two kinds of memory tasks. The correlation between scores was moderately high and statistically significant for her elderly subjects ($r = .59$), but failed to attain significance for her young subjects ($r = .28$).

## Generated Versus Provided Actions

In the everday world, actions are usually self-generated. We see an open safety pin and close it, we unzip a zipper because we need to undress, we sharpen a pencil because the point is dull, and so on. However, on occasion, initiation of an action is provided externally by the request of another person, such as "Close the door, please" and "Open the window, please." The action memory studies we have reviewed so far have all employed provided actions made in response to the experimenter's requests. Conceivably, self-generated actions may be more recallable than provided actions, and they may even be sufficiently recalled to eliminate age deficits in recall.

The generated-versus-provided issue has become an important one in research on verbal episodic memory. In the provided condition subjects read such word pairs as *jacket–coat* and are later asked to recall the second word in each pair. In the generated condition subjects encounter such pairs as *jacket–c*_____ and are asked to give a word beginning with "c" that is a synonym of jacket. A recall test of the generated words follows. The words generated by this procedure are almost certain to be identical to the words read in the provided condition. Nevertheless, young adults are likely to recall more generated than provided words (McFarland, Frey, & Rhodes, 1980; Slamecka & Graf, 1978). Most important, McFarland, Warren, and Crockard (1985) found that the advantage in recallability of generated compared to provided words applies to elderly adults as well as to young adults. However, they also discovered that generating words did not eliminate the age deficit found for provided words (the usual format of verbal memory research). That is, the age difference favoring young adults was as pronounced for generated words as for provided words. In other words, generation served to enhance recallability equally for young and old subjects, leaving the age difference essentially unaffected.

In another part of her study, Lichty (1986) introduced a variation for action memory that closely approximates the generation versus provided variation found in verbal memory research and in the everyday world as well. Subjects were given objects that had a very limited number of possible actions when asked to manipulate them; for example, a cup and a saucer placed apart on a table. Subjects in the provided condition were asked to place the cup on the saucer, while subjects in the generated condition were asked to perform an ordinary, commonplace action with the objects. The action performed by subjects in the generated condition nearly always conformed to the action performed by subjects in the provided condition. In all, 24 actions were performed under either provided or generated conditions, with a recall test of the actions at the end of the series (intentional memory for all subjects). A modestly greater, but statistically nonsignificant, level of recall for generated actions (61%) than for provided actions (53%) was found for her young adult subjects. However, recall of generated actions by her elderly subjects (44%) did not differ from recall of provided actions (also 44%). As a result, the age deficit in recall of actions was, if anything, greater for generated than for provided actions. Why the generation of an action, unlike the generation of a word, does not seem to enhance the later recall of the action is puzzling, but no more so than why some provided actions are more recallable than other provided actions.

# Conceptualization of Activity/Action Memory

## Commonality of Activity Memory and Action Memory

Functional identity means that two phenomena manifest the same relationship with variation in a critical independent variable. As the number of functional identities between the two phenomena increases, our conviction that the two phenomena are really minor variants of the same phenomenon also increases. That is, the two phenomena appear to be governed by the same basic processes. In our case, the two phenomena are activity memory and action memory. Our review of research of these phenomena revealed that their relationships with several important independent variables are strikingly similar. For example, instructional variation expected to alter the extent of rehearsal of task content has little effect on either phenomenon. In addition, input position within a series has similar effects for each phenomenon, namely the presence of a recency effect and the absence of a primacy effect. Moreover, the percentage of tasks recalled is essentially the same, both for young adults and elderly adults, whether the series consists of continuous activities or discrete actions, as is the age difference in the percentage of tasks recalled. The age deficit, in turn, essentially disappears for each form of memory when subjects are given a recognition test of prior task content. Finally, there is evidence indicating that the proficiency of subjects recalling continuous activities correlates positively with their proficiency of recalling discrete actions, especially for elderly adults. Other commonalities remain to be demonstrated, namely those involving frequency estimates, temporal judgments, and reality monitoring. We feel confident that, when these are tested in the laboratory, the results obtained for discrete action tasks will again approximate closely the results obtained previously with continuous activity tasks. Our confidence stems from our belief that the commonality of processes between the two forms of memory must be considerable.

The probable commonality of processes leads us to believe that the distinctions between activity memory and action memory must be relatively minor ones. One such distinction is in the duration of performance—many seconds for activity memory tasks, only a few seconds for discrete action tasks. What is important to subsequent memorability, however, is the fact that the two kinds of tasks require equally the activation of a program that is essential for the initiation of performance. It is the activation of that program that seemingly establishes memorability. Continuation of the program in the form of a sustained performance appears to contribute little to the enhancement of memorability. Our conclusion here is based on our finding that recall of activities is largely unaffected by their durations (see p. 108). The implication is that memory for discrete actions would be similarly unaffected if those actions were to be sustained over time. Such extensions could be accomplished, for example, by altering the nature of the verbal commands given subjects, for example, from "Pick up the pin" to "Pick up the pins" (with a number of pins available) and from "Snap your fingers" to "Snap your fingers until I tell you to stop." In effect, a discrete action becomes a continuous activity under these conditions. As far as we can determine, variation in the number of repetitions of an action, and therefore in the duration of that action, have not been included in studies on action memory. From our perspective, the predicted outcome for a study of this kind is again quite clear—the effect of repeating the action on subsequent recall should be negligible for both young and elderly subjects.

There is another distinction that must be considered between continuous activity memory, at least as far as it has been studied in our laboratory, and discrete action memory. Our tasks employed to study activity memory are admittedly relatively artificial ones in the sense of the lack of their similarity to everyday tasks involving activity memory. By contrast, the laboratory tasks serving to test discrete action memory correspond more closely to everyday tasks. Consequently, the generalizability of our laboratory results on activity memory to everyday memory phenomena (i.e., external validity) may seem to be less than the generalizability of the results obtained in studies on action memory. We believe, however, that the true basis of generalizability rests in the extent to which the processes involved in performances on laboratory tasks are isomorphic with the processes involved in performances on everyday tasks (see Mook, 1983). We are confident that the processes determining memorability of performances on our activity tasks are as generalizable to the everyday world as the processes determining memorability of performances on action tasks; they are, in our opinion, the same basic processes. Thus, a distinction based on veridicality with tasks in the "real world" strikes us as being another superficial one.

## Model of Activity/Action Memory

A single model should be sufficient to conceptualize the processes governing both activity memory and action memory, given their commonalities. The model we propose is suggested by the similarity between the storage of activity/action information and the storage of verbal information via maintenance rehearsal (Craik & Lockhart, 1972). The effects of maintenance rehearsal on verbal memory are nicely demonstrated in a number of experiments (e.g., Glenberg & Bradley, 1979) employing a modification of the Brown–Peterson short-term memory paradigm (Brown, 1958: Peterson & Peterson, 1959). In the modified paradigm, the to-be-remembered items are strings of digits that are presented briefly and then tested for recall after a variable retention interval (e.g., 6 seconds versus 12 seconds) filled with a rehearsal-preventing activity. It is this interpolated activity that is of critical interest. It consists of reading out loud a pair of words repeatedly until the retention interval ends. At the end of the experiment, subjects are given a "surprise" recall test for the distractor words. (i.e., incidental memory). Words read for 12 seconds surely receive more maintenance rehearsal than words read for only 6 seconds. Nevertheless, the added maintenance rehearsal contributes little to the subsequent recallability of the words. Earlier (p. 108) we noted Naveh-Benjamin and Jonides's (1984) explanation of this phenomenon in terms of a two-stage sequence. Briefly, the first stage requires the operationalization of a program for rehearsing (i.e., reading out loud the specific words exposed during a retention interval). It is the activation of this program that transmits memory traces of the words to the episodic long-term store. The second stage consists of maintaining that program by repeating it for successive rehearsals of the words. This "maintenance-of-maintenance rehearsal" is postulated to lead to little further transmission of traces to the store. Consequently, the added rehearsal given to words exposed for longer durations has a negligible effect on their recallability.

We have good reason to believe that a comparable two-stage sequence underlies activity memory and action memory. Note that there is little difference in the recallability of activities performed continuously and actions performed only once. In each case, a program is operationalized, accompanied by the automatic transmission of a memory trace of that program to the episodic long-term store. The memory tasks differ only in that the program must be maintained in working memory while performing a continuous activity (e.g, solving additional anagrams), but the program is terminated as soon as a single action is performed. Maintenance of an activity, however, adds little to memorability, just as maintenance of rehearsal adds little to the memorability of words. Nor does increasing the duration of an activity enhance memorability; again, it is only the initiation of its program that transmits a memory trace to the long-term store.

A schematic representation of this two-stage model (Figure 4.10) depicts the processes as they apply to activity memory under incidental memory conditions, the conditions most likely to be encountered for everyday activities. Input in the form of task instructions is assumed to activate task-relevant knowledge stored in generic, or semantic, memory (Tulving, 1972). This activation transmits to working memory a program that enables performance on the task to begin. Automatically, a memory trace of that program's operationalization is transmitted to and registered in the long-term store. Perpetuation of the program in working memory allows continuing performance on the task at hand, but without further registration of traces in the store. For discrete actions, there is of course no perpetuation of the program in working memory unless repetition of the action is required. Such repetition is viewed here as being irrelevant with respect to the further transmission of traces to the store.

Also present in our model is an expected bypass of the involvement of metamemory. Metamemory consists of self-knowledge about memory functioning, including knowledge about appropriate rehearsal strategies to employ to ensure memorability. Without forewarning of a future memory test, a metamemory bypass is the likely consequence. The rehearsal-independent

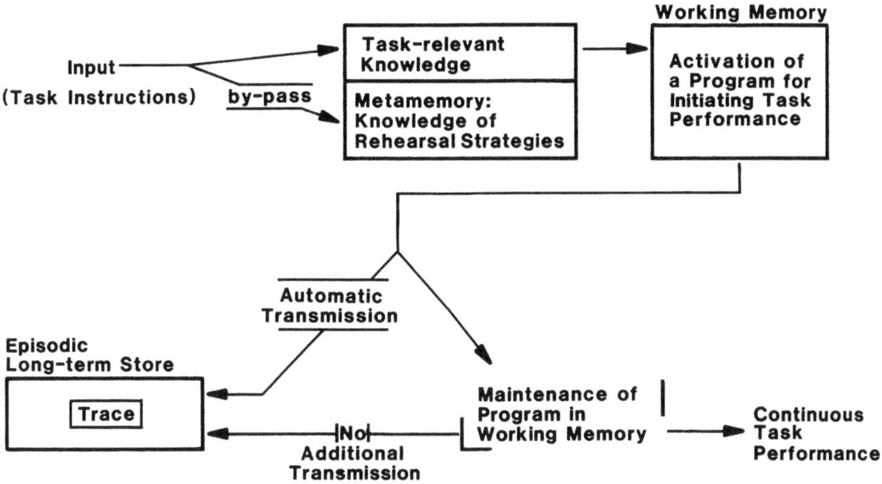


FIGURE 4.10. Two-stage model of activity/action memory.

nature of activity/action memory suggests that even when metamemorial processes are engaged under intentional memory conditions, there is little embellishment of the memory trace transmitted automatically to the store.

Although perpetuation of a program in working memory in order to continue performance on a task is seen as contributing little to memorability, repetition of the same program at a later time is another matter. Each subsequent activation of the program appears to transmit automatically another distinctive trace to the store. It is the presence of these multiple traces that presumably enables subjects to give accurate estimates of their frequencies of performing various activities, just as separate encounters with words in a study list generate multiple traces that enable subjects to estimate fairly accurately the frequencies of those encounters (Hintzman & Stern, 1978). As indicated earlier, we know of no study dealing with frequency estimates for discrete actions performed varying numbers of times within a series. There is a study, however, that reveals an increment in recall for both young and elderly subjects for actions performed twice (widely separated repetitions), relative to actions performed only once (Cohen et al., 1987). The subjects in their study were given a series of 10 actions to perform once and 10 actions to perform twice. Young adults recalled about 48% of their once-performed actions and about 70% of their twice-performed actions; comparable values for their elderly subjects were 34% and 55%, respectively. Thus, the net effect was an age deficit as pronounced for repeated actions as for single actions. Nevertheless, separate traces do seem to be transmitted automatically to the long-term store for separate activations of the same action program. These separate traces provided alternative sources for retrieving information in the store, thereby enhancing recall regardless of age, as well as providing separate traces for mediating estimates of occurrences.

Our model of activity/action memory is intended to apply to adults of all ages. Unanswered, however, is the question of why there are age deficits in the recall of both activities and actions. Earlier (p. 102) we discussed several possible reasons for age-related deficits in recall. One explanation places the blame for age deficits solely on the effortful nature of retrieving episodic information for purposes of recall, regardless of how that information reached the long-term store. Again, according to this hypothesis, the diminished capacity of working memory in late adulthood is the source of the diminished retrieval effort exerted by elderly adults. Acceptance of this explanation has been made difficult, however, by the consistent finding that operational measures of working memory capacity (e.g., digit span, reading span) fail to correlate with measures of recall proficiency for elderly subjects, at least for rehearsal-dependent forms of episodic memory (Hartley, 1986; Light & Anderson, 1985). A second explanation hinted at earlier is that even presumably automatically encoded information may occasionally fail to be transmitted to the long-term store by elderly adults. Here the blame is placed on the breakdown with aging in automaticity, at least to some degree. Our own results with both activity and action memory tasks would seem to rule out this possibility. Recognition scores are essentially as high for elderly subjects as for young subjects, indicating that a trace of each task program is transmitted automatically to the store regardless of age. Moreover, separate traces seem to be transmitted for successive reactivations of a program as effectively for elderly subjects as for young subjects, as witnessed by their comparable performances in estimating frequencies of task participations.

There is another possible explanation that should be given serious consideration. Traces of a program's operationalization may be transmitted automatically at all ages, but the traces may be enhanced by additional information encoded more readily by young than by elderly adults. The additional information may be contextual in nature, consisting of thoughts that accompany the initiation of an activity/action program, such as "I hope I don't stick myself with the stupid pin" for the "Fasten the Safety Pin" task. We observed earlier that age-related decrements in encoding contextual information have been widely employed to explain age-related deficits for many kinds of memory tasks (Burke & Light, 1981). Note that the present hypothesis postulates a different locus of a context effect than the locus considered earlier (pp. 107–108), namely during the activation of a program rather than during ongoing utilization of the program for continuous performance. Although the latter hypothesis appears to be invalid (see p. 108), the former remains feasible. Retrieval of thoughts at the time of recall should result ecphorically in the retrieval of the activity/action information encoded with those thoughts (Tulving, 1983). The ecphoric advantage may account for why recall by young subjects exceeds recall by elderly subjects. The differential encoding of contextual information for different tasks may also account for task differences in recallability. That is, distinctive thoughts are more likely to be elicited by some tasks than by other tasks, giving the former an ecphoric advantage in recall. Discovering ways of testing directly the validity of this variation of the contextual hypothesis presents an important challenge to future research on activity/action memory.

## Summary

Activity memory consists of memory for continuous performances on various tasks (e.g., solving anagrams). Its rehearsal-independent nature is apparent in our studies by the consistent absence of an effect for instructional variation, that is, for memory under incidental versus intentional memory conditions, and by the presence of a recency effect in recall, but not a primacy effect for both young and elderly subjects. Thus, activity memory seems to satisfy a major criterion of automaticity. However, it fails to satisfy a second criterion of automaticity, the absence of adult age differences in proficiency, at least as measured by a recall test. The extent of the age difference, however, is negligible when memory is tested by recognition rather than by recall.

The age deficit in recall of activities is clearly greater for some activities than for other activities. There is evidence to indicate that activities demanding a high degree of mental effort in order to perform them are especially recallable for elderly subjects. However, the age deficit in recall appears to be as pronounced for tasks requiring primarily motor activity as for tasks requiring primarily cognitive activity.

Our research on activity memory has also focused on memory for two noncontent attributes, the frequency with which specific activities were performed in a series and the temporal order in which they were performed. As with memory for activity content, memory for each of these noncontent attributes is unaffected by instructional variation (i.e., incidental versus intentional memory). Frequency estimates were found to be as accurate for elderly as for young subjects. In addition, reality monitoring, defined as the ability to discriminate between the planning of an activity and actually performing the activity, was found to be as proficient for elderly as for young subjects. By contrast, temporal memory for activities, as measured by the accuracy of reconstructing the order in which the specific activities were performed, was found to be substantially more proficient for young than for elderly subjects.

Memory for brief, discrete actions performed in a series, such as picking up a pin, has also been studied in our laboratory and in others. This form of memory displays many of the same characteristics as activity memory, including rehearsal independency; the presence of a recency effect and the absence of a primacy effect in recall; age deficits for recall, but not for recognition; and considerable intertask variability both in overall recallability and in age difference in recallability. In addition, a positive correlation seems to exist between recall scores for a series of activities and recall scores for a series of discrete actions when the series are performed by the same subjects, especially for elderly subjects. A modest generation effect was found for young subjects, but not for elderly subjects.

The functional identity between continuous activity memory and discrete action memory implies that the two forms of memory are governed by the same basic processes. Our model of activity/action memory is patterned after the two-stage model offered by Naveh-Benjamin and Jonides (1984) to explain the effects of maintenance rehearsal on word memory. The first stage consists of the operationalization of a program to perform the requested activity or action. Operationalization of the program in working memory is accompanied by the automatic transmission of a memory trace to the episodic long-term store, regardless of a subject's age. The second stage consists of the perpetuation of that program in working memory in order to sustain either a continuous activity or the repetition of a discrete action. Little, if any, further transmission of traces to the store accompanies the perpetuation of a program. However, separate activations of a program are presumed to transmit separate, multiple traces of that program. Age deficits in recall are presumably the result of young adults being more likely than elderly adults to encode contextual information (thoughts elicited by the task at hand) along with program information. The added contextual information gives young adults an echporic advantage over elderly adults during attempts to recall prior task participations.

## References

Attig, M., & Hasher, L. (1980). The processing of frequency of occurrence information by adults. *Journal of Gerontology, 35,* 66–69.

Bäckman, L. (1985). Further evidence for the lack of adult age differences on free recall of subject performed tasks: The importance of motor action. *Human Learning, 4,* 79–87.

Bäckman, L. (in press). Varieties of memory compensation of older adults in episodic remembering. In L.W. Poon, D.C. Rubin, & B.A. Wilson (Eds.), *Everyday cognition in adult and late life.* New York: Cambridge University Press.

Bäckman, L., & Nilsson, L-G. (1984). Aging effects in free recall: An exception to the rule. *Human Learning, 3,* 53–69.

Bäckman, L., & Nilsson, L-G. (1985). Prerequisites for the lack of age differences in memory performance. *Experimental Aging Research, 11,* 67–73.

Bäckman, L., Nilsson, L-G., & Chalom, D. (1986). New evidence on the nature of the encoding of action events. *Memory & Cognition, 14,* 339–346.

Brainerd, C.J. (1985). Model-based approaches to storage and retrieval development. In C.J. Brainerd & M. Pressley (Eds.), *Basic processes in memory development: Progress in cognitive development research.* New York: Springer-Verlag.

Bromley, D.B. (1958). Some effects of age on short-term learning and remembering. *Journal of Gerontology, 13,* 398–406.

Brown, J.A. (1958). Some tests of the decay theory of immediate memory. *Quarterly Journal of Experimental Psychology, 10,* 12–21.
Burke, D.M., & Light, L.L. (1981). Memory and aging: The role of retrieval processes. *Psychological Bulletin, 90,* 513–546.
Cohen, R.L. (1981). On the generality of some memory laws. *Scandinavian Journal of Psychology, 22,* 267–281.
Cohen, R.L. (1983). The effects of encoding variables on the free recall of words and action events. *Memory & Cognition, 11,* 575–582.
Cohen, R.L., & Bean, G.L. (1983). Memory in educable mentally retarded adults: Deficit in subject or experimenter? *Intelligence, 7,* 287–298.
Cohen, R.L., Peterson, M., & Mantini-Atkinson, T. (1987). Interevent differences in event memory: Why are some events more recallable than others. *Memory & Cognition, 15,* 109–118.
Cohen, R.L., Sandler, S.P., & Schroeder, K. (1987). Aging and memory for words and action events: The effects of item repetition and list length. *Psychology and Aging, 2,* 280–285.
Craik, F.I.M. (1977). Age differences in human memory. In J.E. Birren & K. W. Schaie (Eds.), *Handbook of the psychology of aging.* New York: Van Nostrand Reinhold.
Craik, F.I.M., & Lockhart, R.S. (1972). Levels of processing: A framework for memory research. *Journal of Verbal Learning and Verbal Behavior, 11,* 671–684.
Craik, F.I.M., & Tulving, E. (1975). Depth of processing and the retention of words in episodic memory. *Journal of Experimental Psychology: General, 104,* 268–294.
Ekstrom, R.B., French, J.W., Harman, H.H., & Derman, D. (1976). *Manual for kit of factor-referenced cognitive tests.* Princeton, NJ: Educational Testing Service.
Erber, J.T. (1974). Age differences in recognition memory. *Journal of Gerontology, 29,* 177–181.
Glenberg, A.M., & Bradley, M.M. (1979). Mental contiguity. *Journal of Experimental Psychology: Human Learning and Memory, 5,* 88–97.
Greene, R.L. (1986). Effects of intentionality and strategy on memory for frequency. *Journal of Experimental Psychology: Learning, Memory, and Cognition, 12,* 489–495.
Hartley, J.T. (1986). Reader and text variables as determinants of discourse memory in adulthood. *Psychology and Aging, 1,* 150–158.
Hasher, L., & Zacks, R.T. (1979). Automatic and effortful processes in memory. *Journal of Experimental Psychology: General, 108,* 356–388.
Hasher, L., & Zacks, R.T. (1984). Automatic processing of fundamental information: The case of frequency of occurrence. *American Psychologist, 39,* 1372–1388.
Helstrup, T. (1986). Separate memory laws for recall of performed act? *Scandinavian Journal of Psychology, 27,* 1–29.
Hintzman, D.L., & Stern, L.D. (1978). Contextual variability and memory for frequency. *Journal of Experimental Psychology: Human learning and Memory, 4,* 539–549.
Johnson, M.K. (1977). What is being counted none-the-less? In I.M. Birnbaum & E.S. Parker (Eds.), *Alcohol and human memory.* Hillsdale, NJ: Erlbaum.
Johnson, M.K., Raye, C.L., Hasher, L., & Chromiak, W. (1979). Are there developmental differences in reality monitoring? *Journal of Experimental Child Psychology, 27,* 120–128.
Kausler, D.H. (1974). *Psychology of verbal learning and memory.* New York: Academic Press.
Kausler, D.H. (1982). *Experimental psychology and human aging.* New York: Wiley.

Kausler, D.H., & Hakami, M.K. (1983). Memory for activities: Adult age differences and intentionality. *Developmental Psychology, 19,* 889–894.
Kausler, D.H., Hakami, M.K., & Wright, R.E. (1982). Adult age differences in frequency judgments of categorical representations. *Journal of Gerontology, 37,* 365–371.
Kausler, D.H., Lichty, W., & Davis, R.T. (1985). Temporal memory for performed activities: Intentionality and adult age differences. *Developmental Psychology, 21,* 1132–1138.
Kausler, D.H., Lichty, W., & Freund, J.S. (1985). Adult age differences in recognition memory and frequency judgments for planned activities. *Developmental Psychology, 21,* 647–654.
Kausler, D.H., Lichty, W., & Hakami, M.K. (1984). Frequency judgments for distractor items in a short-term memory task: Instructional variation and adult age differences. *Journal of Verbal Learning and Verbal Behavior, 23,* 660–668.
Kausler, D.H., Lichty, W., Hakami, M.K., & Freund, J.S. (1986). Activity duration and adult age differences for activity performance. *Psychology and Aging, 1,* 80–81.
Kausler, D.H., & Puckett, J.M. (1980). Frequency judgments and correlated cognitive abilities in young and elderly adults. *Journal of Gerontology, 35,* 376–382.
Kausler, D.H., Salthouse, T.A., & Saults, J.S. (in press). Temporal memory over the adult lifespan. *American Journal of Psychology.*
Keppel, G., & Mallory, W.A. (1969). Presentation rate and instructions to guess in free recall. *Journal of Experimental Psychology, 79,* 269–275.
Lichty, W. (1986). Aging and memory for activities. Ph.D. dissertation, University of Missouri, Columbia, Missouri.
Lichty, W., Kausler, D.H., & Martinez, D.R. (1986). Adult age differences in memory for motor versus cognitive activities. *Experimental Aging Research, 12,* 227–230.
Light, L.L., & Anderson, P.A. (1985). Working-memory capacity, age, and memory for discourse. *Journal of Gerontology, 40,* 737–747.
Lowenthal, M.F., Berkman, P.L., Buehler, J.A., Pierce, R.C., Robinson, B. C., & Trier, M.L. (1967). *Aging and Mental disorders in San Francisco.* San Francisco: Freeman.
Maki, R.H., & Ostby, R.S. (1987). Effects of level of processing and rehearsal on frequency judgments. *Journal of Experimental Psychology: Learning, Memory, and Cognition, 13,* 151–163.
Mandler, J.M., Seegmiller, D., & Day, J. (1977). On the coding of spatial information. *Memory & Cognition, 5,* 10–16.
McCormack, P.D. (1981). Temporal coding by young and elderly adults: A test of the Hasher-Zacks model. *Developmental Psychology, 17,* 509–515.
McCormack, P.D. (1982). Temporal coding and study-phase retrieval in young and elderly adults. *Bulletin of the Psychonomic Society, 20,* 242–244.
McFarland, C.E., Jr., Frey, T.J., & Rhodes, D.D. (1980). Retrieval of internally versus externally generated words in episodic memory. *Journal of Verbal Learning and Verbal Behavior, 19,* 210–225.
McFarland, C.E., Jr., Warren, L.R., & Crockard, J. (1985). Memory for self-generated stimuli in young and old adults. *Journal of Gerontology, 40* 205–207.
Mook, D.G. (1983). In defense of external validity. *American Psychologist, 38,* 379–387.
Naveh-Benjamin, M., & Jonides, J. (1984). Maintenance rehearsal: A two-component analysis. *Journal of Experimental Psychology: Learning, Memory, and Cognition, 10,* 369–385.

Naveh-Benjamin, M., & Jonides, J. (1986). On the automaticity of frequency coding: Effects of competing task load, encoding strategy, and intention. *Journal of Experimental Psychology: Learning, Memory, and Cognition, 12,* 378–386.

Perlmutter, M., Metzger, R., Nezworski, T., & Miller, K. (1981). Spatial and temporal memory in 20- and 60-year-olds. *Journal of Gerontology, 36,* 59–64.

Peterson, L.R., & Peterson, M.J. (1959). Short-term retention of individual verbal items. *Journal of Experimental Psychology, 58,* 193–198.

Rankin, J.L., & Kausler, D.H. (1979). Adult age differences in false recognitions. *Journal of Gerontology, 34,* 58–65.

Salthouse, T.A. (1982). *Adult cognition: An experimental psychology of human aging.* New York: Springer-Verlag.

Salthouse, T.A., Kausler, D.H., & Saults, J.S. (1988). Investigation of student status, background variables, and the feasibility of standard tasks in cognitive aging research. *Psychology and Aging, 3,* 29–37.

Slamecka, N.J., & Graf, P. (1978). The generation effect: Delineation of a phenomenon. *Journal of Experimental Psychology: Human Learning and Memory, 4,* 592–604.

Smith, A.D. (1980). Age differences in encoding, storage, and retrieval. In L.W. Poon, J.L. Fozard, L.S. Cermak, D. Arenberg, & L.W. Thompson (Eds.), *New directions in memory and aging.* Hillsdale, NJ: Erlbaum.

Toglia, M.P., & Kimble, G.A. (1976). Recall and use of serial position information. *Journal of Experimental Psychology: Human Learning and Memory, 2,* 431–445.

Tulving, E. (1972). Episodic and semantic memory. In E. Tulving & W. Donaldson (Eds.), *Organization of memory.* New York: Academic Press.

Tulving, E. (1983). *Elements of episodic memory.* New York: Oxford University Press.

Tyler, S.W., Hertel, P.T., McCallum, M.C., & Ellis, H.C. (1979). Cognitive effort and memory. *Journal of Experimental Psychology: Human Learning and Memory, 5,* 607–617.

Wilkinson, A.C., & Koestler, R. (1983). Repeated recall: A new model and tests of its generality from childhood to old age. *Journal of Experimental Psychology: General, 112,* 423–449.

Zacks, R.T., Hasher, L., Alba, J.W., Sanft, H., & Rose, K.C. (1984). Is temporal order encoded automatically? *Memory & Cognition, 12,* 387–394.

# 5. Memory for Prose and Aging: A Meta-Analysis

*Elizabeth M. Zelinski and Michael J. Gilewski*

## Introduction

Research in memory processes in the elderly in the early 1980s was strongly influenced by research in experimental psychology establishing standardized methods for investigating memory for discourses. Previously, memory for prose was not studied; exceptions occurred (Gordon & Clark, 1974; Schneider, Gritz, & Jarvik, 1975; Taub, 1976) in which intuitive or verbatim approaches to scoring recall were used. When more objective methods of prose analysis were developed by various authors, notably Meyer (1975) and Kintsch (1974), investigators in aging began research programs to study memory for discourse.

Their motivations were based on several issues in the aging literature that made prose memory a promising area for research. First, there was some evidence that older adults were better at recalling material they considered meaningful than that considered nonmeaningful (Hulicka, 1967). Texts, therefore, seemed to be especially appropriate for testing memory in older people because they would be much more meaningful than word lists as study material. Any age differences in discourse recall, it was assumed, could then be attributed to memory deficits rather than to methodological problems, such as age, or cohort differences in motivation resulting from task characteristics.

Second, there appeared to be greater ecological validity in recalling discourses compared to lists of words because people are more likely to recall such materials in everyday life (Hartley, Harker, & Walsh, 1980). Further, text recall appeared to be an informative task for evaluating the effects of aging on memory because there was evidence that there were no differences in recall of texts in college-aged adults studying them or reading them for personal interest (Singer, 1982), whereas there was considerable evidence that incidentally learned lists were recalled more poorly than intentionally learned ones (Hasher & Zacks, 1979).Thus, having older adults memorize discourses seemed especially appropriate as a means of simulating everyday memory processes.

Third, the list memory studies conducted before that time had failed to isolate clearly the basis of memory deficits in older people (Burke & Light, 1981). It was assumed because texts were a methodologically sound source of data that conferred ecological as well as construct validity on research efforts in understanding memory and aging, that the conflicting accounts of why older adults remembered less than younger ones would be resolved.

Initial reports of research using prose materials and prose scoring systems indicated that older adults did not differ from younger ones in recall (Harker, Hartley, & Walsh, 1982; Meyer & Rice, 1981). The conclusions of these studies suggested that this approach was a panacea for measuring memory in older adults, because these discourse memory studies had shown, albeit indirectly, that the differences between young and older people in memory for lists of nonsense syllables, unrelated words, categorized words, familiar words, and unfamiliar ones (Craik, 1977; Jerome, 1959) were artifacts of the list memory methodology previously practiced.

Nevertheless, findings of age deficits in prose recall reported in early experiments were replicated with studies using the more sophisticated analysis systems (e.g., Dixon, Simon, Nowak, & Hultsch, 1982; Petros, Tabor, Cooney, & Chabot, 1983; Spilich, 1983; Zelinski, Gilewski, & Thompson, 1980). In their 1984 review of the prose memory literature, Hultsch and Dixon concluded that there were indeed many examples of age-related deficits in memory for discourse. With a loss of optimism about the efficacy of the use of discourse as an ecologically valid paradigm (see also Rice, 1986b), the focus of many researchers in aging shifted to considering why there were inconsistent findings about the reliability of age differences in terms of models of memory in general and of sources of variance in performance within the prose memory paradigm in particular. Both Hultsch and Dixon (1984) and Meyer and Rice (1983, in press) proposed that subject, passage, and task variables interacted, producing age differences in some cases and eliminating them in others.

In this chapter, we review the hypothesized effects of several variables considered by aging researchers to be of importance in predicting the size of age differences in prose recall. Rather than conducting a traditional review of the literature, which has been summarized by Hultsch and Dixon (1984), Meyer and Rice (in press), Hartley (in press-a, in press-b), and Cohen (in press), among others, we report the results of a meta-analysis of those factors suggested to contribute to the variance in age differences across studies. We hope that our findings will clarify the issues in the existing literature and offer suggestions for new directions in research in discourse memory in aging.

## Predictors of Effect Sizes in Memory for Prose and Aging

Several major factors are currently used to explain age differences in memory for discourse. These variables have generally been invoked as *post hoc* explanations for discrepancies in findings (Hartley et al., 1980), but are of interest because the explanations underlying them can be easily applied to the popular theoretical frameworks developed to predict age differences in memory in general. These variables include individual differences in verbal abilities, text genre, the prose analysis scoring system used, and passage length. Verbal ability, as measured by performance on psychometric tests and/or by educational attainment, has been suggested to affect findings, with larger age differences produced for low verbal subjects than high verbal ones.

It has also been argued that text genre, that is, whether narratives or expository material is studied, is influential in the size of age differences produced, with larger differences obtained for narratives than expository prose. Cognitive aging researchers have used different formal scoring systems to devise models representing the text bases of materials studied. It has been suggested that Kintsch's microstructural system (1974) increases the size of age differences relative to Meyer's (1975) more macrostructural system, because scoring in Meyer's system is less likely to produce floor effects as partial credit for material recalled can be given. Finally, it has been argued that long passages produce larger age differences than shorter ones because the increased amount of material to remember increases the difficulty of the memory task for older people to a greater extent than for younger ones.

We discuss each of these factors in turn and evaluate their effects in our meta-analysis of the relative size of age differences in memory for prose. These particular factors are included in the meta-analysis because they can be operationalized in existing studies and their effects can be quantified from published research and analyzed.

Our list, however, is not exhaustive. Other factors discussed by various authors include effects of orienting tasks (Byrd, 1986; Simon, Dixon, Nowak, & Hultsch, 1982), the knowledge bases of subjects (Hultsch & Dixon, 1983), and individual differences in reading practice and their relation to strategies used by subjects in studying and recalling material (Rice 1986a, 1986b; Rice & Meyer, 1986). These latter factors have been addressed by either only one or two studies or cannot be analyzed here because of the limitations of meta-analytic procedures in evaluating published, rather than raw, data.

### Individual Differences in Verbal Abilities

One initial explanation of the discrepancies in results across studies of memory for discourse and aging was that the studies reported by Meyer and

Rice (1981) and Harker et al. (1982) showed no age differences because they compared highly educated younger and older adults with high vocabulary scores. On the other hand, studies showing age-related deficits (e.g., Simon et al., 1982; Zelinski et al., 1980) compared samples of less educated, less verbally skilled individuals. Furthermore, Meyer and Rice (1983) selected individuals for a series of comparisons, which they claimed represented the kinds of populations tested previously. They obtained large age differences with people whose vocabulary score were low, but the size of the age deficits were reduced and even eliminated when comparing people whose scores were high.

These findings correspond to other work in cognitive psychology. Psychometric studies have shown that individuals who have good verbal skills are better at remembering and verbal coding than those with poorer skills (Hunt, 1978). In addition, those with good verbal abilities are also more efficient at reading than their less verbally skilled counterparts (Perfetti, 1985). An individual differences model would thus predict that older adults who are highly skilled in verbal abilities would be better at recalling discourse than those less skilled.

Age differences among like-skilled people could vary to the extent that highly verbal older people do not differ from highly verbal younger ones in prose recall. Alternatively, age differences could be substantial between low verbal younger and older people. This prediction, suggested by Meyer and Rice (1983, in press; Rice & Meyer, 1986) is based on the notion that highly verbal elderly individuals maintain their reading skills by utilizing them more frequently than do their less verbal age mates. Younger low-skilled individuals would be more practiced in reading for recall because they have been in school more recently. Thus, Meyer and Rice's suggestion is based on a model of recency of practice in verbal tasks interacting with skill level, which is essentially a strategy or production deficiency explanation (discussed later). Other models of memory and aging, which we discuss shortly, make identical predictions about the effect size of age differences in discourse recall as a function of verbal and other cognitive abilities but for different reasons.

Studies examining individual differences have evaluated patterns of age differences based on scores on vocabulary tests, education levels, practice with reading and recall, and/or multivariate measures of various verbal and other cognitive skills. Indeed, verbal-ability-by-age interactions in discourse recall have followed the pattern suggested here (Dixon, Hultsch, Simon, & von Eye, 1984; Hartley, 1986; Taub & Kline, 1978) but other research has found larger age differences with high verbal groups than low verbal ones (Hultsch, Hertzog, & Dixon, 1984) and in two experiments, parallel age differences with subjects at different vocabulary levels were reported (Petros et al., 1983). In our meta-analysis, we will attempt to resolve the question of whether effect sizes for age differences vary in studies employing highly educated adults scoring highly on vocabulary tests compared to those in which less educated. less verbally skilled adults participated.

## Discourse Genre

It has been suggested by Hartley et al. (1980) and Meyer and Rice (in press) that the genre of the discourse studied can differentially affect results of prose recall studies with the young and old. Their claim is that age differences should be larger with stories or narratives than with essays or expository prose. This hypothesis served as an explanation for why studies with highly verbal, highly educated young and older adults (which, according to Meyer and Rice, should have produced small, if any age differences) reported large and significant age-related deficits (Cohen, 1979, Experiment. 3; Gordon & Clark, 1974). According to this explanation, such studies resulted in age differences because they involved study and recall of stories, whereas those with no differences involved recall of expository prose (Harker et al., 1982).

Differences in the proportion of recall as a function of passage genre occur in young people. Graesser, Haupt-Smith, Cohen, and Pyles (1980) found that college-aged adults recalled more from narratives than from expository discourses. One explanation for this comes from work done by Smith (1985), who found that expository text and narratives consist of genre-appropriate clauses with expository material containing an orientation without reference to either particular individuals or chronological ordering, whereas narratives contain references to both agents and temporal sequencing. These differences lead to the hypothesis that narratives are easier to remember because temporal sequencing and causal chains are critical to the organization and retrieval of discourse (Nezworski, Stein, & Trabasso, 1982), and these are more clearly defined in narratives than in expository tests (see also Graesser, Higginbotham, Robertson, & Smith, 1978).

Relevant to the question of whether discourse genre produces different effect sizes in aging comparisons is the issue of text readability and its impact on recall. Miller and Kintsch (1980) investigated how well subject-related variables (such as the number of inferences and the number of reinstatements of previously presented information required for comprehension) and text-related variables, (such as word frequency and sentence length) predicted readability and recallability of expository prose. They found that many of the same variables accounted for readability and recallability, and that the significant predictors included both text- and subject-related variables. This suggests that there is an interaction between the text and the reader in terms of what will be recalled. Thus, it would not be surprising that older adults who may process text material less efficiently than younger adults (see following) might be more deficient in recalling narratives than expository material.

The only study in which a direct test of an Age × Text genre interaction has been made was conducted by Hartley (1986). She found, contrary to the predictions made here, that subjects recalled more from expository versions of four texts than narratives derived from those passages. Nevertheless, age did not interact with genre, although older people recalled less reliably than younger ones.

In our meta-analysis, we will construct effect sizes for age differences in studies in which discourses are narratives (stories) with those of expository prose (essays). The specific predictions about these vary with the theoretical position one takes on the nature of the age differences in discourse memory, a topic we take up shortly.

## Prose Analysis Systems

As mentioned, the development of prose analysis systems was the pivotal factor in encouraging investigators in aging to study memory for discourse. The systems used by aging researchers reported to date are those developed by Kintsch (1974), Meyer (1975), Brown and Smiley (1977), Mandler and Johnson (1977), and Johnson (1983). The former three can be applied to any type of discourse, including expository prose, stories, and instructions whereas the latter two are story grammars, and therefore can only be applied to narratives. The discourse analysis systems vary somewhat in their approaches.

Kintsch's system (1974) is the most atomistic of the four; it evaluates the microstructure of the text by decomposing sentences into basic ideas or propositions. Relations between propositions within sentences are determined, and those which are repeated most frequently are considered to be the most important or central to the discourse. Centrality is therefore a function of local factors, not the overall organization of the text.

Meyer's system (1975) is more oriented toward text macrostructure; that is, the organization of idea units (propositions + their relations) and less toward microstructure than Kintsch's. Important idea units are determined by the investigator because the thematic statement is identified (by the investigator) with other idea units within and between sentences subordinate to it, their level of subordination being determined by the nature of the semantic interrelationships between idea units. Meyer's system is focused on identifying semantic roles and relations between idea units as a means of reflecting structurally what the author was trying to express. Because this system requires that the investigator identify thematic information, it is less objective and more difficult to apply than Kintsch's.

Brown and Smiley's (1977) approach is to have judges identify the relative importance of information in texts and assign hierarchical levels to propositions across the entire text. Consensus among judges is the basis for determining the text structure. This system is the only one that is based purely on empirical data and not on a predetermined theoretical model of text structure and its comprehension.

The two story grammars of Mandler and Johnson (1977) and Johnson (1983) involve the use of rewrite rules that identify the role of the proposition in terms of its semantic content in a schema universal to stories. Relative importance of propositions is determined by their roles; thematic information and goals of the characters are at the top of the hierarchy, and attempts and subgoals are subordinate to top-level propositions. As in Meyer's system ,the theme statement is identified by the investigator, so it is not completely objectively determined.

Comparisons of the sensitivity of some of these systems to memory processes have been made for young adults (Cofer, Scott, & Watkins, 1978; Meyer, 1985) and to developmental differences in memory in children (Bieger & Dunn, 1984). Cofer et al. reported that, for three subjects, there were no differences in overall recall between Kintsch's and Meyer's analyses. In an evaluation of seven recall protocols, Meyer (1985) found that agreement was high between the two systems for the total percent recalled when protocols of individuals with high proportions of recall, which were also accurate, were examined. Discrepancies in scoring were greater for situations in which a lower proportion of recall was obtained, and when what was recalled was less accurate. Situations in which recall met this description included delayed recall and recall by an elderly individual, with the Meyer system producing a higher total recall score in all cases. Meyer therefore suggested that the Kintsch system is more efficient for scoring accurate and relatively complete recall, and that hers is more appropriate for work in which recall is sketchy and relatively inaccurate, because credit can be given for partially correct recall and floor effects can thereby be reduced.

Bieger and Dunn (1984) also found that the Meyer system produced somewhat better recall scores and higher $F$ ratios than Kintsch's for reading ability and grade level differences in recall in a sample of 212 children. However, given the large $N$ in this study, the effect sizes (estimated from reported probability levels for the $F$s) for the analyses reported appear not to differ significantly across scoring methods.

It is unclear whether the different scoring systems that have been used by cognitive aging researchers might affect the relative size of age differences. For example, as Meyer has suggested, there might be larger age differences for studies utilizing Kintsch's system because it relies on recall accuracy and older people are less accurate in recall. Older people, who are more likely than younger persons to forget verbatim information, might be more penalized in recall scores when the Kintsch system, compared to the Meyer analysis, is applied.

In the meta-analysis, we test whether effect sizes of age differences in discourse recall vary as a function of the recall scoring system by comparing studies using the Meyer system with those using the Kintsch approach. A second analysis focuses on whether Kintsch's system, with its focus on microstructure, produces different effect sizes than other formal analysis systems that use macrostructure analyses; it is possible that it is the emphasis on microstructure that may penalize older subjects.

### Formal Scoring and Gist Scoring of Recall

It was the original assumption of cognitive aging researchers that formal approaches to evaluating recall are preferable to intuitive scoring of gist remembering. There were two major reasons for this assumption. First, analysis systems systematically represent the structure of texts. Second, they can produce variables that can be tested to evaluate qualitative aspects of recall, namely, recall as a function of the relative importance of information.

The prose analysis systems described here designate the hierarchical structure of texts by assigning propositions to levels. High level propositions (typically levels 1 and 2) are thematic statements or those most referred to (and therefore repeated) in the text; lower level propositions (level 3 and lower) often supply details and other subordinate information (Kintsch, 1974). It has been suggested that older adults are less sensitive to levels effects in discourse recall than younger ones (Meyer & Rice, 1981). However, some findings cast doubt on the reality of this proposed interaction of age with levels in recall. Rubin (1985) reported a meta-analysis evaluating the effect size of interactions of age with levels effects based on raw data from five experiments. He found that 0% of the recall variance was accounted for by the interaction in four of the five experiments; only Meyer and Rice's experiment accounted for more, with 4%.

Because of Rubin's negative findings, we do not pursue the interaction of age with levels in this chapter. A second reason is that the limitations of the meta-analytic approach we are using, which is based on obtaining summary statistics from the literature, makes this examination impossible. (The specific limitation is that effect sizes estimated from summary statistics can only contain 1 degree of freedom in the numerator of the *F* ratio, which rules out all studies evaluating Age × Levels interactions.)

We assume in this chapter, based on Rubin's meta-analysis, that the crucial issue in discourse memory in aging is a quantitative rather than qualitative age difference in recall. Because of this assumption, we will test whether formal prose analysis systems are as critical to evaluating age differences in memory for discourse as researchers have believed. This is accomplished by comparing effect sizes of all studies involving formal scoring systems with effect sizes of studies utilizing gist recall only. The results will indicate whether prose analysis systems, with their greater objectivity, have any impact on the relative size of quantitative age differences in recall. If there are no differences in effect size as a function of formal versus gist scoring, this finding would suggest that when quantitative age differences are investigated, the additional work required to analyze texts and to score recall according to the analysis might not be warranted, relative to gist scoring. If there are larger effect sizes for age differences with formal systems, it would suggest that formal systems penalize older adults. If smaller effect sizes are observed for formal systems than gist scoring, we would conclude that it is worthwhile to use the former because they reduce variance in recall data; thus, as had been assumed, they are a most appropriate approach to evaluating memory for discourse in the elderly.

### Passage Length

A final issue related to the memorability of discourse is the length of the text. Hartley et al. (1980) suggested that longer texts should produce larger age differences than shorter ones, just as word lists do (Craik, 1968) because older adults have difficulty acquiring or retrieving the additional information when more material has been studied. On the other hand, Meyer (in press) has argued that the general finding in the literature is that age differences are exacerbated when short texts are studied.

In one of our experiments, we examined recall for summaries of two passages (which averaged 212 words) and compared it with recall for their unabridged versions (which averaged about 640 words); we found no interaction of passage length with age (Zelinski, Light, & Gilewski, 1984, Experiment 3).

As with the question of relative age differences as a function of text genre, there are specific predictions that vary with the model of memory and aging invoked. In our meta-analysis, we compare studies in which the passages studied were relatively short (299 words or less) with those in which the passages are longer (300 words or more). This is a fairly arbitrary split for passage length, but results were the same regardless of how we divided studies.

## Predictions of Models of Memory and Aging for Subject and Text Variables

Three models of memory processing in aging are relevant to the question of effect size as a function of individual differences as well as the memorability of passages. In evaluating the efficacy of these models, we will look at patterns of differences in effect sizes for the two text variables we are studying, namely passage genre and length. All three models make identical predictions about individual differences in verbal abilities and age differences in prose recall, so we cannot differentiate among them. The same problem exists for evaluation of the processing resource deficit and working memory capacity models in predicting the effects of the two text variables, but we can compare their hypotheses with those of the production deficiency explanation.

The production deficiency hypothesis predicts that older adults use inadequate mnemonic strategies in studying and remembering. They are assumed to be capable of using appropriate strategies, but choose not to do so, possibly because they are less likely to be as strategy-oriented as the college students with whom they are typically compared or because they simply do not know appropriate strategies (Kausler, 1970). If individual differences in verbal skills and recall occur because of practice and/or application of good memorization strategies, as suggested by Meyer and Rice (1983, in press; Rice & Meyer, 1986), we would expect age differences to be larger for people low in verbal skills because presumably low verbal young people would use strategies and similarly skilled older ones would not. Younger and older adults with high scores on vocabularly tests would show smaller differences because both groups would be likely to use strategies. In the case of genre, more memorable material should encourage good strategy use in the young but not the old, and the model would predict that narratives would have larger effect sizes than expository material and that shorter texts would exacerbate age differences relative to longer ones.

The processing resource deficit hypothesis suggests that older adults are unable to process material to a deep semantic level and cannot therefore utilize the rich relationships between concepts in encoding and/or at retrieval (Craik, 1977; Craik & Simon, 1980). As a result, older adults may not remember prose as well as younger ones because they cannot as thoroughly encode the complex connections between propositions (Craik & Byrd, 1982). If resources vary across individuals, and those with greter resources are more verbally skilled (Perfetti, 1985), we would expect smaller age differences with highly skilled, highly verbal adults than with those low in verbal skills.

The processing resource deficit model predicts that effect sizes should be larger for expository prose than for narratives because material that is less readable/recallable should be more difficult for older adults to comprehend and remember. However, passage length should not differentially affect effect sizes, as the problem for older adults is qualitative, not quantitative, and amount to recall would not be as important as the depth of semantic processing.

The working memory capacity deficit hypothesis argues that older adults have difficulties comprehending and remembering prose when the processes underlying comprehension place an excessive burden on working memory (Cohen, 1979, 1981). Problems in recall, according to this perspective, should occur as a function of the cognitive capacity required to comprehend and remember the texts. Using the same logic as for the resource deficit hypothesis, the prediction for individual differences would be based on the notion that highly verbally skilled older people also have greater working memory capacity than less skilled ones.

In developing predictions about text variables and age differences based on a capacity model, there is evidence that easy texts require more capacity to comprehend than difficult ones (Britton, Westbrook & Holdredge, 1978), and that having prior knowledge of a topic is related to increased use of cognitive capacity while reading about that topic (Britton & Tesser, 1982). Thus easy-to-remember texts such as stories, which require more capacity, should produce larger age differences than essays. Long texts should not require more working memory capacity than short ones, as only several propositions at a time are processed and then stored in long-term memory. Thus, we would predict no differences in effect size as a function of passage length.

# Methodology

The purpose of meta-analysis is to evaluate the relative size of certain effects or results found in the extant literature in an objective way. Traditional reviews of research are often colored by the perspective of the reviewer, and because findings in psychology are often mixed, it is difficult to determine systematically which findings are reliable. Indeed, an examination of chapters reviewing discourse memory in the aged will show that authors devote a great deal of space to cataloging the differences across studies and attempt to develop a meaningful set of explanatory principles to predict (actually to postdict) discrepant results. By mathematically combining the findings of a body of research, we can use significance tests to identify which findings are most reliable. Following the methods outlined by Rosenthal (1984), we used two basic approaches: combining probabilities to test whether the age differences reported over the studies evaluated differ significantly from an effect size of zero, which would reflect the null hypothesis, and comparing effect sizes from studies by using analysis of variance to examine the predictions about the relevant factors hypothesized to account for age differences in discourse recall.

## Criteria for Inclusion of Studies

We surveyed the aging and cognition literature for papers focusing on recall of prose in younger and older adults. Criteria for selection for the meta-analysis included publication of means and standard deviations for young and elderly subjects, indices of statistical tests (most typically $F$ ratios and correlation coefficients), or probability levels. When results were nonsignificant, and none of these values was given in the publication, we used $F$ of 1.00 and the number of subjects minus the degrees of freedom ($df$) to estimate effect size.

Meta-analysis of summary statistics is meaningful only for comparisons between groups involving 1 $df$ in the numerator of the $F$ ratio. The reason for this is that $F$s involving comparison of three or more groups cannot index the specific differences between pairs of groups. As a result, the amount of variance accounted for by a particular comparison between two groups cannot be indexed in indicators of effect size. We therefore could not examine effects involving more than two groups or multiple factors with more than two groups each.

Comparisons between young and older adults only were included, so those studies that investigated differences among young, middle-aged, and old adults had to be eliminated unless other data, such as probabilities given for contrasts of young versus old individuals, had been published. Papers with multiple experiments or comparisons were treated as separate studies, provided that the individual studies met the criteria for inclusion. Studies with conditions not conforming to normal prose (i.e., scrambled sentences) in a standard study-recall paradigm were also excluded, as were those in which recall was scored only at the verbatim, rather than gist, level. A total of 36 studies met our criteria for inclusion. They are documented in Table 5.1.

## Coding of Variables

In meta-analysis, the results of individual studies are the unit of analysis, and the variables or factors to be evaluated are those common to the studies that can be operationally defined and coded. In our analysis, we coded for verbal ability level of the comparison groups, discourse genre, the scoring system, and passage length.

Verbal ability was coded as high if both age groups averaged a minimum of 3 years of college. If they did not, their mean vocabulary scores were at least 70% of the total correct score. We elected to use schooling as our primary criterion because the vocabulary tests used across studies vary considerably in difficulty, and as vocabulary and education correlate well, this appeared to be a reasonable method for classification. Verbal ability was coded as low if both groups averaged 1 year of college education or less, or if they had vocabulary scores below the 70% cutoff. This approach is quite crude, but even when we included only those studies in which older subjects had mean education levels greater than 16 years, and compared them with studies testing young and old subjects who were low in verbal ability, the results remained the same.

If the study made specific comparisons between high and low vocabulary subjects in both age groups, and effect sizes were available for the age main effect, verbal ability was coded as mixed (e.g., Dixon et al., 1984). It was also coded as mixed in studies in which verbal ability was treated as a continuous variable and education was low (e.g., Hultsch et al., 1984). Finally, a mixed code was assigned to studies in which only one of the two age groups could be classified as high or low. We did not enter studies with a mixed classification into the analyses of effect sizes and vocabulary level.

Discourse genre was coded by the kind of materials reported, with stories coded as narratives and essays or newspaper articles as expository materials.

The scoring system was coded either as the system reported (e.g., Kintsch's, Mandler & Johnson's) or as gist, which involved no formal system but not verbatim scoring.

Passage length was coded: passages less than 299 words were considered as short and those with more than 300 as long. We had also varied the coding

TABLE 5.1. Studies Included in the Meta-Analysis of Age Differences in Memory for Discourse

| Study | Verbal Ability | Discourse Genre | Scoring System | Passage Length | $N$ | $r$ | $Z$ |
|---|---|---|---|---|---|---|---|
| Zelinski et al. (1984); Exp. 2, second text | High | Narrative | Meyer | Short | 124 | .42 | 4.91 |
| Zelinski et al. (1984); Exp. 2, *The Old Farmer and His Stubborn Animals* | High | Narrative | Meyer | Short | 45 | .40 | 2.75 |
| Zelinski et al. (1984); Exp. 2, The Old Farmer/Circle Island version | High | Narrative | Meyer | Short | 42 | .48 | 3.23 |
| Zelinski et al. (1984); Exp. 2, *Queen Island* | High | Narrative | Meyer | Short | 39 | .45 | 3.20 |
| Gordon & Clark (1974) | High | Narrative | Gist | Short | 44 | .53 | 5.27 |
| Light & Anderson (1983); Exp. 2 | High | Narrative | Gist | Short | 48 | .30 | 2.04 |
| Smith et al. (1983); normal story only | High | Narrative | Mandler & Johnson | Short | 24 | −.21 | −.98[a] |
| Spilich (1983); normal old subjects versus young only | High | Narrative | Kintsch | Long | 32 | .68 | 5.08 |
| Cohen (1979); Exp. 3, highly educated old versus highly educated young only | High | Narrative | Gist | Long | 40 | .51 | 4.49 |
| Hess, Donley, & Vandermas (1986) | High | Narrative | Gist | Long | 48 | .39 | 2.73 |
| Mandel & Johnson (1984) | High | Narrative | Johnson | Long | 80 | .13 | 1.21 |

TABLE 5.1 *Continued*

| Study | Verbal Ability | Discourse Genre | Scoring System | Passage Length | $N$ | $r$ | $Z$ |
|---|---|---|---|---|---|---|---|
| Zelinski et al. (1984); Exp. 3, *Treatment of Psychological Disorders* (summary version) | High | Expository | Meyer | Short | 77 | .29 | 2.52 |
| Zelinski et al. (1984); Exp. 3, *Parakeets: Ideal Pets* (summary version) | High | Expository | Meyer | Short | 81 | .26 | 2.38 |
| Hartley (1986) | High | Narrative & Expository | Kintsch | Short | 48 | .44 | 6.89 |
| Hartley (in press b) | High | Expository | Kintsch | Short | 72 | .23 | 1.96 |
| Zelinski et al. (1984); Exp. 3, *Treatment of Psychological Disorders* (complete version) | High | Expository | Meyer | Long | 81 | .23 | 2.07 |
| Zelinski et al. (1984); Exp. 3, *Parakeets: Ideal Pets* (complete version) | High | Expository | Meyer | Long | 77 | .27 | 2.34 |
| Meyer & Rice (1981) | High | Expository | Meyer | Long | 32 | .18 | .98 |
| Meyer & Rice (1983); comparison of high verbal old versus high verbal young | High | Expository | Meyer | Long | 100 | −.22 | −2.18 |
| Meyer & Rice (1983); comparison of high verbal old versus "random" young | High | Expository | Meyer | Long | 100 | .10 | 1.00 |

| | | | | | | | |
|---|---|---|---|---|---|---|---|
| Harker et al. (1982); Study 1 | High | Expository | Kintsch | Long | 70 | .12 | .99 |
| Harker et al. (1982); Study 2 | High | Expository | Kintsch | Long | 48 | .13 | 1.10 |
| Byrd (1985) | High | Expository | Kintsch | Long | 50 | .61 | 2.86 |
| Zelinski et al. (1984); Exp. 1 | Low | Narrative | Meyer | Short | 104 | .54 | 5.84 |
| Cohen (1979); Exp. 3 (low educated old versus low educated young only) | Low | Narrative | Gist | Long | 40 | .51 | 4.49 |
| Surber et al. (1984) | Low | Narrative | Mandler & Johnson | Long | 60 | .56 | 4.52 |
| Hultsch & Dixon (1983) | Low | Narrative | Kintsch | Short | 48 | .14 | .99 |
| Taub & Kline (1978) | Low | Expository | Gist | Short | 36 | .37 | 1.88 |
| Meyer & Rice (1983); comparison of low verbal old versus "matching" young | Low | Expository | Meyer | Long | 100 | .30 | 3.07 |
| Meyer & Rice (1983); comparison of low verbal old versus "matching" young | Low | Expository | Meyer | Long | 100 | .55 | 5.92 |
| Petros et al. (1983); Exp. 1 | Mixed | Narrative | Brown & Smiley | Long | 53 | .38 | 2.74 |
| Petros et al. (1983); Exp. 2 | Mixed | Narrative | Brown & Smiley | Long | 40 | .56 | 3.61 |
| Zelinski et al. (1980) | Mixed | Expository | Meyer | Short | 196 | .21 | 2.96 |
| Dixon et al. (1984) | Mixed | Expository | Kintsch | Short | 72 | .23 | 1.96 |
| Taub (1979) | Mixed | Expository | Gist | Short | 54 | .56 | 4.27 |
| Rice & Meyer (1986) | Mixed | Expository | Meyer | Long | 305 | .24 | 1.03 |

[a]A minus sign preceding an $r$ or $Z$ indicates that the results were in the direction of older subjects recalling more than younger ones.

for passage length in different ways, but those results were identical to those using the binary coding, which essentially involved a median split of passage lengths in the texts used in the studies analyzed.

### Effect Size Calculations

The effect size for age differences in discourse recall and age, $r$ (the product-moment bivariate correlation coefficient), was calculated from $F$ ratios as

$$r = \sqrt{\frac{F}{F + df\ \text{error}}}\ .$$

If probabilities were used to calculate effect size from studies in which $F$ was not reported, the probabilities reported were used to determine $Z$, from the standardized normal distribution, with $r$ calculated from

$$r = \frac{Z}{\sqrt{N}}\ .$$

To analyze the effect sizes, we used $z$, Fisher's transformation, to normalize them. For the analyses involving combining probabilities, $Z$ was calculated as

$$Z = \sqrt{\frac{df\ (\log_e{}^{(1+F)})}{df}}\ \sqrt{1 - \frac{1}{2\ df}}$$

where $df$ is the $df$ error for $F$ ratios or $N - 2$ for $t$ tests (with $t^2$ substituted for $F$). The value of $Z$ is interpreted as a score in a standardized normal distribution; for example, a $Z$ of 1.96 is significant at $p < .05$. The $r$ and $Z$ associated with each study, along with their coded characteristics, are given in Table 5.1.

## Results

### Overall Age Differences

The evaluation of whether there are significant age differences in memory for prose as reported in the literature involved calculating the mean $r$, which was .35. To determine whether this effect size differed significantly from an $r$ of zero, we calculated the combined probability of $r$ using the formula:

$$\text{overall } Z = \frac{\sum Z_j}{\sqrt{K}}$$

where $K$ = the number of studies. The overall $Z$ was 16.68 at $p < .0000001$. It is thus clear that older adults recall significantly less than younger ones when prose is studied.

## Focused Predictions

The next set of analyses tested specific predictions of effect sizes as a function of verbal ability level, discourse genre, scoring system, and passage length by entering $z_r$ in several analyses of variance (ANOVA). We did not conduct multifactor ANOVAs because coding on the four factors was not evenly distributed over cells, and because ANOVA essentially tested interactions of age with each of the factors. With multiple factors,we would have been evaluating three-way and higher order interactions, which would have been difficult to interpret. Along with the $F$ ratios, we report the overall $Z$ associated with each mean $r$, to determine whether the mean effect sizes differed from zero.

### Verbal Ability

The first hypothesis we tested was whether studies with high verbal subjects had produced smaller age differences than those with low verbal ones. There were 23 studies meeting the high verbal ability criteria, and 7 meeting the low ability criteria. The mean $r$ for high verbal ability studies was .31 and for low verbal ability studies was .44. The combined probabilities for each were also highly significant: $Z = 11.85$ and 10.09, respectively, both at $p < .0000001$, for studies testing high verbal and low verbal subjects. The $F$ test comparing differences in effect sizes was not reliable, however; $F\ (1, 28) = 2.03, p < .17$. Because of the discrepancy in $n$, we performed a weighted analysis, weighting $z_r$ for high verbal studies by $-7$ and $z_r$ for low verbal studies by 23. The results were now significant: $Z = 2.92, p < .03$. Thus, as predicted, effect sizes were reliably larger for studies comparing low verbal subjects than for those comparing high verbal ones.

### Discourse Genre

The next analysis examined differences in the effect size for age as a function of text genre. Results showed that there was a significant effect for discourse type, $F\ (1, 34) = 6.16, p < .02$, with age differences larger for narratives than for expository texts. The mean $r$ for age differences in the studies testing recall of narratives was .43 ($n = 16$), and it was .26 for essays ($n = 20$). $Z$ was 13.78 and 8.73 for narratives and expository passages, respectively, with $p < .0000001$.

### Scoring System

We first tested differences in effect sizes between studies using Kintsch's system and those using Meyer's. There were 16 experiments in which Meyer's system was used, yielding a mean $r$ of .31, and 8 using Kintsch's, with a mean $r$ of .35. The combined probabilities were also significant, with $Z = 10.50$ and

7.72, both $p < .0000001$, for the studies using Meyer's system and Kintsch's, respectively. Results indicated no differences in effect size, $F < 1$. A weighted analysis similar to the one for verbal ability was also conducted, with nonsignificant results: $Z = .32, p < .38$.

The second ANOVA compared effect sizes of studies using macropropositional scoring systems with Kintsch's micropropositional one. The mean $r$ for the 21 studies involving macropropositional systems was .31, $Z = 11.59, p < .0000001$: for the comparison with Kintsch's system, $F < 1$. A weighted analysis also yielded a nonsignificant $Z$ of .23. The third analysis contrasted 29 studies that used formal scoring systems with the 7 that used a gist criterion. Mean $r$ was .35 ($Z = 13.92, p < .0000001$) for studies using formal systems and .49 ($Z = 9.51, p < .0000001$) for those using gist scoring. This difference was marginally reliable ($F\ (1,34) = 2.93, p < .10$), but significant when a weighted analysis was applied ($Z = 2.59, p < .01$).

### Passage Length

Analysis of passage length did not reveal any reliable differences in the effect size for age ($F < 1$). Mean $r$ for the 17 studies evaluating recall of short passages was .36 ($Z = 12.63, p < .0000001$), and for the 19 long ones it was .37 ($Z = 11.65, p < .0000001$).

## Discussion

In our meta-analysis, three patterns of effect size differences across studies were observed. First, there were overall age deficits in recall, as determined by combining the probability levels for age effects across all studies. Second, verbal ability, as measured by education and vocabulary test performance, did mediate recall differences between younger and older adults, with larger effect sizes obtained for studies in which individuals were designated as low in verbal ability than those in which people high in verbal ability participated. Third, text genre had reliable effects, with studies involving narratives producing larger age effects than those with expository texts. An additional reliable effect was that of formality of scoring system, with studies using informal gist scoring reporting significantly larger effect sizes than those in which formal prose analysis systems were used to score recall. On the other hand, there were no difference in age effects as a function of the formal scoring systems used. Finally, passage length was unrelated to the effect size of age differences.

### Variables Predicting Effect Sizes in Memory for Discourse

These findings serve to clarify some of the major issues in aging and memory for discourse. It is obvious from our analysis of the overall size of age differences that older adults do recall reliably less than younger ones. Thus, the reports that memory for prose did not follow the same recall functions for older adults that memory for other verbal materials did (Hartley et al., 1980; Meyer & Rice, 1981) appear to have been premature. The age deficits we have observed in this meta-analysis replicate those of Rubin's (1985) analysis, which also resulted in the conclusion that memory functions did not differ much across verbal materials ranging from paired-asociates lists to discourses. We therefore conclude that, in general, older people do have a deficit in memory for prose.

However, we have found that there appear to be factors that mediate the relative size of the age difference. As predicted by Hultsch and Dixon (1984) and Meyer and Rice (1983, in press), several different classes of variables account for some of the variance in recall for discourse. Hultsch and Dixon had suggested that a model of the interaction of subject and materials variables along with orienting and criterial tasks was more useful than a univariate approach to explaining age differences in memory for prose. Meyer and Rice, in a similar vein, argued that the factors of learner, text, and task variables interacted in accounting for variance in age differences. We observed that the subject variable of verbal ability, the text variable of passage genre, and the measurement variable of formality of recall scoring system each interacted with age in accounting for recall variance in the extant literature. Thus, the suggestions that age interacts with certain methodological factors have been confirmed by our analysis.

Two other factors, the features of the formal prose analysis system and passage length, did not however, interact with the relative size of age differences. Thus, Meyer's (1985) clain that her system would be more appropriate for evaluating recall protocols of older adults than Kintsch's was not confirmed. This suggests that Meyer's system is no more but also no less effective than Kintsch's, and that scoring systems based on an analysis of macrostructure are also equivalent in the size of age differences obtained as Kintsch's, which is based on an analysis of text microstructure.

The suggestion that age differences would be exacerbated with long passages (Hartley et al., 1980) was not confirmed here. Our findings thus suggest that not all measurement or text factors account for age-related differences in discourse recall.

Our findings are also at variance with the assumptions of the reviews of Hultsch and Dixon and of Meyer and Rice, in which it was claimed that age differences would disappear under the appropriate circumstances. In no case were the combined probabilities for age differences reported for any levels of the factors we examined nonsignificant. Indeed, in all cases the combined probabilities exceeded $p < .0000001$. We therefore see that certain variables can reduce but not eliminate age differences when we combine the results of studies.

It remains possible, however, that there are circumstances under which age differences in prose recall may be consistently very small or nonexistent.

For example, Byrd (1986) found that older people who had to organize sentences that told a story but were in scrambled order at the outset recalled as much as younger ones in an incidental memory task. Hultsch and Dixon (1983) found that older adults actually recalled more than younger ones when the text was a biography of someone with whom they were more familiar. Meyer and her colleagues (Meyer, Young, & Bartlett, 1986) found that older adults and younger ones improved recall of expository texts after a series of sessions designed to teach them the basic principles of how authors present information in prose and how to remember it efficiently, and that age differences at pretest were eliminated after training. Thus, older adults may not differ from younger ones in discourse recall when they have had extensive experience with the material, its theme, or with related tasks.

## Implications for Accounts of Age Differences in Discourse Memory

Our findings have some implications for theoretical accounts of the relative size of age differences in memory for discourse. First, our finding that the size of age deficits increased with subjects low in verbal ability confirm Meyer and Rice's (1981, 1983) prediction, and conflicts with the Hultsch and Dixon's (1984) claim, that age differences might be larger with highly verbal adults than with less verbal ones. It is possible that by using mean vocabulary test scores and educational attainment (as we have in selecting high and low verbal groups), we did not define verbal ability adequately (see Hartley, 1986; Hultsch et al., 1984). However, our results are based on the data of 30 experiments, and so we believe that they reflect reliable phenomena.

As indicated earlier, variation in the effect size of age differences as a function of individual differences is predicted by the three models of aging and memory that are currently popular. Following a production deficiency hypothesis, Meyer and Rice (1983, in press) have given a practice explanation for this finding, namely, that highly verbal adults have more experience participating in verbal activities, which makes remembering discourse a rather familiar task for them. Based on a processing resource deficiency/working memory deficit model Hartley (in press-b) has instead suggested that people who have good verbal skills are more likely to pursue activities that utilize those skills. Regardless of the causal origin of our finding, it is clear that memorial skills are apparently retained in highly verbal adults to a greater extent than less verbally skilled individuals, and that individual differences in cognitive abilities do in fact predict the relative size of age differences in discourse recall.

We had made several focused predictions about models of memory and aging for evaluating both passage length and text genre. The production deficiency model predicted that age differences would vary as a function of passage length and genre. The processing deficit and working memory capacity hypotheses predicted genre but not length differences. Our findings verify that these two latter hypotheses do indeed account for the findings. The processing deficit/working memory models are therefore probably better suited than the production deficiency one in providing theoretical accounts for memory for prose in aging, which confirms conclusions drawn by Burke and Light (1981) from the word recall literature. However, it should be noted that our findings cannot differentiate which of these two models more adequately accounts for age differences in recall. Moreover, there is growing discontent with either explanation as a model of the mechanisms of age differences in both the discourse literature (e.g., Hartley, 1986; Light & Anderson, 1985; but see Cohen, in press, for a different conclusion), as well as the general aging literature (see Salthouse, this volume).

In an exploratory analysis, we found that studies using formal prose analysis systems produced smaller effect sizes of age differences than those using gist scoring. This suggested that the effort involved in analyzing texts and applying those analyses to recall protocols is beneficial in evaluating recall performance in older adults because the likelihood of obtaining floor effects is reduced.

## Disadvantages of Meta-Analysis

In general, we are satisified that the more objective approach inherent in evaluating the literature through meta-analysis reduces the bias that reviewers (including ourselves) bring to their summaries of the literature. Nevertheless, there are some limitations to our meta-analysis that we would like to address here.

Unless raw data are obtained from authors, higher order interactions between variables that have been predicted by different reviews (Hultsch & Dixon, 1984; Meyer & Rice, in press) cannot be evaluated. As Rosenthal (1984) pointed out, the state of understanding of various phenomena in the social sciences is sufficiently vague as to preclude evaluating complex interactions meaningfully. We echo that sentiment, and offer as evidence the fact that there are currently no adequate models that can unify the plethora of conflicting findings in the area of discourse memory and aging without resorting to complicated *post hoc* explanations.

A second issue involves the lack of comparability across studies on text materials, the number of texts studied, vocabulary tests, and procedures. This can make categorization of studies difficult. In the case of the present meta-analysis, the reader can take issue with our categorization of experiments for verbal ability and passage length as being fairly arbitrary. As noted earlier, we tried several different approaches to coding these factors but obtained the same results.

A final problem is that the specific manipulations of studies are lost in the data analysis because experiments are the unit of analysis, and in some cases there are too few individual studies to investigate particular factors.

## Conclusions

Despite these limitations, we believe our results confirm that verbal ability, text genre, and formal scoring systems are important in predicting the effect size of age differences in memory for discourse. Our findings on the interaction of verbal ability and age also suggest that the recent approach of evaluating individual differences in the component abilities believed to underlie memory for discourse including vocabulary ability, reasoning, processing speed, working memory capacity, and other measures (Dixon et al., 1984; Hultsch et al., 1984; Hartley, 1986; in press-a; in press-b) appears to be promising in extending our understanding of age differences in memory in general and in memory for discourse in particular. Also, the next generation of prose memory studies, which are directed at determining when older adults show no or small recall deficits relative to the young (see above) and at developing interventions to improve their recall (Meyer et al., 1986), will give us new insights into the complexities of the relationships among individual differences, text variables, and task variables in aging.

In sum, discourse memory studies have not proven to be the panacea that cognitive aging researchers had envisioned in their attempts to test age differences in memory with measures high in construct and ecological validity, which would also help identify the sources of any age deficits. They have, however, played a significant role in spurring research in the direction of reevaluating current models of memory and aging and may be important in developing more adequate models in the future.

*Acknowledgments.* Preparation of this chapter was funded in part by grant R01 AG4114 from the National Institute on Aging to E.M. Zelinski.

## References

Bieger, G.R., & Dunn, B.R. (1984). A comparison of the sensitivity of two prose analysis models to developmental differences in free recall of text. *Discourse Processes, 7,* 257–274.

Britton, B.K., & Tesser, A. (1982). Effects of prior knowledge on use of cognitive capacity in three complex cognitive tasks. *Journal of Verbal Learning and Verbal Behavior, 21,* 421–436.

Britton, B.K., Westbrook, R.D., & Holdredge, T.S. (1978). Reading and cognitive capacity usage: Effects of text difficulty. *Journal of Experimental Psychology: Human Learning and Memory, 4,* 582–591.

Brown, A.L., & Smiley, S.S. (1977). Rating the importance of structural units of prose passages: A problem of meta-cognitive development. *Child Development, 48,* 1–8.

Burke, D.M., & Light, L.L. (1981). Memory and aging: The role of retrieval processes. *Psychological Bulletin, 90,* 513–546.

Byrd, M. (1985). Age differences in the ability to recall and summarize textual infor-

mation. *Experimental Aging Research, 11,* 87-91.
Byrd, M. (1986). The use of organizational strategies to improve memory for prose passages. *International Journal of Aging and Human Development, 23,* 257-265.
Cofer, C.N., Scott, C., & Watkins, K. (1978, August). *Scoring systems for the analysis of passage content.* Paper presented at the annual meeting of the American Psychological Association, Toronto, Canada.
Cohen, G. (1979). Language comprehension in old age. *Cognitive Psychology, 11,* 412-429.
Cohen, G. (1981). Inferential reasoning in old age. *Cognition, 9,* 59-72.
Cohen, G. (in press). Age differences in memory for texts: Production deficiency or processing limitations? In L.L. Light and D.M. Burke (Eds.), *Language, memory and aging.* Cambridge: Cambridge University Press.
Craik, F.I.M. (1968). Short-term memory and the aging process. In G.A. Talland (Ed.), *Human aging and behavior* (pp. 131-168). New York: Academic Press.
Craik, F.I.M. (1977). Age differences in human memory. In J.E. Birren & K.W. Schaie (Eds.), *Handbook of the psychology of aging* (pp. 384-420). New York: Van Nostrand Reinhold.
Craik, F.I.M., & Byrd,M. (1982). Aging and cognitive deficits: The role of attentional processes. In F.I.M. Craik & S. Trehub (Eds.), *Aging and Cognitive Processes* (pp. 191-211). New York: Plenum Press.
Craik, F.I.M., & Simon, E. (1980). Age differences in memory: The roles of attention and depth of processing. In L.W. Poon, J.L. Fozard, L.S. Cermak, D. Arenberg, & L.W. Thompson (Eds.), *New directions in memory and aging: Proceedings of the George A. Talland Memorial Conference* (pp. 95-112). Hillsdale, NJ: Erlbaum.
Dixon, R.A., Hultsch, D.R., Simon, E.W., & von Eye, A. (1984). Verbal ability and text structure effects on adult age differences in text recall. *Journal of Verbal Learning and Verbal Behavior, 23,* 569-578.
Dixon, R.A., Simon, E.W., Nowak, C.A., & Hultsch, D.F. (1982). Text recall in adulthood as a function of level of information, input modality, and delay interval. *Journal of Gerontology, 37,* 358-364.
Gordon, S.K., & Clark, W.C. (1974). Application of signal detection theory to prose recall and recognition in elderly and young adults. *Journal of Gerontology, 29,* 64-72.
Graesser, A.C., Haupt-Smith, K., Cohen, A.D., & Pyles, L.D. (1980). Advanced outlines, familiarity, text genre, and retention of prose. *Journal of Experimental Education, 48,* 281-290.
Graesser, A.C., Higginbotham, M.W., Robertson, S.P., & Smith, W.R. (1978). A natural inquiry into the National Enquirer: Self-induced versus task-induced reading comprehension. *Discourse Processes, 1,* 355-372.
Harker, J.O., Hartley, J.T., & Walsh, D.A. (1982). Understanding discourse: A life-span approach. In B. Hutson (Ed.), *Advances in reading/language research* (pp. 155-202). Greenwich, CT: JAI Press.
Hartley, J.T. (in press-a). Individual differences in memory for written discourse. In L.L. Light and D.M. Burke (Eds.), *Language, memory and aging.* Cambridge: Cambridge University Press.
Hartley, J.T. (in press-b). Memory for prose: Perspectives on the reader. In L.W. Poon, D. Rubin, & B. Wilson (Eds.), *Everday cognition in adulthood and old age.* Cambridge: Cambridge University Press.
Hartley, J.T. (1986). Reader and text variables as determinants of discourse memory

in adulthood. *Psychology and Aging, 1,* 150–158.
Hartley, J.T., Harker, J.O., & Walsh, D.A. (1980). Contemporary issues and new directions in adult development of learning and memory. In L.W. Poon (Ed.), *Aging in the 1980's: Some contemporary issues in the psychology of aging* (pp. 239–252). Washington, DC: American Psychological Association.
Hasher, L., & Zacks, R.T. (1979). Automatic and effortful processes in memory. *Journal of Experimental Psychology: General, 108,* 356–388.
Hess, T.M., Donley, J. & Vandermas, M.O. (1986). *Aging-related changes in the processing and retention of script information.* Manuscript submitted for publication.
Hulicka, I.M. (1967). Age differences in retention as a function of interference. *Journal of Gerontology, 22,* 180–184.
Hultsch, D.F., & Dixon, R.A. (1983). The role of pre-experimental knowledge in text processing in adulthood. *Experimental Aging Research, 9,* 17–22.
Hultsch, D.F., & Dixon, R.A. (1984). Text processing in adulthood. In P.B. Baltes & O.G. Brim (Eds.), *Life-span development and behavior (Vol. 6,* pp. 77–108). New York: Academic Press.
Hultsch, D.F., Hertzog C., & Dixon, R.A. (1984). Text recall in adulthood: The role of intellectual abilities. *Developmental Psychology, 20,* 1193–1209.
Hunt, E. (1978). Mechanics of verbal ability. *Psychological Review, 85,* 109–130.
Jerome, E.A. (1959). Age and learning—Experimental studies. In J.E. Birren (Ed.), *Handbook of aging and the individual* (pp. 655–699). Chicago: University of Chicago Press.
Johnson, N.S. (1983). What do you do if you can't tell the whole story? The development of summarization skills. In K.E. Nelson (Ed.), *Children's language* (Vol. 4, pp. 315–383). Hillsdale, NJ: Erlbaum.
Kausler, D.H. (1970). Retention-forgetting as a nomological network for developmental research. In L.R. Goulet & P.B. Baltes (Eds.), *Life-span developmental psychology: Research and theory* (pp. 306–353). New York: Academic Press.
Kintsch, W. (1974). *The representation of meaning in memory.* Hillsdale, NJ: Erlbaum.
Light, L.L., & Anderson, P.A. (1983). Memory for scripts in young and older adults. *Memory & Cognition, 11,* 435–444.
Light, L.L., & Anderson, P.A. (1985). Working-memory capacity, age, and memory for discourse. *Journal of Gerontology, 40,* 737–747.
Mandel, R.G., & Johnson, N.S. (1984). A developmental analysis of story recall and comprehension and recall. *Journal of Verbal Learning and Verbal Behavior, 23,* 643–659.
Mandler, J.M., & Johnson, N.S. (1977). Remembrance of things parsed: Story structure and recall. *Cognitive Psychology, 9,* 111–151.
Meyer, B.J.F. (1975). *The organization of prose and its effect on recall.* Amsterdam: Elsevier North-Holland.
Meyer, B.J.F. (1985). Prose analysis: Purposes, procedures, and problems. In B.K. Britton & J.B. Black (Eds.), *Understanding expository text: A theoretical and practical handbook for analyzing explanatory text* (pp. 11–64). Hillsdale, NJ: Erlbaum.
Meyer, B.J.F. (in press). Reading comprehension and aging. In K.W. Schaie (Ed.), *Annual review of gerontology and geriatrics* (Vol. 7) New York: Springer.
Meyer, B.J.F., & Rice, G.E. (1981). Information recalled from prose by young, middle, and old adult readers. *Experimental Aging Research, 7,* 253–268.
Meyer, B.J.F., & Rice, G.E. (1983). Learning and memory from text across the

adult life span. In J. Fine & R.O. Freedle (Eds.), *Developmental issues in discourse* (pp. 294–306). Norwood, NJ: Ablex.

Meyer, B.J.F., & Rice, G.E. (in press). Prose processing in adulthood: The text, the learner, and the task. In L.W. Poon, D. Rubin, & B. Wilson (Eds.), *Everyday cognition in adulthood and old age.* Cambridge: Cambridge University Press.

Meyer, B.J.F., Young, C.J., & Bartlett, B.J. (1986). *A prose learning strategy: Effects of instruction on young and older adults* Unpublished manuscript. Seattle: University of Washington.

Miller, J.R., & Kintsch, W. (1980). Readability and recall of short prose passages: A theoretical analysis. *Journal of Experimental Psychology: Human Learning and Memory, 6,* 335–354.

Nezworski, T., Stein, N.L., & Trabasso, T. (1982). Story structure versus content in children's recall. *Journal of Verbal Learning and Verbal Behavior, 21,* 196–206.

Perfetti, C.A. (1985). *Reading ability.* New York: Oxford Univeristy Press.

Petros, T., Tabor, L., Cooney,T., & Chabot, R.J. (1983). Adult age differences in sensitivity to semantic structure of prose. *Developmental Psychology, 19,* 907–914.

Rice, G.E. (1986a). The everyday activities of adults: Implications for prose recall—Part I. *Educational Gerontology, 12,* 173–186.

Rice, G.E. (1986b). The everyday activities of adults: Implications for prose recall—Part II. *Educational Gerontology, 12,* 187–198.

Rice, G.E., & Meyer, B.J.F. (1986). Prose recall: Effects of aging, verbal ability, and reading behavior. *Journal of Gerontology, 41,* 469–480.

Rosenthal, R. (1984). *Meta-analytic procedures for the social sciences.* Beverly Hills, CA: Sage.

Rubin, D.C. (1985). Memorability as a measure of processing: A unit analysis of prose and list learning. *Journal of Experimental Psychology: General, 114,* 213–238.

Schneider, N.G., Gritz, E.R., & Jarvik, M.E. (1975). Age differences in learning, immediate, and one week delayed recall. *Gerontologia, 21,* 10–20.

Simon, E.W., Dixon, R.A., Nowak, C.A., & Hultsch, D.F. (1982). Orienting task effects on text recall in adulthood. *Journal of Gerontology, 31,* 575–580.

Singer, M. (1982). Comparing memory for natural and laboratory reading. *Journal of Experimental Psychology: General, 111,* 331–347.

Smith, E.L. (1985). Text type and discourse framework. *Text, 5,* 229–247.

Smith, S.W., Rebok, G.W., Smith, W.R., Hall, S.E., & Alvin, M. (1983). Adult age differences in the use of story structure in delayed free recall. *Experimental Aging Research, 9,* 191–195.

Spilich, G.J. (1983). Life-span components of text processing: Structural and procedural differences. *Journal of Verbal Learning and Verbal Behavior, 22,* 231–244.

Surber, J.R., Kowalski, A.H., & Pena-Paez, A. (1984). Effects of aging on the recall of extended expository prose. *Experimental Aging Research, 10,* 25–28.

Taub, H.A. (1976). Method of presentation of meaningful prose to young and old adults. *Experimental Aging Research, 2,* 469–474.

Taub, H.A. (1979). Comprehension and memory of prose materials by young and old adults. *Experimental Aging Research, 5,* 3–13.

Taub, H.A., & Kline, G.E. (1978). Recall of prose as a function of age and input modality. *Journal of Gerontology, 33,* 725–730.

Zelinski, E.M., Gilewski, M.J., & Thompson, L.W. (1980). Do laboratory memory tasks relate to everyday remembering and forgetting? In L.W. Poon, J.L. Fozard, L.S. Cermak, D. Arenberg, & L.W. Thompson (Eds.), *New directions in memory and aging: Proceedings of the George A. Talland Memorial Conference* (pp. 519–544). Hillsdale, NJ: Erlbaum.

Zelinski, E.M., Light, L.L. & Gilewski, M.J. (1984). Adult age differences in memory and prose: The question of sensitivity to passage structure. *Developmental Psychology, 20,* 1181–1192.

# Part II Cognitive and Performance Factors

# 6. Analysis and Synthesis in Problem Solving and Aging

*David Arenberg*

In the literature on aging, the amount of research in problem solving is far less than that in other areas of cognition such as memory and intelligence, and this has been true for many years. No experimental research in problem solving was included in a review of intelligence and problem solving by Jones in 1959, although a few studies from the Nuffield Unit at Cambridge were reported about the same time (Welford, 1958). Even 14 years later it was possible to be virtually exhaustive in reviewing problem solving in a small segment of a chapter on cognition and aging (Arenberg, 1973).

Fortunately, that is no longer true today. Recent broad-scope reviews of problem solving and aging by Charness (1985) and by Reese & Rodeheaver (1985) were, of necessity, highly selective. This chapter is much narrower in scope, focusing on a few related issues in problem solving and aging and emphasizing the analytic and synthetic aspects of problem solving.

The term "analysis" is used to describe information gathering; "synthesis" is used to describe attempts to integrate pieces of information to reach a solution. In the pioneer efforts by John (1957) to devise logical problems that would maximize observable problem-solving behavior, one important goal was to obtain measures of analytic and synthetic performance. Subsequently, both Jerome (1962) and Young (1966) used John's problems in studies comparing young and old adults. Age differences were found, but separate measures of analysis and synthesis were not reported.

A major portion of this chapter is devoted to a longitudinal study of men over a broad range of age, emphasizing analytic and synthetic performance on problems similar to those used by Jerome and Young. Unfortunately, these terms rarely appear in the recent literature on problem solving or on aging in that domain. The terms have emerged in Sternberg's (1985) triarchic theory of intelligence, but with somewhat different meanings. It is argued here that analysis and synthesis are significant components of problem solving, and that age studies of these components will enhance our understanding of aging and this extremely important aspect of cognition.

## Analysis and Aging

Analysis, as used in this chapter, is a major component of several types of problem solving, such as 20 questions and its variations, troubleshooting, and concept identification with a selection paradigm, that have been studied in aging (Arenberg, 1982; Denney, 1980; Bernardelli as cited in Welford, 1958; Wetherick, 1964). Typically, such studies have found cross-sectional age differences with the oldest groups showing the poorest performance (see Denney, 1982; Charness, 1985; and Reese & Rodeheaver, 1985 for recent reviews, and Botwinick, 1973 for a review of the earlier studies).

Several studies of aging (Arenberg, 1982; Hartley & Anderson, 1983a, 1983b; Hybertson, Perdue, & Hybertson, 1982; Kesler, Denney, & Whitely, 1976; and Young, 1971) are described here in some detail because they all included measures of analytic performance based on the information value of each inquiry during a problem. In all these studies, the measure of analytic efficiency was determined by the potential reduction of uncertainty of each inquiry.

Hybertson et al. (1982) characterized the problems they used as "... essentially a visual 20-questions game." (p. 110). Pictures and names of 20 characters were displayed. One of the characters was the solution, and the task was to identify that solution with as few questions as possible. Only questions that could be answered "yes" or "no" were permitted. It was possible to ask categorical questions because the characters varied in such attributes as sex, race, occupation, clothing, and accessories. Each question could be quantified in terms of the amount of potential information it could yield. The measure was "... the ratio of the minimum number of characters that could be eliminated by the question to the total number of remaining characters." (p. 111). An optimal question divided the viable solutions at that point in the problem into two equal parts.

Three age groups (45–50, 60–65, and 75–80 years) of subjects with high mean WAIS (Wechsler Adult Intelligence Scale) vocabulary scores were included. The oldest group had the lowest mean efficiency measure on the first problem but the two other groups did not differ. On two subsequent problems in which additional information about categorizing was provided, all three age groups improved; but the oldest group continued to solve problems less efficiently than did the two younger groups.

Three age groups (40s, 50s, and 60+) were also included in the study by Young (1971), but superficially the problems appeared to be quite different. The display for each problem consisted of 8 or 16 buttons, each labeled with a consonant. A question consisted of lighting any subset of the buttons, and the answer was a light that turned one color if the solution button had been on and another color if it had been off. The efficiency of each question was determined using the number of buttons that could be eliminated and the number of viable buttons at that point in the problem. As in the study by Hybertson et al. (1982), the measure of efficiency was based on potential rather than actual information gain of each question. A weighted average of these individual measures for ten problems is the measure reported here.

The results were different for men and women. For the men, the oldest group solved both the 8-button and the 16-button problems least efficiently, but the two younger groups did not differ. For the women, however, no statistically significant age differences were found. A major difference in procedure between this study and the study of Hybertson et al. (1982) was the use of notes; in the latter study, subjects were encouraged to take notes. Note taking was not mentioned in the paper by Young. It should be pointed out, however, that the rectangular array of buttons in that study provided a memory aid for those subjects who used a systematic approach to the problems. Rows, columns, and blocks of buttons may be easier to keep track of than sex, race, occupation, clothing, and accessories (as in the study by Hybertson et al.).

Kesler et al. (1976) included the 16-button problems used by Young (1971) in their study of several problem-solving procedures. Using Young's information measure, they found small differences between middle-aged (30–50 years old) and elderly (65–81 years old) men and women favoring the younger groups. Unlike the results of Young's study, small gender differences favoring the men were found for both age groups.

The data reported by Arenberg (1982) were from preliminary analysis of a study of concept problem solving that began in 1967 and is still in progress in the Baltimore Longitudinal Study of Aging (Shock, Greulich, Andres, Arenberg, Costa, Lakatta, & Tobin, 1984). A selection paradigm is used providing "questions" that can be evaluated on the basis of potential information gain similar to the measures used in the studies described. When a selection paradigm is used in a concept study, the problem solver attempts to identify the concept (the solution to the problem) by selecting instances. These instances contain a value for each dimension in a problem, and each instance is designated either positive (an exemplar) or negative (a nonexemplar). It is much easier to describe such problems as poisoned-food problems (as they are in this study). The solution to the simpler problems is one poisoned food. Instances are meals, dimensions are courses, and values are specific foods available in each course. In this study, a meal consists of four courses, and two choices are available for each course. Subjects select meals, one at a time; and each meal is designated "died" if the poisoned food is included or "lived" if the poisoned food is not included in that meal. Meals are selected until one of the eight foods is identified as the poisoned food.

In addition to the one-food problems described above, two types of two-food problems are presented: conjunctive and inclusive disjunctive. In the conjunctive problems, two foods are poisoned; and both foods must be included for a meal to be fatal. If either poisoned food is in a meal without the other, that meal is designated "lived." In the disjunctive problems, two foods are poisoned; and either is fatal. Only if neither poisoned food is in a meal is it designated "lived." Participants are instructed about the concept rule, and that information is displayed throughout the problems. Conjunctive and disjunctive problems are presented under two different conditions: high and low initial information. In the high-initial-information condition, the first meal is designated "died" in conjunctive problems and "lived" in disjunctive problems. That eliminates 18 of 24 possible solutions. In the low-initial-information condition, the first meal is designated "lived" in conjunctive problems and "died" in disjunctive problems. That eliminates 6 of the 24 possible solutions. Also, fortuitous actual gains in information are prevented (see Arenberg, 1970).

Twelve problems are presented: 2 one-food followed by 2 conjunctive and 2 disjunctive (in one of four orders), and those 6 problems are repeated (in the same order). Subjects are required to write each meal and its designation so they can review all the information at any time. They are also encouraged to write notes if they find that helpful. All problems are subject paced; no time limits are imposed.

Results from 1967 to 1986 are presented for the men who attempted all 12 problems. The mean number of problems solved correctly is shown for seven age groups in Table 6.1. The means decrease monotonically from the youngest to the oldest group, and the correlation between the number of problems correct and age is −.45.

As in the studies just described, each input can be evaluated on the basis of potential information gain. The number of viable solutions at that point in the problem and the minimum number that could be eliminated by that meal are determined for each meal (after the first, which is determined by the

TABLE 6.1. Mean Number of Concept Problems Correct

| Age | *N* | Mean |
|---|---|---|
| <30 | 99 | 10.4 |
| 30s | 169 | 9.8 |
| 40s | 162 | 9.0 |
| 50s | 150 | 8.3 |
| 60s | 124 | 8.0 |
| 70s | 126 | 6.6 |
| 80+ | 36 | 5.7 |

type of problem). Those numbers are converted to bits of information. The ratio of the bits for a meal and the bits for an optimal selection is the measure of efficiency for that meal. The mean of these measures for each problem is the measure of analytic efficiency.

The means of the efficiency measures for each of three types of problems are shown in Tables 6.2–6.4 for seven age groups of men. In the one-food problems, the means decreased virtually monotonically with age, and the correlation was −.40. The means also declined monotonically for the two-food problems with high initial information; the correlation for those problems was −.37. The pattern of results was similar for the two-food problems with low initial information as well. The decline in means was virtually monotonic, and the correlation with age was −.38.

The analysis of the data for the women in this study is incomplete. On the basis of preliminary results, however, the gender difference in the age pattern reported by Young (1971) is not emerging in this study. The age differences for the women are quite similar to those of the men.

Hartley and Anderson (1983a) used variants of 20 questions and information measures to test the hypothesis that "... older persons may be balancing the need to solve the problem efficiently against the cognitive demands of the strategies they select." The hypothesis was based, in part, on Denney's (1980) finding that the old improved their efficiency when the amount of information (number of possibilities) was very large. Hartley and Anderson manipulated the cognitive demands of the task in three ways: amount of information (size of the array), time pressure, and using two solutions simultaneously. The requirement that the problem be solved in 1 minute had no effect on either age group (14–35 and 60–83 years). Increasing the array size from an 8-by-8 to a 16-by-16 board resulted in reduced analytic efficiency for the older group but not for the young. The requirement to identify two solutions simultaneously reduced efficiency for both groups. The hypothesis was not confirmed. Also, no gender difference was found.

In another study, Hartley and Anderson (1983b) used even larger arrays to determine whether the elderly improve their analytic efficiency when the difficulty of the task is increased. They used 8-by-8 and 100-by-100 arrays and

TABLE 6.2. Mean Analytic Efficiency: One-Food Problems

| Age | *N* | Mean |
|---|---|---|
| <30 | 99 | .80 |
| 30s | 169 | .80 |
| 40s | 160 | .75 |
| 50s | 150 | .73 |
| 60s | 123 | .69 |
| 70s | 125 | .62 |
| 80+ | 36 | .55 |

TABLE 6.3. Mean Analytic Efficiency: High Initial Information

| Age | *N* | Mean |
|---|---|---|
| <30 | 99 | .83 |
| 30s | 166 | .82 |
| 40s | 155 | .78 |
| 50s | 141 | .75 |
| 60s | 118 | .71 |
| 70s | 114 | .66 |
| 80+ | 35 | .63 |

TABLE 6.4. Mean Analytic Efficiency: Low Initial Information

| Age | *N* | Mean |
|---|---|---|
| <30 | 99 | .68 |
| 30s | 167 | .64 |
| 40s | 160 | .61 |
| 50s | 145 | .61 |
| 60s | 115 | .56 |
| 70s | 122 | .54 |
| 80+ | 32 | .50 |

found only an age difference. The size of the array and whether it was physically or mentally represented had no effect on efficiency for either age group.

The results of the cross-sectional studies in which the analytic efficiency of each inquiry throughout a problem could be measured are quite clear. Analytic efficiency is diminished in the elderly. In addition, preliminary longitudinal data indicate declines in analytic efficiency even after only six years among the oldest groups (Arenberg, 1982).

## Synthesis and Aging

Compared with analysis, relatively few studies of aging and problem solving have used problems which require predominantly synthetic performance. Anagrams, water-jar problems, syllogistic reasoning, experimental series completion, and concept identification with a reception paradigm are examples of such problems that have been studied in cross-sectional aging research (e.g., Arenberg, 1968; Hayslip & Sterns, 1979; Heglin, 1956; Nehrke, 1972; Salthouse & Prill, 1987; Wetherick, 1966). Although many of those studies found age differences in performance favoring the younger adult age groups, a few did not (e.g., anagrams in Hayslip & Sterns, 1979; Wetherick, 1966).

The two studies described here in some detail were designed to provide information about where in a problem an error or difficulty in synthesis arose. Arenberg (1968) compared two groups of men (17–22 and 60–77 years) with concept problems using a reception paradigm. They were presented as poisoned-food problems. Nine foods were listed for each problem, and one of the foods was poisoned. Meals consisting of three of the foods were presented sequentially and each meal was designated "died" if it included the poisoned food or "lived" if the poisoned food was not in the meal. After each meal and designation, subjects were required to cross out the foods listed that could be eliminated and to write all foods that were still possibly poisoned. In that way, it was possible to identify the meal that resulted in an error in synthesis. Five different sequences of positive instances (meals designated "died") and negative instances (meals designated "lived") were used to determine whether negative information or covertly redundant information (providing no new information) were especially difficult for the older men. The five different problem sequences were presented and then repeated in a different order.

The young men solved more problems correctly in each subset of five problems. Redundant information resulted in many more errors for the older men than the young group. Nine of 21 older men committed such an error; none of the 21 young men committed this type of error. The older men, however, were not more susceptible to errors than the young when negative information followed positive information. That result was surprising, because Wetherick (1966) had reported that such errors were prevalent among the elderly. It should be noted that, in Wetherick's study, the previous instances and their designations had to be remembered; in Arenberg's study, however, all of that information plus the results of the reasoning to that point were available for review. It may be that negative information following positive information is especially difficult for the elderly only under a memory load.

Hartley (1981) also used poisoned-food concept problems and obtained responses after each instance (with its designation). The task and the responses, however, were quite different from those in Arenberg's (1968) study. Rather than identify the specific food that was poisoned, subjects were instructed to identify which two courses had been adulterated. After each meal and its designation, subjects were "... asked, for each course in turn, to say whether or not it was one of the two that had been tampered with." (p. 702). Furthermore, a confidence rating was required for each judgment. Meals consisted of three courses and there were four possible foods in each course. The inclusive disjunctive rule was used, that is, any meal that included either of the two poisoned foods was a positive instance, but subjects were not informed of what rule was operating. Information about which courses had been tampered with had to be gleaned from changes in foods and designations from previous meals to the current meal. The sequence of meals provided information of four types: uninformative, uncertain, certain, and redundant in that order. All previous meals and designations remained in view, and subjects were encouraged to make notes.

There were four groups of participants: three highly educated (18–24, 36–51, and 56–72 years old) and one somewhat less educated older group (58–87 years old). The numbers of successful problem solvers were 33 of 39 in the young group, 28 of 36 in the middle group, 20 of 36 in the highly educated older group, and 17 of 36 in the less educated older group.

In the analyses of the confidence ratings, solvers and nonsolvers were separated. Old solvers were indistinguishable from younger solvers on confidence ratings for the four types of information. Nonsolvers were also similar across age groups, but they were quite different from solvers at critical points in the problem. For the relevant course that had no uncertain information provided, solvers were quite confident about their judgments immediately after the meals containing the certain information were presented. Nonsolvers were far less confident about their judgments immediately after the meals containing the certain information were presented. Nonsolvers were far less confident about their judgments even after those meals that confirmed that information redundantly. Similarly, for the irrelevant course, solvers became rather confident at the point in the problem when that deduction could be made, whereas nonsolvers continued to judge that course to be relevant. Surprisingly, solvers and nonsolvers were not different in confidence ratings for the relevant course that had uncertain information provided. Hartley interpreted the different results for the two relevant courses in this way: "It is as though the uncertain information drew the attention of the nonsolvers so that when the dimension was confirmed as relevant, they noticed. When their attention had not been drawn to a relevant dimension, they missed the information that it was relevant." (p. 705).

Similar to the results of Arenberg (1968), age differences in synthesis performance were clear as evidenced by the proportion of solvers in the different age groups. In addition, results of the confidence ratings suggest that, when memory demands are relatively low, successful solvers synthesize information in much the same way regardless of age.

## Logical Problem Solving: Cross-Sectional Studies

Two studies compared a young and an old group on the logical problems devised by John (1957). In both studies (Jerome, 1962; Young, 1966), the same apparatus and types of problems were used. All problems were displayed on a board with nine numbered lights in a circle and one light in the center. Adjacent to each light on the periphery was a pushbutton to turn that light on. The light in the center was the goal light; it had no button. Each problem was displayed on a disk with arrows between lights that were directly related.

Each arrow indicated one of three possible logical relations and the direction of the causal effect. The task was to light the goal light in a way that will be explained shortly.

In order to solve the problem, it was necessary to understand the meanings of the arrows on that disk. Every arrow was assigned one of three meanings (causal relations): (1) effector, (2) combinor, or (3) preventor. An effector arrow meant that one light was sufficient to result in another light. Combinor arrows came in pairs and meant that two lights combined in the same input (but neither alone) resulted in a common target light. A preventor arrow meant that one light prevented another light from resulting. The display in Figure 6.1 is similar to those in the studies of Jerome and Young. To help the reader, the arrows are labeled. Effector arrows are designated "1"; combinor arrows are designated "½"; and preventor arrows are designated "0". These labels never appeared on any problem disk, but they demonstrate the pieces of information needed to synthesize the solution to a problem.

While analyzing the meanings of the arrows, subjects were permitted to press any buttons. When they were synthesizing a solution sequence, however, only the buttons for the three lights at the bottom of the display were permitted. That is, a solution was defined as a sequence of inputs that culminates in the goal light, and throughout that sequence only buttons at the bottom of the display are pressed. The color of those three lights was dif-

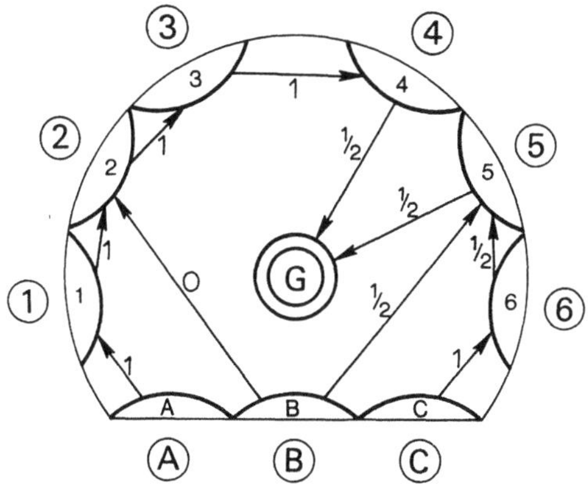


FIGURE 6.1. Sample problem. The solution sequence is:

A →1 →2 →3 →4 } →G
C →6 }
B } →5

where A, B, and C represent lights that were activated by button presses, and 1, 2, 3, 6, 4, 5, and G represent lights that resulted as outcomes of the previous input. 0 = preventor; ½ = combinor; 1 = effector.

ferent from the color of the other six lights on the periphery. Subjects were not only instructed about the procedures but were urged to use a backward solution strategy in every problem. This strategy consisted of identifying the meanings of the arrows directly related to the goal light. After the "subgoal" condition was determined, the sequence required to result in each light of the subgoal was determined by repeated application of the backward solution strategy. This strategy was demonstrated at many points during the several sessions of the experiments.

When John (1957) originally designed the apparatus to administer these problems in an automated format, periodically (every 3 seconds) the lights that were on were extinguished and the results of those lights came on. That feature was retained in the apparatus used by Jerome (1962) and by Young (1966). Also, in both studies, subjects were urged to make notes to reduce memory demands.

In Jerome's study, performance of 12 women in the young group (mean age 23 years) was compared with that of 11 men and women in the older group (60–85 years). Most of the participants were college educated. The problems were designed with four levels of difficulty. When a problem was not solved in 30 minutes, it was interrupted, and the specific stumbling block was identified. At that time and again at the beginning of the next session, the backward solution of that problem was demonstrated. Then the second problem at the same level was presented. Whenever a subject failed to solve either of the two problems at one level of difficulty, the sessions were terminated.

All 12 young women solved a problem at the first three levels of difficulty, and 11 solved a problem at the most difficult level. Only 8, 6, and 1 of the 11 older subjects solved a problem at the first three levels, respectively; none solved a problem at the most difficult level. The older group made many more inquiries (inputs) than the young, and most of those were redundant inputs. This was true even for the problems successfully solved by the older group. The typical performance of the older group was described as "a lack of order in the search plan" (p. 819). Jerome concluded that "... the patterns of heuristic behavior, so laboriously built up during youth through formal education and emulation of skillful acquaintances, decay with age." (p. 822). He advocated that "... a strong effort should be made to study the possibility of reeducating the aged in the heuristic principles that seem so clearly to have decayed." (p. 822).

A few years later, Young (1966) attempted to follow Jerome's suggestion. She administered three problems at the same four levels of difficulty used by Jerome. Whenever a problem was unsolved at the end of the 30-minute period, a special procedure was initiated "... designed to impose order on the search for information." (p. 506). This procedure involved transparencies to demonstrate the backward solution strategy and note-taking at each step in that strategy. Each transparency contained one of the arrows of the failed problem. The overlays were placed on the display one on top of another in an order adhering to the backward solution strategy. For each overlay, the subject "... pressed the appropriate buttons to identify the relation shown and made notes of the information obtained." (p. 506). After all the overlays had been placed on the display, the subject had a complete set of notes showing all the information obtained and the temporal sequence for a solution. All three problems at each level of difficulty were presented.

The two age groups were 54 to 76 and 29 to 45 years old. The median education for each group was 12 years. All 10 young subjects solved the third problem at the first three levels of difficulty, and 9 solved the third problem at the most difficult level. This result was virtually identical to that for Jerome's (1962) young group. Also similar to Jerome's results, only 4, 6, 6, and 3 of the 10 older subjects solved the third problem at the four levels of difficulty, respectively. Even with the carefully designed procedure for training the backward solution strategy and accurate notes, the older group made many more inquiries than the young, and almost all those additional inquiries were redundant. Although a few more older subjects were able to solve the most difficult problems with the training and note-taking procedures, the general picture remained the same. Typically the old group was "... able to identify the goal (to turn on the center light) and soon learned to identify the immediate subgoal (the relation of each of the lights with arrows pointing to the goal light), but they were unable to trace back a step at a time in a systematic way the activation chain for these subgoal lights to the starting point..." (Young, 1966, pp. 508–509).

## Logical Problem Solving: Longitudinal Studies

In 1962, a study of logical problem solving was initiated in the Baltimore Longitudinal Study of Aging (Shock et al., 1984). In that study, not only were cross-sectional age differences found, but some evidence of intraindividual declines was found for the men initially over 70 years old when they were remeasured at least 6 years later (Arenberg, 1974). When that study was designed, it was expected to yield indices of both analytic and synthetic aspects of performance. That expectation was overly optimistic, however. The current longitudinal study, also from the Baltimore Longitudinal Study of Aging (BLSA), was designed specifically to provide measures of analytic and synthetic performance. This was accomplished by presenting each problem in two separate parts. In the first part, the task was to obtain all the relevant pieces of information—the analytic aspect of the problem. In the second part, the task was to use that information to create a solution sequence—the synthetic aspect of the problem. The study was designed not only to determine which aspects of logical problem solving were age related cross-sectionally, but to remeasure the same men 6 years later to obtain individual measures of change.

The procedures were modifications of the problems devised by John (1957). He also devised a method for separating each solution into predominantly analytic and predominantly synthetic phases. The current procedure of presenting each problem in two separate parts in somewhat artificial; it constrains (and masks) the more natural tendencies of individuals to shift from analysis to synthesis when they choose to do so. Although this shift is fixed by the procedure in the current study (thereby sacrificing such behavior), the gain was independent measures of analytic performance and synthetic performance that could be used to assess age differences and changes. The difficulty with the John procedure was that an error in analysis could result in much wasted synthetic activity; this has the appearance of poor synthetic performance, but is totally attributable to an error in analysis. Put another way, it is difficult (perhaps even impossible) to reach a solution effectively (synthesis) with incorrect information (faulty analysis). This state of affairs could be avoided by separating each problem into two parts and providing all of the correct "pieces" of information in the second part (synthesis) as was done in the current study.

## The New Study

All participants in the BLSA who were available from 1966 through 1974 and who had not participated in the first study of logical problem solving were included in the second study. The resulting group consisted of 305 men who ranged in age from 22 to 85 years at their first time of measurement. The longitudinal sample consisted of the 180 men who returned for repeated measurement at least 6 years after their first. Most men in the BLSA are educated, of high socioeconomic status, and working in or retired from positions as scientists, professionals, or managers. Mean WAIS Vocabulary raw scores and the proportion of men with at least one earned degree are shown for each age decade in Table 6.5 for all men who participated in this study.

The three problems were logically identical to those in Arenberg (1974) and the first three levels of difficulty in Jerome (1962) and Young (1966). The three possible meanings of arrows were explained and demonstrated in the instructions. During the first part of each problem (analysis), the specific meanings of the arrows were investigated by inputs that consisted of one light or a combination of two or three lights. Participants were instructed to make inputs to obtain enough information to identify all the arrow meanings, but to do this with as few inputs as they could.

In the second part of the problem (synthesis), all the correct meanings of the arrows were displayed. The task was to create a sequence of inputs that would culminate in the goal light. (In a sequence of inputs, the outcome of each input becomes part of the next input.) In this part of the problem, however, only a subset of three buttons (A, B, and C) could be used. The task was to create a solution sequence with as few inputs as possible.

TABLE 6.5. Mean WAIS Vocabulary and Proportion With Earned Degree

| Sample | 20s | 30s | 40s | 50s | 60s | 70s | 80s | Total *N* |
|---|---|---|---|---|---|---|---|---|
| Total | | | | | | | | |
| *N* | 19 | 29 | 67 | 70 | 52 | 58 | 10 | 305 |
| Mean vocabulary | 62.4 | 62.2 | 63.7 | 66.3 | 66.6 | 66.6 | 61.1 | |
| Proportion with degree | .68 | .83 | .75 | .79 | .81 | .79 | .70 | |
| Cross-Sectional | | | | | | | | |
| *N* | 19 | 27 | 64 | 69 | 49 | 46 | 5 | 279 |
| Mean vocabulary | 62.4 | 62.8 | 64.8 | 66.3 | 67.0 | 68.5 | 66.6 | |
| Proportion with degree | .68 | .81 | .75 | .80 | .82 | .83 | .80 | |
| Longitudinal | | | | | | | | |
| *N* | 12 | 25 | 48 | 49 | 24 | 22 | 0 | 180 |
| Mean vocabulary | 62.1 | 62.1 | 65.5 | 66.7 | 66.8 | 68.5 | — | |
| Proportion with degree | .75 | .80 | .81 | .86 | .88 | .91 | — | |

The sample problem is displayed in Figure 6.1, which shows: (1) the 10 lights (A, B, C, 1, 2, 3, 4, 5, 6, and G) common to all problems; (2) the disk with the arrows unique to that problem; and (3) a code to show the specific meanings of those arrows (1, ½, or 0). Those meanings were never displayed in that way at any time, but are provided in Figure 6.1 to help describe the sample problem here. Effector arrows (designated "1") meant that 1 light was sufficient to result in another light. Combinor arrows (designated "½") came in pairs and meant that 2 lights in the same input were necessary to result in a light. Preventor arrows (designated "0") meant that a light prevented another light from resulting. The solution to the sample problem is shown in the legend of Figure 6.1.

The sample problem shown in Figure 6.1 was used to introduce the many rules and procedures involved in this type of problem. Included were demonstrations of input–outcome transitions emphasizing that at the subject's command (and only then) outcome lights replaced input lights, explanations of the three possible meanings of arrows, and instructions about restrictions on button pressing for the two parts of each problem. In addition, the notation used by the experimenter to record all inputs and their outcomes was shown. These records provided a complete log that could be reviewed at any point in a problem to minimize the memory aspects of the task and to maximize the reasoning components. Furthermore, unlike the earlier cross-sectional studies of similar problems (Jerome, 1962; Young, 1966), in this study, the tasks were completely subject paced. The apparatus was not automated. No transition from current lights on the display (input) to the lights resulting from that input (outcome) occurred until the subject indicated to the experimenter that he wanted the results of the current lights.

Following the sample problem, the two parts of the practice problem were administered. Questions about rules and procedures were encouraged. Whenever help was needed in solving the practice problem, the experimenter attempted to elicit the source of the difficulty in order to maximize the subject's understanding of the tasks and the permissible operations. Questions about rules and procedures were permitted throughout both parts of each problem.

All participants attempted both parts of the first problem and also attempted the second and third problems if time permitted. At least 6 years after the first set of problems was administered, a set of logically identical problems was administered to those men who continued in the study.

In the first part of each problem, the analytic task, subjects attempted to identify the meanings of the arrows with as few inputs as possible. Two dependent measures were derived: (1) the number of arrows identified correctly; and (2) the number of inputs that provided no new information about the meanings of arrows at that point in the problem. Two dependent measures were also derived from the synthetic task during which subjects attempted to construct a solution sequence: (1) the number of inputs exceeding the minimum required; and (2) whether a correct sequence was constructed.

## Cross-Sectional Results

Of the total sample, 26 men did not provide usable data. As a result, there were 279 men in the cross-sectional sample (see Table 6.5). Most of these losses were men over 70 who either quit before the first problem or could not understand the instructions.

### Analysis

Means for age decades are shown in Table 6.6 for the two dependent measures of analytic performance, that is, the number of arrows correctly identified and number of uninformative inputs. In the first problem, the mean number of correctly identified arrows tended to decrease with age; the correlation of this measure with age was −.26 ($p < .01$). Similarly, the mean number of uninformative inputs increased with age; the correlation was .21 ($p < .01$).

For the men who reached the second problem, similar results were found. Although few errors were made in identifying the meanings of arrows, those errors did increase with age, and the correlation between number of arrows correctly identified and age was −.13 ($p < .05$, one-tailed). The mean number of uninformative inputs tended to increase with age; the correlation was .28 ($p < .01$).

Similar results were found for the men who reached the third problem. Although the number of errors in identifying the meanings of arrows was quite low, the correlation between number of arrows correctly identified and

TABLE 6.6. Cross-Sectional Means of Analytic Performance

| | Problem 1 | | | | Problem 2 | | | | Problem 3 | | | |
|---|---|---|---|---|---|---|---|---|---|---|---|---|
| | Correct Identification | | Uninformative Inputs | | Correct Identification | | Uninformative Inputs | | Correct Identification | | Uninformative Inputs | |
| Age | $N^a$ | Mean | $N^a$ | Mean | $N$ | Mean | $N$ | Mean | $N$ | Mean | $N$ | Mean |
| 20s | 19 | 10.9 | 19 | 1.5 | 19 | 9.8 | 19 | 1.0 | 17 | 12.0 | 17 | 1.2 |
| 30s | 27 | 10.3 | 27 | 1.6 | 24 | 9.8 | 24 | 1.5 | 20 | 11.5 | 20 | 1.1 |
| 40s | 64 | 9.7 | 63 | 3.0 | 57 | 9.7 | 57 | 2.4 | 40 | 11.1 | 40 | 1.6 |
| 50s | 69 | 10.3 | 69 | 3.3 | 63 | 9.7 | 63 | 2.2 | 46[a] | 10.9 | 45[a] | 1.8 |
| 60s | 49 | 9.2 | 46 | 3.2 | 33 | 9.6 | 33 | 2.7 | 21 | 11.0 | 21 | 2.2 |
| 70s | 46 | 9.3 | 45 | 4.3 | 29 | 9.2 | 29 | 4.8 | 13 | 10.9 | 13 | 4.5 |
| 80s | 5 | 5.8 | 4 | 3.5 | 0 | — | 0 | — | 0 | — | 0 | — |

[a]The difference in $N$ within a problem resulted from subjects who quit during a problem; it was possible to obtain a measure for correct identification but not for uninformative inputs.

age was $-.15$ ($p < .05$, one-tailed). In addition, the mean number of uninformative inputs increased with age; correlation with age was .33 ($p < .01$).

All cross-sectional results were consistent, with a decline in analytic performance with age.

### Synthesis

Results for the two dependent measures of synthetic performance are shown in Table 6.7. In the first problem, the mean number of extra inputs to create a solution sequence tended to increase with age, and the correlation was .15 ($p < .05$). In addition, the proportion of correct solutions decreased with age.

For the men who reached the second problem, the mean number of extra inputs again tended to increase with age. The two youngest groups had the fewest extra inputs and the two oldest groups had the most. The correlation with age was .32 ($p < .01$). Also, the proportion of correct solutions decreased with age.

Although the men who reached the third problem were a very select group, the number of extra inputs tended to increase with age; the youngest group had the fewest, and the oldest group the most. The correlation with age, however, was only .12, which was not statistically significant. Very few men who reached the third problem failed to solve it.

As in the cross-sectional results for analytic performance, synthetic performance generally declined with increasing age.

## Longitudinal Results

### Analysis

Of 180 men who returned at least 6 years after their first problem-solving session, 161 produced usable data from both sessions that could be compared. On one measure in the first problem, number of correct arrow identifications, only the oldest group (men in their seventies at their first session) showed a substantial mean decline. The correlation of individual change with age was $-.16$ ($p < .05$). On the other measure of analysis, number of uninformative inputs in identifying arrow meanings, the means tended to decline with age at both times of measurement; but the total group changed very little, and the magnitude of change was not related to age. The means of these measures are shown in Table 6.8.

On the second problem, 136 men had usable data at both sessions. Although few errors were made in identifying arrows, the correlation of age with change in number correct again was $-.16$ ($p < .05$, one-tailed). Uninformative inputs tended to increase with age in both sessions, but the total group changed very little, and the magnitude of change was not related to age.

TABLE 6.7. Cross-Sectional Results of Synthetic Performance

| | Problem 1 | | | | Problem 2 | | | | Problem 3 | | | |
|---|---|---|---|---|---|---|---|---|---|---|---|---|
| | Extra Inputs | | Correct Solutions | | Extra Inputs | | Correct Solutions | | Extra Inputs | | Correct Solutions | |
| Age | $N^a$ | Mean | $N^a$ | Proportion | $N^a$ | Mean | $N^a$ | Proportion | $N^a$ | Mean | $N^a$ | Proportion |
| 20s | 19 | 1.6 | 19 | 1.00 | 18 | 1.6 | 19 | .95 | 17 | 1.1 | 17 | 1.00 |
| 30s | 28 | 3.9 | 28 | 1.00 | 23 | 1.3 | 25 | .92 | 21 | 2.2 | 21 | 1.00 |
| 40s | 60 | 4.0 | 64 | .94 | 54 | 3.4 | 58 | .93 | 41 | 2.1 | 41 | 1.00 |
| 50s | 64 | 4.9 | 68 | .94 | 55 | 3.4 | 62 | .89 | 44 | 2.2 | 45 | .98 |
| 60s | 41 | 4.1 | 48 | .85 | 27 | 9.1 | 33 | .82 | 21 | 2.2 | 21 | 1.00 |
| 70s | 39 | 6.1 | 46 | .85 | 20 | 8.6 | 29 | .69 | 12 | 3.7 | 13 | .92 |
| 80s | 0 | — | 5 | .00 | 0 | — | 0 | — | 0 | — | 0 | — |

[a]The difference in $N$ within a problem resulted from subjects who quit during a problem; when that occurred, the problem was considered "incorrect," but no measure of "extra inputs" was available.

TABLE 6.8. Longitudinal Means of Analytic Performance

Correct Identifications

| Initial Age | Problem 1 | | | Problem 2 | | | Problem 3 | | |
|---|---|---|---|---|---|---|---|---|---|
| | | Means | | | Means | | | Means | |
| | N | First | Second | N | First | Second | N | First | Second |
| 20s | 12 | 11.0 | 10.4 | 12 | 9.8 | 10.0 | 10 | 12.0 | 11.6 |
| 30s | 23 | 10.3 | 10.3 | 20 | 9.9 | 10.0 | 17 | 11.6 | 11.6 |
| 40s | 46 | 10.2 | 10.4 | 44 | 9.8 | 9.5 | 31 | 11.3 | 11.0 |
| 50s | 47 | 10.4 | 9.2 | 38 | 9.8 | 9.9 | 26 | 11.2 | 11.0 |
| 60s | 21 | 10.1 | 9.8 | 15 | 9.8 | 9.3 | 10 | 10.7 | 10.4 |
| 70s | 12 | 9.6 | 7.3 | 7 | 9.9 | 9.1 | 2 | 12.0 | 8.0 |

Uninformative Inputs

| Initial Age | Problem 1 | | | Problem 2 | | | Problem 3 | | |
|---|---|---|---|---|---|---|---|---|---|
| | | Means | | | Means | | | Means | |
| | N | First | Second | N | First | Second | N | First | Second |
| 20s | 12 | 1.9 | 1.7 | 12 | 1.1 | 1.4 | 10 | 1.4 | 0.4 |
| 30s | 23 | 1.3 | 1.5 | 20 | 1.5 | 0.9 | 17 | 0.9 | 0.4 |
| 40s | 46 | 2.5 | 2.1 | 43 | 2.4 | 1.8 | 31 | 1.8 | 1.3 |
| 50s | 43 | 2.8 | 3.3 | 38 | 1.5 | 2.7 | 26 | 1.4 | 2.9 |
| 60s | 20 | 2.6 | 3.2 | 15 | 1.9 | 2.3 | 10 | 2.3 | 3.8 |
| 70s | 10 | 3.9 | 3.5 | 7 | 2.7 | 3.1 | 2 | 6.0 | 2.5 |

Only 96 men had usable data on the third problem both times. The number of correct arrow identifications declined very little, and the correlation between magnitude of change and age was not statistically significant. Change in uninformative inputs, however, was related to age ($r = .26$; $p < .05$).

SYNTHESIS

The results for the two measures of synthesis appear in Table 6.9. On the first problem, although only the oldest group substantially increased their number of extra inputs in constructing a solution sequence, the correlation of change on this measure with age was .14 ($p < .05$, one-tailed). In the lower half of Table 6.9, the number of men who correctly solved a problem the first time and attempted to solve that problem the second time are shown together with the proportion of those men who solved that problem correctly the second time. The lowest proportions were found for the two oldest groups.

On the second problem, although the number of extra inputs increased with age at both times of measurement, change in this variable was not

TABLE 6.9. Longitudinal Results of Synthetic Performance

Extra Inputs

| | Problem 1 | | | Problem 2 | | | Problem 3 | | |
|---|---|---|---|---|---|---|---|---|---|
| | | Means | | | Means | | | Means | |
| Initial Age | N | First | Second | N | First | Second | N | First | Second |
| 20s | 11 | 1.6 | 0.8 | 11 | 1.5 | 0.6 | 10 | 0.8 | 0.8 |
| 30s | 24 | 4.3 | 3.5 | 19 | 0.7 | 1.4 | 18 | 1.4 | 1.1 |
| 40s | 44 | 3.4 | 3.3 | 42 | 2.9 | 2.4 | 31 | 1.5 | 2.1 |
| 50s | 42 | 4.5 | 5.8 | 36 | 3.6 | 6.3 | 27 | 1.8 | 3.3 |
| 60s | 19 | 3.3 | 4.2 | 12 | 9.8 | 5.3 | 8 | 1.8 | 12.3 |
| 70s | 9 | 5.1 | 9.7 | 4 | 9.5 | 8.5 | 2 | 4.5 | 15.0 |

Correctness

| Age | N[a] | Proportion Correct[b] | N[a] | Proportion Correct[b] | N[a] | Proportion Correct[b] |
|---|---|---|---|---|---|---|
| 20s | 12 | .92 | 11 | 1.00 | 10 | 1.00 |
| 30s | 24 | 1.00 | 19 | 1.00 | 18 | 1.00 |
| 40s | 45 | .98 | 42 | 1.00 | 31 | 1.00 |
| 50s | 43 | .98 | 37 | .97 | 27 | 1.00 |
| 60s | 21 | .90 | 13 | .92 | 10 | .80 |
| 70s | 11 | .82 | 5 | .80 | 2 | 1.00 |

[a]*N*, Number who solved correctly at Time 1 and attempted that problem at Time 2.
[b]Proportion, of that *N*, proportion who solved correctly at Time 2.

related to age. Very few men who solved this problem correctly the first time failed to solve it the second time; again, the proportions who solved correctly the second time declined with age.

On the third problem, not only was the number of extra inputs related to age the second time, but the magnitude of change was substantially related to age ($r = .40$; $p < .01$). Only two men who had solved this problem correctly the first time failed to solve it the second time; both men were in their sixties initially.

In summary, although not all measures on all problems showed a relationship between magnitude of decline and age, the preponderance of the longitudinal evidence was in that direction for both analysis and synthesis. Despite the fact that vocabulary scores were highest for the oldest men (see Table 6.1), in general both their analytic and synthetic performance declined.

One of the general strategies for solving complex problems is to subdivide them into smaller problems. With regard to subdividing, it may be instructive to compare the procedures in the current study with those in the earlier study in the BLSA in which the same problems were used. Each of the problems used in the earlier study was presented in two separate parts in the current study. In a sense, each problem was subdivided for the problem solver. Although the studies were not designed to compare performance between studies, it is possible to sum two variables in the current study and compare that combined variable with a similar variable in the previous study. The two variables that were summed were the uninformative inputs in the analysis part of a problem with the extra inputs in the synthesis part of that problem.

Means of those sums are shown in Table 6.10 with the comparable means from the previous study by age group for each problem. In the first problem, there was no apparent advantage from partitioning the problem into two parts. A substantial advantage, however, resulted from the partitioning in the second problem for the groups under 60 years old, and in the third problem for all age groups. An unsystematic review of the raw data indicated that, in the earlier study, some of the repetitious attempts to solve problems seemed to result from incomplete or erroneous information about specific arrow meanings; these attempts were eliminated by the procedures in the current study. In this study, complete and correct information about the meanings of the arrows were provided in the synthesis part of each problem. Because the studies were not designed to answer questions about the effects of subdivision, those effects were confounded with the effects of having complete and correct information provided during synthesis. These findings, however, suggest that subdivision improves problem-solving performance for both old and young, and that the effects may be stronger in more complex problems and/or for better performers.

TABLE 6.10. Mean Extra/Uninformative Inputs

| | | Problem 1 | | Problem 2 | | Problem 3 | |
|---|---|---|---|---|---|---|---|
| Age | | Previous | Current | Previous | Current | Previous | Current |
| <40 | *N* | 43 | 46 | 39 | 40 | 37 | 37 |
| | Mean | 5.1 | 4.5 | 7.4 | 2.5 | 8.9 | 2.9 |
| 40s | *N* | 74 | 59 | 71 | 53 | 60 | 40 |
| | Mean | 7.4 | 7.0 | 10.4 | 5.8 | 9.1 | 3.6 |
| 50s | *N* | 73 | 64 | 66 | 55 | 51 | 44 |
| | Mean | 6.9 | 8.1 | 10.7 | 5.4 | 10.3 | 4.0 |
| 60s | *N* | 37 | 41 | 27 | 27 | 18 | 21 |
| | Mean | 8.5 | 7.2 | 11.0 | 11.4 | 16.3 | 4.4 |
| 70s | *N* | 36 | 39 | 24 | 20 | 13 | 12 |
| | Mean | 8.5 | 10.3 | 14.0 | 13.1 | 14.1 | 7.8 |

In virtually all the studies cited in this chapter, the problems were selected to minimize familiarity. Even the variants of 20 questions were presented in forms different from the way the parlor game is typically played. Experienced problem solvers may not show the same age differences or changes as novices. Charness (1985), in his review of aging and problem solving in familiar domains, provided an excellent summary of his research on aging and skilled performance in chess and bridge (Charness, 1979, 1981a, 1981b, 1981c, 1982, 1983). He concluded that "... as bridge players and chess players age they may become slower at encoding information about the problem, but once the problem space has been represented, they search it as effectively as their level of acquired skill permits." (p. 250). He did caution his readers that, because the oldest players in his studies were in their sixties or early seventies, nothing can be said about performance of players even older.

It should be noted here that Sternberg's (1985) triarchic theory of intelligence (see Trotter, 1986 for a popularized description), which has gained much attention recently in both the scientific community and the lay press, uses the terms "analysis" and "synthesis" somewhat differently from their meanings in this chapter. Sternberg's componential "Alice-type" intelligence, described as analytic, apparently includes both analysis and synthesis as used here. His experiential "Barbaresque" intelligence, described as synthetic, seems highly weighted with insight and creativity. No claims are made here that what we refer to as synthesis includes creativity, although the temporal aspect of the synthetic task in the longitudinal study reported here may have some of the characteristics of insight.

Sternberg and his colleagues are making progress in measuring analysis and synthesis as he uses those terms. It is encouraging but at the same time somewhat disappointing that these important components of problem solving, which were introduced by John (1957) in his attempts to study process variables, are virtually absent in current problem-solving research but are reemerging in the intelligence domain where the emphasis is typically on products rather than processes.

Are the age differences and changes in problem solving in analysis or in synthesis? The answer at this point is that both are implicated. Elderly individuals apparently have difficulty identifying the pieces of information needed to solve problems; furthermore, when the pieces of information are provided, the old typically encounter difficulty putting them together to reach a solution to a problem. As in virtually all cognitive research in aging, however, there is much variability in performance among people of the same age, and performance of some old individuals is indistinguishable from that of young adults.

Reese and Rodeheaver (1985) concluded their extensive review of research in problem solving and aging with "... although older adults have been shown to respond differently from young adults in many problem situations, few significant steps have been taken toward understanding the nature of the differences." It is hoped that future research, including further componential efforts beginning with analysis and synthesis, will provide such steps and thereby enhance our understanding of problem solving as well as this extremely important aspect of cognition and aging.

*Acknowledgments.* Among those who have contributed to the studies of problem solving in the Baltimore Longitudinal Study of Aging by administering and scoring the procedures with great care are Karen Douglas, Judy Friz, Darrell Gray, Pat Hawthorne, Barbara Hiscock, Joan King, Judith Plotz, Don Reynolds, Susan Robinson, and Marcia Schwartz. Judith Plotz handled all the computer analyses. Their many contributions are gratefully acknowledged.

# References

Arenberg, D. (1968). Concept problem solving in young and old adults. *Journal of Gerontology, 23,* 279–282.

Arenberg, D. (1970). Equivalence of information in concept identification. *Psychological Bulletin, 74,* 355–361.

Arenberg, D. (1973). Cognition and aging: Verbal learning, problem solving and memory. In C. Eisdorfer & M.P. Lawton (Eds.), *The psychology of adult development and aging.* American Psychological Association, Washington, D.C.

Arenberg, D. (1974). A longitudinal study of problem solving in adults. *Journal of Gerontology, 29,* 650–658.

Arenberg, D. (1982). Changes with age in problem solving. In F.I.M. Craik & S. Trehub (Eds.), *Aging and cognitive processes* (pp. 221–235). New York: Plenum Press.

Botwinick, J. (1973). *Aging and behavior.* New York: Springer.

Charness, N. (1979). Components of skill in bridge. *Canadian Journal of Psychology, 33,* 1–16.

Charness, N. (1981a). Aging and skilled problem solving. *Journal of Experimental Psychology: General, 110,* 21–38.

Charness, N. (1981b). Search in chess: Age and skill differences. *Journal of Experimental Psychology: Human Perception and Performance, 7,* 467–476.

Charness, N. (1981c). Visual short-term memory and aging in chess players. *Journal of Gerontology, 36,* 615–619.

Charness, N. (1982). Problem solving and aging: Evidence from semantically rich domains. *Canadian Journal on Aging, 1,* 21–28.

Charness, N. (1983). Age, skill, and bridge bidding: A chronometric analysis. *Journal of Verbal Learning and Verbal Behavior, 22,* 406–416.

Charness, N. (1985). Aging and problem-solving performance. In N. Charness, (Ed.), *Aging and human performance* (pp. 225–259). New York: Wiley.

Denney, N.W. (1980). Task demands and problem-solving strategies in middle-aged and older adults. *Journal of Gerontology, 35,* 559–564.

Denney, N.W. (1982). Aging and cognitive change. In B.B. Wolman & G. Stricker (Eds.), *Handbook of developmental psychology* (pp. 807–827). Englewood Cliffs, NJ: Prentice-Hall.

Hartley, A.A. (1981). Adult age differences in deductive reasoning processes. *Journal of Gerontology, 36,* 700–706.
Hartley, A.A., & Anderson, J.W. (1983a). Task complexity and problem-solving performance in younger and older adults. *Journal of Gerontology, 38,* 72–77.
Hartley, A.A., & Anderson, J.W. (1983b). Task complexity, problem representation, and problem-solving performance by younger and older adults. *Journal of Gerontology, 38,* 78–80.
Hayslip, B., & Sterns, H.L. (1979). Age differences in relationships between crystallized and fluid intelligences and problem solving. *Journal of Gerontology, 34,* 404–414.
Heglin, H.J. (1956). Problem-solving set in different age groups. *Journal of Gerontology, 11,* 310–317.
Hybertson, D., Perdue, J., & Hybertson, D. (1982). Age differences in information acquisition strategies. *Experimental Aging Research, 8,* 109–113.
Jerome, E.A. (1962). Decay of heuristic processes in the aged. In C. Tibbitts & W. Donahue (Eds.), *Social and psychological aspects of aging* (pp. 808–823). New York: Columbia University Press.
John, E.R. (1957). Contributions to the study of the problem-solving process. *Psychological Monographs, 71,* 1-39.
Jones, H.E. (1959). Intelligence and problem-solving. In J.E. Birren (Ed.), *Handbook of aging and the individual.* Chicago: University of Chicago Press.
Kesler, M.S., Denney, N.W., & Whitely, S.E. (1976). Factors influencing problem solving in middle-aged and elderly adults. *Human Development, 19,* 310–320.
Nehrke, M.F. (1972). Age, sex, and educational differences in syllogistic reasoning. *Journal of Gerontology, 27,* 466–470.
Reese, H.W., & Rodeheaver, D. (1985). Problem solving and complex decision making. In J.E. Birren & K.W. Schaie (Eds.), *Handbook of the psychology of aging* (2nd ed., pp. 474–495). New York: Van Nostrand Reinhold.
Salthouse, T.A., & Prill, K.A. (1987). Inferences about age impairments in inferential reasoning. *Psychology and Aging, 2,* 43–51.
Shock, N.W., Greulich, R.C., Andres, R., Arenberg, D., Costa, P.T., Jr., Lakatta, E.G., & Tobin, J.D. (1984). *Normal human aging: The Baltimore Longitudinal Study of Aging.* NIH Publication No. 84-2450. Washington, DC: U.S. Government Printing Office.
Sternberg, R.J. (1985). *Beyond IQ.* New York: Cambridge University Press.
Trotter, R.J. (1986, August). Three heads are better than one. *Psychology Today,* pp. 56–62.
Welford, A.T. (1958). *Ageing and human skill.* London: Oxford University Press.
Wetherick, N.M. (1964). A comparison of the problem-solving ability of young, middle-aged and old subjects. *Gerontologia, 9,* 164–178.
Wetherick, N.M. (1966). The inferential basis of concept attainment. *British Journal of Psychology, 57,* 61–69.
Young, M.L. (1966). Problem-solving performance in two age groups. *Journal of Gerontology, 21,* 505–509.
Young, M.L. (1971). Age and sex differences in problem solving. *Journal of Gerontology, 26,* 330–336.

# 7. The Role of Processing Resources in Cognitive Aging

*Timothy A. Salthouse*

The goal of this chapter is to examine and elaborate a theoretical perspective on cognitive aging, based on the concept that at least some age-related impairments in cognition are attributable to a reduction in a critical processing resource required for the successful completion of many cognitive tasks. Because the chapter is rather lengthy, a brief outline of its organization is presented. The initial section specifies the scope of phenomena to be addressed, and the second section briefly documents the existence and approximate magnitude of these phenomena with several types of comparisons. Categories of possible explanations for these age differences in cognition are then discussed, followed by a review of previous application of the processing resources concept in explanations of cognitive aging phenomena. Methods of investigating the nature and role of processing resources in cognitive aging are discussed next, followed by a report of three new research studies designed to analyze the contribution of processing resources to age differences in cognitive functioning. The final sections consist of a reappraisal of the resources construct and a critical examination of alternative methods of subjecting it to investigation.

## Restriction of Scope

When attempting to formulate a theoretical explanation of a phenonenon so complex as the effects of aging on human cognition, it is essential to be very explicit at the outset in specifying the scope of the exposition. Indeed, it could be argued that there have not been more previous attempts at providing theoretical interpretations of age-related cognitive differences in adulthood because potential theorists have been overwhelmed by the breadth and diversity of the findings to be explained by a successful theory. An obvious means of reducing the problem to manageable proportions is to restrict one's theoretical coverage to only certain types of cognitive phenomena.

This restriction strategy is employed here by deliberately excluding those aspects of cognition that can be presumed to be heavily dependent on cumulative experience. Of course the degree of experiential influence can seldom be determined directly, and it is probably unreasonable to expect that any cognitive measure will fail to exhibit at least some improvements as a function of practice or specific experience. Nevertheless, it seems plausible that certain cognitive measures are much more dependent on one's experiential history than are other measures (cf., the distinction between crystallized and fluid intellectual abilities; Horn [1978, 1982]; Horn & Cattell [1967]). For example, a score on a vocabulary test is almost certainly influenced by the number or variety of words to which one has been exposed, and thus it would be expected to vary greatly depending on the nature and quantity of one's experiences. On the other hand, there may be little influence of general experience (as opposed to specific practice) on performance of certain tests of abstract reasoning or rote memorizing, particularly if the task contents or stimulus material are highly familiar to all members of the population being examined.

This distinction between measures with high and low degrees of sensitivity to general experience (i.e., experience presumably common to most members of the population) is particularly important in research on aging because older adults, simply by virtue of their greater ages, have generally had 40 or more years of additional exposure opportunity to acquire the relevant experience than young adults. This inevitably introduces a confounding in that general experience will tend to be positively correlated with age, and therefore "true" aging effects may, depending on the nature of the variables, be minimized, exaggerated, or completely masked by the uncontrolled effects of experience. For this reason, the perspective examined here is only concerned with accounting for the effects of aging on fluid cognitive abilities that can be presumed to be relatively independent of variations in experience.

## Documenting the Decline

Before examining hypotheses that might account for the effects of aging on fluid cognitive abilities, it is first desirable to document the general nature of these effects. This section therefore summarizes the magnitude of aging effects on measures derived from tasks assessing memory, spatial ability, and reasoning. These categories are rather broad, and distinctions across different types of tasks within each of the categories will be ignored. Although this type of all-inclusive characterization of age effects on cognitive abilities is undoubtedly oversimplistic and runs the risk of neglecting potentially important variables, it may provide an overview of what needs to be explained by any satisfactory theory of cognitive aging.

The domains of memory ability, spatial ability, and reasoning ability are best described by listing the types of tasks contained within each general category. Memory abilities have been assessed in studies of cognitive aging with tasks ranging from the serial recall of randomly arranged digits, to free (unordered) recall of lists of unrelated words, to the recall of information from meaningful paragraphs. Tests designed to evaluate spatial abilities include assorted embedded figures and spatial manipulation tests, the Hooper Visual Organization Test, and several subtests in omnibus intelligence batteries such as the Picture Completion, Picture Arrangement, Object Assembly, and Block Design subtests from the Wechsler Adult Intelligence Scale (WAIS). Reasoning abilities have been evaluated with a variety of different tests, but the two most common with adult subjects have been some form of series completion test and the Raven's Progressive Matrices test.

Two different approaches can be taken to document the amount of age-related decline found in these categories of mental ability. One approach is to examine correlation coefficients between age and the relevant performance measure. [Although correlation coefficients will underestimate the magnitude of age effects if the relationships between age and performance are not linear, the data summarized in Figures 4.1 through 4.14 of Salthouse (1982) indicate that the average trends closely approach linearity for many variables.] To be directly comparable, all samples should be relatively large and involve adults between approximately 18 and 80 years of age. Salthouse (1985a, Tables 11.1, 12.1, and 13.1) has tabulated 54 such correlations from 24 different studies assessing memory, spatial, and reasoning abilities. The overall median of these correlations was −.36, and the correlations were of similar magnitude across the different abilities: the medians were −.33 for the 22 memory correlations, −.38 for the 18 spatial correlations, and −.35 for the 14 reasoning correlations.

The second approach to assessing the magnitude of age-related cognitive decline involves determining the location, in standard deviation units, of the average older adult in the distribution of young adult scores. There will necessarily be some variability in the range of ages defining the young and old samples, but because many research studies have employed generally similar selection criteria (i.e., young samples tend to average between 18 and 30 years of age and old samples between 60 and 75 years of age), the degree of imprecision should not be too great. Once again, data summarized in Tables 11.1, 12.1, and 13.1 of Salthouse (1985a) can be used to quantify the magnitude of the decline with this procedure. A total of 111 values derived from 52 separate studies are contained in these tables, with the overall median being −1.35. As was true with the correlational data, variation across ability domains in the amount of age difference was relatively small; the medians were −1.26 for the 67 memory values, −1.27 for the 22 spatial values, and −1.60 for the 22 reasoning values.

These two different types of data converge in portraying a picture of rather substantial age-related declines in cognitive abilities. The correlation with age averages about −.36, and the average 65-year-old can be estimated to fall between the 5th and the 12th percentile of the distribution of 20-year-olds. Expressing results in this fashion obviously ignores the contribution of many potentially important variables, and may lead to confusion unless properly interpreted. In particular, it is essential to note that these data are derived from fluid ability tasks and do not reflect the crystallized or experience-influenced abilities that may be of much greater importance in most daily activities. It is also important to point out that the declines represent relative losses and not complete impairments. By no means do these data indicate that normal aging, at least between the ages of 20 and about 75, results in a complete inability to perform tasks of this type. Finally, it should be emphasized that these results correspond to average levels of performance observed in cross-sectional studies, and consequently the trends could conceivably be quite different when aging effects are examined longitudinally within particular individuals. Despite these important qualifications, the data summarized in this section indicate that there is considerable evidence of cross-sectional decline in fluid ability aspects of cognitive functioning.

If one accepts the conclusion that moderately large age differences do exist in a variety of cognitive abilities concerned with memory, spatial integration and manipulation, and simple reasoning, these differences must be explained. What mechanisms are responsible for the progressive declines associated with increased age in the effectiveness of memory, spatial, and reasoning tasks?

## How Are Age Differences to Be Explained?

The information-processing approach to cognition provides three general categories of explanation that might be used to account for individual differences in cognitive functioning when variations in amount of experience or degree of knowledge are assumed to be minimal: (a) differences in component efficiency; (b) differences in strategy effectiveness; and (c) differences in the quantity of relevant processing resources. Variations in the efficiency or effectiveness of an information-processing component or process postulated to be critical for successful completion of a task could obviously contribute to individual differences in performance on that task. Several sets of components have been proposed which, when properly combined, have been presumed to account for performance of a large number of cognitive tasks (e.g., Carroll, 1976; Newell & Simon, 1972; Rose, 1980). For example, Rose (1980) suggested the list consists of components responsible for encoding, constructing, transforming, storing, retrieving, searching, comparing, and responding. To the extent that two individuals differ in the duration, or in the quality of the product, of any of these component operations, it is reasonable to expect that they will also differ in the overall performance of tasks involving those operations.

Strategies can be defined in the information-processing perspective as particular sequences of processing components. Certain component sequences may be more effective than others at accomplishing the goals of a given task, and hence it is clearly possible that at least some individual differences in cognitive performance could be attributable to variations across individuals in the strategy used to perform the task. Because strategies, like the performance they are intended to explain, can be considered a type of behavior, this is not a particularly satisfying type of explanation until an account has been provided for the hypothesized differences in strategy. It would nevertheless constitute a distinct explanatory category if the strategy differences were demonstrated to be independent of possible differences in component efficiency or in the quantity of relevant processing resources.

A third potential source of individual differences from the information-processing perspective is the amount of a general-purpose entity, designated by Norman and Bobrow (1975) as a processing resource. These authors suggested that "Resources are such things as processing effort, the various forms of memory capacity, and communication channels" (Norman & Bobrow, 1975, p. 45). Navon (1984) subsequently provided a definition that may better capture the generality of the resources concept as it is currently used in the cognitive psychology literature:

> ... the concept of a resource would be broadly defined as any internal input essential for processing (e.g., locations in storage, communication channels) that is available in quantities that are limited at any point in time. (p. 217)

If individuals vary in the quantity of the available resource, one might expect people with lesser quantities of the resource to perform at lower levels on tasks making demands on those resources than people with greater quantities of the resource.

Although explanations from each of these three categories have appeared, the component efficiency and strategy effectiveness interpretations are at a disadvantage in accounting for age differences in cognition because the pervasiveness of the aging effects seems to require the postulation of many specific, and presumably independent, age-sensitive components or strategies. That is, because components are concerned with a particular type of processing, and because strategies refer to specific sequences of components applied to the solution of a limited set of tasks, each distinct task in which age differences are observed may necessitate hypothesizing the existence of a new impaired component or another inefficient strategy.

This limited applicability of hypotheses generated to account for phenomena within a single restricted topical area is a natural consequence of what has been called "issue isolationism" (Salthouse, 1985a) or "research sectarianism" (Birren & Renner, 1977). Although often necessary, particularly in the early stages of research, the strategy of pursuing interpretations of select aging phenomena while ignoring the existence of many other phenomena also exhibiting substantial age-related performance differences leads to an unintegrated and chaotic research literature in which each phenomenon has a separate and independent interpretation. Even in the best of circumstances, in which each "explanation" is reasonably well supported by empirical data, the field is left with a potentially enormous number of specific age-affected processes or strategies because of the great diversity of tasks that exhibit age-related differences in performance. Indeed, in an unsystematic survey, Salthouse (1985a, Table 7.1) recently identified 47 "explanations" for cognitive aging phenomena which, if not completely independent, at least employed different phrasing or terminology.

In addition to this proliferation, reliance on postulated differences at the component or strategy level also provides little basis for integrating hypotheses derived from different research areas. For example, an interpretation of adult age differences in memory that has been popular in recent decades is that increased age primarily affects memory processes concerned with retrieval. This speculation has seemed plausible because age differences are often found to be smaller in recognition tests, in which retrieval processes are presumably not very important, than in recall tests, in which retrieval of the information is critical for successful performance. However, a limitation of this type of theorizing is that such interpretations are applicable only to tasks containing a retrieval component (or whatever components or strategies are thought to be critical), and consequently there may be little generality to similar tasks not involving that component, and even less to quite different tasks.

It should be emphasized that the preference for a small number of general causes rather than a multitude of specific causes is not necessarily dictated by empirical observations but is only a theoretical bias, and one that may eventually have to be abandoned if no unifying causal mechanisms can be identified. The goal of seeking a few common principles that might serve to integrate the causes of many different phenomena is clearly more ambitious than the alternative of pursuing independent explanations of each presumably separate phenomenon, but the potential benefits of parsimony and unification justify such efforts. This chapter examines the rationale behind, and evidence for, interpretations of cognitive aging phenomena based on the postulation of general-purpose processing resources presumed to decline in quantity or effectiveness with increased age.

## Review of Resource Interpretations in Cognitive Aging

Reliance on the processing resources concept in explanations of adult age differences in cognition has been both ubiquitous and, in many respects, vacuous. Ubiquitousness of the construct is easy to establish by simply citing a sample of the studies in which age differences in some aspect of cognition have been interpreted in terms of a resource-like concept. For example, an age-related reduction in "processing capacity," "processing resources," "cognitive capacity," "cognitive resources," "intellectual resources," "attentional capacity," "mental energy," or "working-memory capacity" has been mentioned as a potential explanation for age differences in various studies: memory for individual words or their characteristics (Attig & Hasher, 1980; Bromley, 1958; Craik & Byrd, 1982; Craik & Simon, 1980; Duchek, 1984; Howe, this volume; Inman & Parkinson, 1983; Kausler, Hakami, & Wright, 1982; Kausler & Puckett, 1980, 1981; Macht & Buschke, 1983; Parkinson, Inman, & Dannenbaum, 1985; Parkinson, Lindholm, & Urell, 1980; Rabinowitz & Ackerman, 1982; Rabinowitz, Ackerman, Craik, & Hinchley, 1982; Rabinowitz, Craik, & Ackerman, 1982); memory for connected discourse (Arbuckle & Harsany, 1985; Byrd, 1985; Cohen, 1979; Hartley, J., 1986; Hess, 1985; Light & Anderson, 1983, 1985; Petros, Tabor, Cooney, & Chabot, 1983; Spilich, 1983, 1985; Zelinski & Gilewski, this volume); memory for activities (Kausler & Hakami, 1983; Kausler & Lichty, this volume; Kausler, Lichty, & Davis, 1985); reasoning or problem solving (Arenberg, this volume; Arenberg & Robertson-Tchabo, 1985; Charness, 1985; Cohen, 1981; Hartley & Anderson, 1983; Hess, 1982; Hess & Slaughter, 1986; Light, Zelinski, & Moore, 1982; Wright, 1981); and attention and perception (Hoyer & Plude, 1980, 1982; Plude & Hoyer, 1985, 1986; Plude, Hoyer, & Lazar, 1982, Puglisi, 1986). Numerous studies also have focused on the examination of age effects in processes thought to be automatic, a term that is meaningful only if one accepts the existence of some type of general processing resource. That is, automaticity refers to the absence of limitations imposed by a restricted processing resource, and thus investigation of automaticity implies at least tacit acceptance of the concept of processing resources.

Despite its pervasiveness in the contemporary literature, the processing resources concept can be considered vacuous because it has never been explicitly defined in a manner that would allow empirical investigation. Some problems with the resources concept, particularly with respect to the lack of diagnosticity of evidence claimed to justify the processing resources concept, were recently discussed by Navon (1984). However, Navon seemed to accept the sufficiency (as distinct from the necessity) of the resource interpretation for certain nondevelopmental phenomena, and he was relatively unconcerned about the absence of any direct measures of resource quantity. Different concerns appear to be important when resource theory is applied to developmental phenomena. For example, the question of the exclusivity of the resource interpretation as opposed to some alternative interpretation of cognitive aging phenomena is not yet very meaningful, because there are presently no other proposals in the research literature with the breadth and scope of the resource perspective. Moreover, it is still an open question whether the resource interpretation is sufficient to account for cognitive aging phenomena because all resource interpretations are dependent on completely unverified assumptions about resource quantity, both with respect to the amount needed for a task and with respect to the amount available to an individual.

This argument can be elaborated by examining one of the most prominent resource theories in the cognitive aging literature, that proposed by Hasher and Zacks (1979). These theorists relied on an attentional conceptualization of resources by defining attention as "a nonspecific resource for cognitive processing... necessary in varying amounts for carrying out mental operations" (p. 363). They also proposed two hypotheses: first, that encoding operations or tasks vary in their attentional requirements; and second, that attentional capacity varies both within and among individuals, and of particular relevance in the present context, declines in quantity with increased age.

Unfortunately, none of these three critical premises was subjected to investigation. That is, there was no empirical evaluation of the following assumptions: (1) that cognitive performance is influenced by the quantity of processing resources; (2) that cognitive tasks vary in their resource requirements; and (3) that increased age is associated with a reduction in the amount of available resources. Without some means of verifying these assumptions, or at least establishing their general plausibility, the meaningfulness of the resources construct in explanations of age differences in cognitive functioning can be questioned (cf. Salthouse, 1982). Under some circumstances, the reasoning becomes completely circular because the existence of age differences in performance is attributed to a reduction in the quantity of processing resources, and the reduction in amount of processing resources is inferred on the basis of the age differences in performance. This type of usage of the processing resources concept may even impair progress, because as Navon (1984) has warned, it may "divert... attention from the absence of substantive explanations for behavior" (p. 232).

Baddeley (1981) expressed similar reservations about the concept of working memory, which can be considered one particular type of processing resource:

> Given almost any poorly understood performance decrement, it is possible to attribute it to the inadequate performance of... (working memory). Hence, if the concept is to be useful, it is important that an attempt is made to ensure that it is not simply used as a label for one's ignorance of the underlying cause of a given decrement. (p. 18)

As Baddeley implies, the way to make an explanatory construct meaningful is to subject it to empirical investigation. This is a primary goal of this chapter, especially with respect to examining the assumptions that processing resources decline with increased age and this reduction is responsible for many age differences in cognitive functioning.

## Investigating Processing Resources

Although one's first impression is that it should be easy to obtain evidence relevant to the existence of a general age-related factor influencing performance across a variety of different cognitive tasks, closer examination reveals considerable difficulties with this endeavor. For example, one might expect that if the age differences in an assortment of tasks result from reduction in the amount of some critical processing resource, then performance on all tasks requiring that resource should be impaired to a similar degree. A further expectation might be that scores from different resource-dependent tasks should all be highly correlated. However, this reasoning fails to consider that there are multiple determinants of performance on virtually every task, and thus the absolute level of performance may not be predictable from knowledge of a single determinant. It is also unlikely that the variance attributable to nonresource factors will change simply because the quantity of the resource has declined. Therefore while the overall level of performance should be lower among the individuals thought to have smaller amounts of the critical resource, the scores from those individuals need not exhibit higher intercorrelations than those from a group with greater amounts of the resource.

Moreover, because the magnitude of a correlation is affected by the range of the scores involved in that correlation, the size of the correlations may be influenced by what might be considered rather uninteresting nonresource factors. For example, the correlations could increase with age if the interindividual variability (and hence the range of scores) increases because some individuals experience losses in the resource while others do not. On the other hand, the correlations could decrease with age if the lower overall level of performance reduces the interindividual variability because of a measurement floor. Mere inspection of the pattern of correlations is therefore not a satisfactory means of investigating the existence of general-purpose processing resources because a pattern of higher average correlations is neither necessary nor sufficient to infer a general factor.

Another possible means of investigating the influence of general-purpose processing resources in cognitive age differences relies on secondary task methods to infer the amount of processing resources available to different individuals. Most secondary task procedures involve performance assessment in a secondary task performed alone and concurrent with a primary task, and then use an index of the difference in performance as a reflection of the processing demands of the primary task. The logic of the approach is straightforward and based on two assumptions: (a) the primary and secondary tasks compete for the same type of processing resource; and (b) performance on the secondary task reflects the quantity of processing resources remaining after the amount required by the primary task has been allocated.

Although the secondary task procedure could be extended to individual difference comparisons by using performance on the secondary task as a reflection of the total amount of processing resources available to the individual, application of this procedure in research on individual differences has several complications. One is that there is no means of determining that the demands for processing resources by the primary and secondary tasks are equivalent in different individuals. Misleading inferences about the relative amounts of processing resources would result if one or both tasks required more processing resources for successful execution in some individuals than in others.

A second potential problem is that individuals might vary in the proportion of their available resources allocated to the two tasks or in the concurrence cost associated with performing two simultaneous activities. To illustrate, consider the difficulty of inferring the quantity of resources in two individuals if one person allocates only 80% of his or her total resources while another allocates 100%, or if one person can coordinate two simultaneous activities only by using an additional 5% of the total resources while another can coordinate them without any additional resource requirements.

Still another complication with the secondary task procedure for estimating the quantity of processing resources in individuals is that people might differ in the relation between resource quantity and secondary task performance. That is, one unit of resource might correspond to a change of three units of secondary task performance in one individual, but to a change of five units of secondary task performance in another individual. Without some means of ensuring equivalent mapping of resource quantity to task performance, it may be meaningless to estimate the amount of available processing resources on the basis of secondary task performance.

The large number of unverified assumptions needed to make relevant inferences about the quantity of processing resources available to an individual clearly weakens the confidence one could have in any conclusions derived from the secondary task procedure. Therefore, in light of these and other problems (cf. Salthouse, 1982, 1985a), it is desirable that alternative procedures for assessing the amount of available processing resources should be pursued.

A more promising approach to investigating the contribution of processing resources to cognitive aging phenomena examines the pattern of age differences across tasks presumed to differ in the amount of resources required for successful performance. The rationale underlying this approach can be illustrated with the aid of Figures 7.1 and 7.2 portraying hypothesized relations among available resources, resource demands, and performance. Small to nonexistent variations in performance across different amounts of resource availability are postulated when the resource demands are low, but

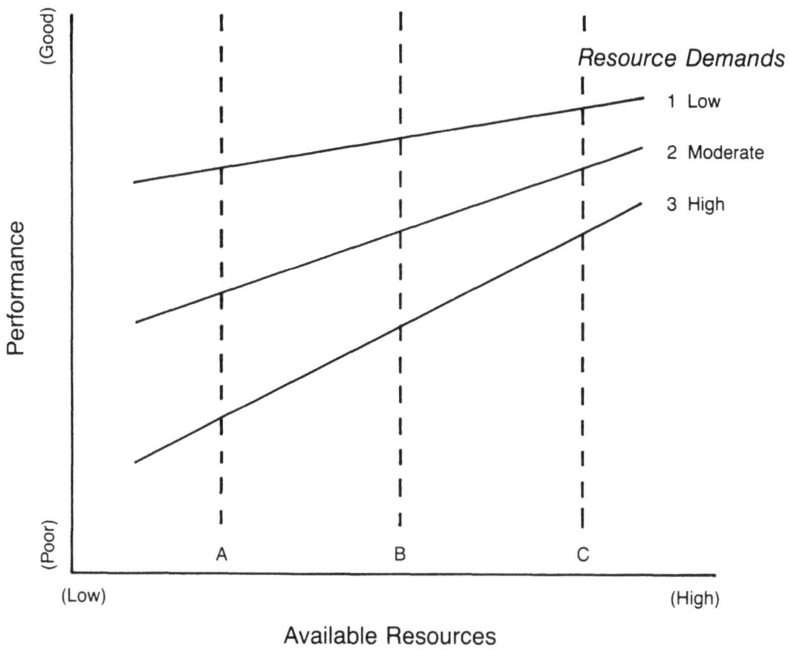


FIGURE 7.1. Hypothesized relations between performance and amount of available resources for different levels of resource demands.

progressively larger effects of resource availability on performance are expected as the resource demands increase (Figure 7.1). A complementary perspective on the relations among these variables is illustrated in Figure 7.2. Here resource demands are postulated to have relatively small effects on performance when there are many resources available, but performance is expected to decline dramatically with increased resource demands when available resources are low.

Figures 7.1 and 7.2 are relevant to the current discussion if one assumes that increased age leads to a reduction in the amount of available resources, and that an increase in the complexity of the task is often associated with an increased demand for resources. Viewed from this perspective, the preceding arguments provide an explanation for the well-established "Complexity Effect Phenomenon," that is, the tendency for the magnitude of age differences in performance to increase as the task becomes more complex (Botwinick, 1978; Cerella, Poon, & Williams, 1980; Crowder, 1980; Salthouse, 1982, 1985a, 1985b). In the representations of Figures 7.1 and 7.2, older adults can be considered analogous to A and young adults to C, while simple tasks are represented by the number 1 and complex tasks represented by the number 3. According to the resource interpretation, the complexity effect (i.e., a larger

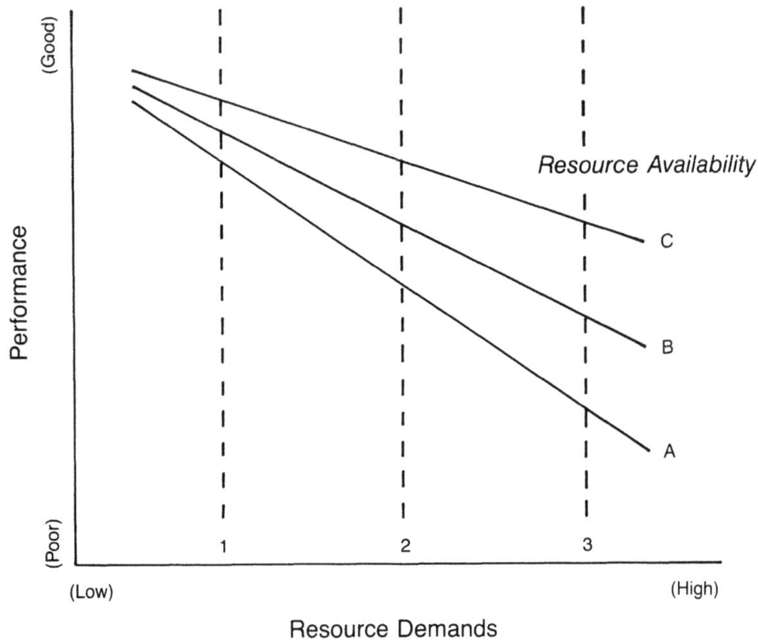


FIGURE 7.2. Hypothesized relations between performance and level of resource demands for different amounts of available processing resources.

difference between conditions 1 and 3 at the A level of resources than at the C level of resources) is attributable to the more complex tasks demanding more of the resources that are in lower supply with increased age.

The resource interpretation of the complexity effect would be particularly compelling if it could be demonstrated that the complexity or resource demands in the experimental situation could be increased without introducing any new processes or operations, but instead by simply increasing the number of repetitions of the same processes or operation. A qualitative interpretation of the complexity effect phenomenon, in which the reduced performance is attributed to a new operation or different strategy that is particularly age sensitive, would presumably be inadequate to account for the phenomenon if it was evident when the resource demands were increased without changing the identity of the required operations. Notice, however, that this argument is not symmetrical in that a quantitative (resource) interpretation could still apply even when complexity is increased by the introduction of a qualitatively new processing component, because the total resource demands can be assumed to increase by the addition of any new operation.[1]

[1]Although it is frequently convenient to express the differences between resource and nonresource theories in terms of a quantitative–qualitative distinction, it should be recognized that this is somewhat misleading because quantitative variations could easily be responsible for what appear to be qualitative differences (Salthouse, 1982, 1985a).

A further expectation from the resources interpretation is that if the quantity of available processing resources determines the amount by which increases in the processing requirements of the task affects performance, then the slopes of the complexity functions from different tasks should be positively correlated with one another. In other words, if a steep slope of the function relating performance to task complexity or processing demands is an indication that necessary processing resources are in short supply, then an individual who has a steep slope in one task should also have a steep slope in another task requiring the same type of processing resources. Correlations among slope parameters derived from quantitative manipulations of complexity across different tasks can therefore be examined to evaluate the construct validity of the notion of general-purpose processing resources. Very low correlations would weaken confidence in the meaningfulness of the construct, while moderate to high correlations should enhance one's belief in the existence of general-purpose processing resources.

Although the concept of general-purpose processing resources has been presumed to have wide applicability, it is important to realize that resources are not the only determinant of cognitive performance. Interpretations of age differences in cognition from the resource perspective must therefore be sensitive to factors such as data-limited influences, strategic and experiential variation, and a variety of measurement-related characteristics. Failure to appreciate the contribution of nonresource factors in cognitive aging has sometimes led to the misperception that resource interpretations lead to the expectation of a proportionally equivalent, nonmodifiable, decrement across virtually all cognitive tasks. These extreme claims clearly do not pertain to resource-based theories in which both the amount of resource dependence, and the influence of a variety of other factors, are postulated to vary across and within different cognitive tasks.

The distinction between resource-limited and data-limited processes was introduced by Norman and Bobrow (1975), who postulated that performance could be restricted either by the amount of resources or by the availability of data, with the latter broadly interpreted as the material on which the resource-limited processes operate. Therefore, if increased age results in a reduction in the quality of data, then at least some of the age differences in performance might result from data limitations rather than resource limitations.

Because some processing strategies may be more resource efficient than others, inferences about resource quantity should be made only when one is fairly confident that all comparisons involve the same strategy of performing the task. Although this goal is theoretically well-justified, it may be quite difficult to achieve in practice because some strategies may require more resources than are presently available, and the supply of available resources could influence the selection of particular strategies.

Degree of experience or level of expertise is also a potentially important consideration; the amount of processing resources needed to perform a task successfully may decrease as experience increases and the task presumably becomes more automated. Comparison of individuals from different ages without attempting to control amount of relevant experience may therefore be so confounded as to preclude meaningful inferences.

Measurement characteristics, such as floor and ceiling effects in one or more age groups, may also distort the relation between resources and performance, and could result in misleading inferences if not recognized and properly interpreted.

The preceding discussion can be summarized in terms of Eq. (1), in which P represents performance on a cognitive task, R represents the quantity of available resources, and D indicates the demand for resources placed by that task at a given stage of practice or experience:

$$P = R/D + \text{Other Determinants.} \tag{1}$$

This equation makes explicit the assumption that cognitive performance is influenced by the quantity of resources relative to the demands upon those resources, plus a variety of other determinants. Therefore, only if those other determinants are held relatively constant could one successfully investigate the contribution of processing resources to performance.

One means of minimizing the influence of nonresource determinants is to systematically vary the hypothesized resource demands while keeping all other aspects of the task the same. An index of the differences in performance across variations in resource demands, such as the slope of functions like those in Figure 7.2, might then serve as a measure of resource-dependent performance. This is only one possible procedure, but it is essential that some analytical strategy be used to distinguish between resource and nonresource determinants of performance if one is attempting to investigate only the former and not a combination of both.

If one can assume that nonresource determinants of the performance measure are minimal, Eq. (1) can be simplified to Eqs. (2) and (3) for young and old adults, respectively:

$$P'y = Ry/Dy \tag{2}$$

$$P'o = Ro/Do \tag{3}$$

where the prime indicates that the performance measures are 'purified' from nonresource influences. By further assuming that the task demands for processing resources are comparable in young and old adults,[2] the D terms in the equations become identical and provide a basis for rearranging the terms into Eq. (4). That is, because

[2]This assumption derives from the basic premise of resource theories that an age-related reduction in resource quantity is responsible for most of the observed age differences in performance. Because P = R/D, an equivalent assumption is that resource quantity remains constant and resource demands increase. However, if both resource quantity declined and resource demands increased, then the computational equations that follow would lead to overestimates of the amount of resource reduction.

$$Dy = Ry/P'y \text{ and } Do = Ro/P'o$$

when Dy = Do = D, then

$$D = Ry/P'y = Ro/P'o. \quad (4)$$

One more rearrangement of terms results in Eq. (5):

$$Ro/Ry = P'o/P'y, \quad (5)$$

which indicates that the ratio of (a resource-dependent measure of) the performance of old adults to (a resource-dependent measure of) the performance of young adults provides an estimate of the amount of resources available to old adults compared to that available to young adults. However, because performance is often scaled with higher numbers indicating poorer performance (e.g., time or errors), while a greater quantity of resources is always postulated to lead to better performance, it is frequently convenient to represent the P'o and P'y terms as the reciprocals of actual performance. Moreover, because the ratio of reciprocals is equivalent to exchanging the numerator and denominator in the initial ratio, Eq. (6) will apply in situations in which better performance is represented by smaller numbers:

$$Ro/Ry = P'y/P'o. \quad (6)$$

The reasoning culminating in Eq. (6) suggests it might be possible to obtain an estimate of the relative amount of processing resources available to young and old adults by examining the ratio of the complexity-function slopes in the two age groups. That is, if an index of performance is determined by the ratio of the supply of processing resources to the demand for those resources, and if the demand can be assumed to be equivalent across young and old adults, then the quantity of resources available to old adults relative to that available to young adults can be estimated from the reciprocal of the ratio of the performance of young adults to the performance of old adults.

To summarize, three techniques are proposed to investigate issues related to the role of processing resources in age differences in cognitive performance. First, the plausibility of invoking a general explanatory construct such as processing resources will be addressed by determining if the complexity effect phenomenon can be demonstrated with quantitative manipulations of complexity. A result of this type will suggest that age differences are influenced by *how much* processing is required, and not necessarily *which kind* of processing. Second, the validity of the resources construct will be strengthened if moderate to high positive correlations are obtained among the slopes of complexity-performance functions from different tasks, suggesting that a common entity is involved in each of the functions. Third, the relative amount of resources available to young and old adults will be estimated from the ratio of an index of resource-dependent performance in the two groups.

## What Is the Nature of the Processing Resource?

The question of the specific type of processing resource (as opposed to the questions of whether there is any processing resource, or how much of whatever resource) involved in cognitive age differences might be answerable by correlational analyses. Three alternative models of the interrelations of age, resource quantity, and performance are summarized in Table 7.1 along with predictions derived from each model concerning the relative magnitudes of specified correlations. Model 1 is the strongest and purest form of a processing resource model; the age-related reduction in resource quantity is assumed to be directly and completely responsible for observed age-related differences in cognitive performance. If this causal path is correct, one should find that statistical control of the resource factor by means of partial or semipartial[3] correlations should eliminate, or at least greatly attenuate, the relation between age and performance, but that comparable control of the age variable should have relatively little effect on the magnitude of the resource-performance correlation.

Model 2 differs from Model 1 in that the quantity of processing resource is not assumed to be the only age-related determinant of performance. In this respect, Model 2 is a weak version of the resource interpretation. Because age is presumed to have a direct (or at least not resource-mediated) influence on cognitive performance in addition to the indirect one mediated by the processing resources, statistical control of the resources should reduce, but not completely eliminate, the association between age and performance. Statistical control of age should disrupt the nonresource linkage between age and performance, and thus the variance common to the resource and perfor-

TABLE 7.1. Three Alternative Conceptualizations of the Interrelations of Age, Cognitive Performance, and Resource Quantity

| Model[a] | Predictions | |
|---|---|---|
| $A \rightarrow R \rightarrow P$ | AP.R = 0 | RP = RP.A |
| $A \rightarrow R \rightarrow P$ | AP > AP.R > 0 | RP > RP.A > 0 |
| └────────↑ | | |
| $R \leftarrow A \rightarrow P$ | AP = AP.R | RP.A = 0 |

[a]A = age, R = resource quantity, and P = cognitive performance.

[3]The method of statistical control employed in the present studies was partial correlation. Horn (1982; Horn, Donaldson, & Engstrom 1981) has suggested that partial or semipartial correlations might be preferable, but because the goal is to remove the age-resource relation from the age-performance relation, and not simply to remove the influence of the resource on the performance variable, the partial correlation procedure seems more appropriate in the present case (Salthouse, 1985a). In fact, however, the same qualitative pattern was evident with both part and partial correlations, although the former were generally smaller in magnitude than the latter.

mance variables should be reduced by the amount of their joint variance also shared by the age variable.

Model 3 differs in representing the resource and performance variables as separate correlates of age rather than as one mediating the other. According to this model, therefore, there should be little if any reduction in the age-performance correlation by statistically controlling for the amount of resource, but a substantial reduction in the resource-performance correlation by controlling for age.

The predictions summarized in (Table 7.1) suggest a means of investigating the nature of the processing resource presumed to be responsible for age-related differences in cognition, because different resource indices should be differentially successful in their degree of fit to the strong resource interpretation represented by Model 1. The major obstacle in conducting this type of investigation is identifying suitable measures to serve as markers for different types of processing resources. It is obviously difficult to subject the resources perspective to empirical investigation without operational definitions of what one means by a processing resource, and it is simply impossible to attempt a comparative evaluation of several alternative resource candidates without suitable procedures to estimate the quantity of each.

One means of identifying appropriate measures of different types of resources is to categorize the ways in which the processing resources concept has been employed in the research literature, and then to select optimal measures from each category. Salthouse (1985a) suggested the major usages of the processing resources construct in cognitive psychology can be classified into three broad categories roughly analogous to the concepts of space, energy, and time. The space conceptualization of resources is based on the notion of a finite working-memory capacity that serves as the storage and computational workspace for most of one's cognitive work. Because this space is presumed to be the region where cognitive operations are performed and intermediate products are temporarily stored, its size or area could be a very important processing resource. Moreover, if the size of the workspace becomes smaller with increased age, then most processes requiring access to that critical area will be impaired, in terms either of reduced accuracy because of loss of information or of increased time because of the need to perform many more time-consuming operations moving information to and from long-term memory.

The conceptualization of resources as energy can be traced to Spearman (1927), who introduced the term "mental energy" to account for individual differences in his g factor, but it has been more recently popularized by Kahneman (1973) in the guise of attentional capacity or mental effort. An energistic conceptualization is implied by the usage of such terms in discussions of processing resources as "resource reservoir," "pool of capacity," and the "draining," "channeling," or "expenditure" of capacity or resources. The exact nature of the energy has never been explicitly identified, but virtually anything would be considered an energy-like resource if it functioned as a "fuel" for information processing. Furthermore, if the amount of this "mental energy" available to allocate to cognitive processes declines with age, then it is reasonable to expect age-related declines in all tasks that normally require that energy for their successful performance.

The conceptualization of resources in terms of time is rather new, although it has been used in a related sense by researchers such as Jensen (1982) and Eysenck (1967) in the field of psychometric intelligence. The fundamental premise is that individuals who take longer to perform elementary cognitive operations are frequently less accurate than faster individuals, either because the relevant information from the environment has changed, because the products of earlier operations have been lost by the time later operations requiring that information are completed, or because a combination results in an inability to execute more abstract levels of processing based upon the products of lower level processing. In these respects time is a processing resource because the quicker or faster operations are executed, the more likely it is that other operations can be initiated and completed. To the extent that increased age is associated with a progressive slowing in the time to process information, therefore, many of the cognitive deficits associated with aging may be attributable to this decrease in the rate at which basic cognitive operations are executed.

It should be emphasized that this tripartite classification scheme is intended only as a first approximation, and neither the number of categories nor the boundaries between them should be interpreted as fixed and rigid. In some respects the classification scheme might be considered unduly precise because certain conceptualizations of processing resources may fit in two or more categories. For example, working memory might be hypothesized to be limited by space factors, in the sense that there is a maximum number of items that can be maintained, and by either energy or time factors because expenditure of energy or rapid execution of operations may be needed to keep that maximum number of items active. On the other hand, it could also be argued that the distinction among only three categories is too gross and unrefined. That is, there is currently considerable controversy about whether there are single or multiple forms of working memory (e.g., Baddeley, 1981; Brainerd & Kingma, 1985; Reisberg, Rappaport, & O'Shaughnessy, 1984) and whether there is only one or many pools of attentional capacity (e.g., Navon & Gopher, 1979; Wickens, 1980), and thus it could be argued that more than three distinct categories are necessary.

Despite these limitations, the classification of processing resources in terms of space, energy, and time is useful in providing an initial categorization of a concept that has heretofore resisted precise definition and investigation. The next logical step is to identify variables that might be used to index the quantity of processing resources corresponding to the contructs of space, energy, and time. Unfortunately, there is currently little consensus on this issue, even among proponents of a particular type of processing resource.

(There has also been considerable debate regarding the number of distinct types of resources that must be postulated to coexist within an individual, but unless there are only a few general-purpose resources the resource interpretation becomes functionally indistinguishable from the perspective postulating multiple independent determinants of cognitive aging phenomena.) To select promising indices of each type of resource, criteria are proposed that could be used to evaluate alternative candidate measures of resource quantity.

One essential criterion is that the potential processing-resource measure should be very reliable in terms of consistency of measurement and with respect to the stability of the underlying phenomenon. Unless one is confident that the variable is consistent in assessing the resources construct, and that the quantity of resources does not change substantially across time, then it may be fruitless to attempt to interpret any results involving that variable.

The second and third criteria are also related to classical issues in testing, and concern the convergent and discriminant validity of the measure. Convergent validity is important because unless the measure is correlated with other measures presumed to reflect the same construct, the variable may not really assess what it is proposed to measure. It is also important to establish that the variable is not merely providing another assessment of some other construct by demonstrating that the variable is not highly correlated with variables postulated to reflect different constructs.

The fourth proposed criterion for a suitable resource index is that the variable should exhibit a moderately large negative correlation with adult age. A negative relation between resource quantity and age is required if the resource is assumed to be responsible for age-related performance differences, because it is obviously impossible for age declines in cognitive performance to be mediated by age reductions in resource quantity if there is no evidence that the amount of resources does in fact decline with age.

The final criterion presumed necessary for an index of processing resources is that the variable should have at least a moderately large positive correlation with cognitive performance. Unless there is evidence that greater quantities of the resource are associated with better performance on cognitive tasks, it is unreasonable to attempt to explain age differences in cognition in terms of a reduction in the quantity of that resource (cf. Horn's [1982] discussion of this topic which he refers to as "the missing-link issue").

The three studies that follow were designed to identify suitable measures to index the space (working-memory) and time (processing speed) conceptualizations of processing resources and to then use them in investigating the role of processing resources in cognitive aging. No attempt was made to evaluate the energy conceptualization of processing resources because of the difficulty of identifying measures that have plausibility as indices of the quantity of mental or attentional energy.

## Study 1

The purpose of the first study was to examine several candidate measures of the speed and working-memory conceptualizations of processing resources in terms of the evaluation criteria previously identified. It would have been desirable to use factor-analytically defined measures as the resource indices, but limitations on time available for testing after administration of the primary tasks in subsequent studies dictated that each resource be assessed with a single measure. Thus, this study attempted to identify a single best measure for each relevant resource. Tasks selected to assess speed of processing consisted of very simple repetitive activities such as substituting symbols for digits, comparing numbers or pictures, and locating specified targets. Because working memory is often assumed to involve the active manipulation or transformation of information and not simply its passive maintenance (Craik & Rabinowitz, 1984; Daneman & Carpenter, 1980), these tasks required some type of operation to be performed on the to-be-remembered material. In different tasks, all involving random digit stimuli, the subjects (a) repeated the digit sequence in a reversed order; (b) repeated the digits after first subtracting two from each digit; (c) identified the missing digit when the sequence was repeated in a random order; and (d) remembered digits while simultaneously performing arithmetic operations on them.

### Method

*Subjects.* Sixteen women[4] and 4 men aged 18 to 26 years (mean, 19.2), and 17 women and 3 men aged 58 to 75 years (mean, 69.6), participated in a single experimental session of approximately 1 hour. Self-reported health status on a 5-point scale (1 = Excellent, 5 = Poor) averaged 1.6 for the young adults and 1.9 for the older adults, with 100% of each group reporting themselves to be in average or better-than-average health (i.e., a rating of 3 or less on the scale). The young subjects averaged 12.6 years of education (range, 11 to 14), and the older subjects 16.3 (range, 10 to 22).

*Procedure.* The same sequence of eight tasks was administered to each subject twice in a counterbalanced order. Four tasks were designed to assess the speed of performing simple activities, and four to provide estimates of the capacity of working memory. The speed tasks were a specially constructed Digit Symbol Substitution test very similar to that employed in the WAIS, the

[4]Although an attempt was made to balance the ratio of males and females in the young and old age groups in this and subsequent studies, no analyses of the sex differences are discussed in the text: sex differences were evident only in the Digit Symbol scores among the young subjects (females were faster than males), and were not apparent in any of the other measures in any study for either age group.

Finding A's test, the Number Comparison test, and the Identical Pictures test. These last three tests are from the ETS Cognitive Reference Battery (French, Ekstrom, & Price, 1963), and have been postulated to index a factor of perceptual speed. The time limits were 90 seconds to write the symbols associated with digits in the Digit Symbol Substitution test, 120 seconds to locate all words containing the letter 'a' in the Finding A's test, 90 seconds to determine whether sets of digits were the same or different in the Number Comparison test, and 90 seconds to select identical pictures from sets of five alternatives in the Identical Pictures test. Performance on each task was represented by the number of items correctly completed in the designated time.

The four memory tests were the Backwards Digit Span from the WAIS, and specially devised procedures termed the Subtract Two Span, the Missing Digit Span, and the Computational Span. In the Backwards Digit Span task the subjects were instructed to repeat an orally presented digit sequence in the reverse order of presentation. In the Subtract Two Span task, subjects attempted to repeat the original sequence of orally presented digits after first subtracting 2 from each digit. In the Missing Digit Span task, the subject heard two random strings of digits in different sequential orders, with the first string containing one digit not present in the second string. The task for the subject was to identify the digit from the first string missing from the second. The Computational Span task consisted of the subject attempting to remember the last digit in each of a series of orally presented arithmetic problems while concurrently solving these problems. All arithmetic problems involved one addition operation and one subtraction operation, and resulted in a digit different from the to-be-remembered digit in that problem.

Each of the memory tasks started with a series length of two digits and increased by one digit when the subject was correct on at least one of two attempts at that sequence length. The tasks were terminated after two failures at a given sequence length, and the span then identified as the number of digits in the previous (successful) sequence. If a subject was unsuccessful at both attempts with the two-digit sequence, the procedure was repeated with only a single digit to be remembered.

## Results and Discussion

The major results of this study are summarized in Tables 7.2 and 7.3. Table 7.2 displays the means and standard deviations of the performance measures, averaged across the two administrations of each task, for the 20 young subjects and the 20 older subjects. Also presented in this table are three indices of the magnitude of the age differences for each variable: (a) average performance of the older subjects expressed as a percentage of the average performance of the subjects; (b) the number of standard deviations (from the distribution of young scores) separating the average older subject from the mean of the younger subjects; and (c) the correlation between age and level

TABLE 7.2. Mean Levels of Performance and Three Indices of the Age Differences for the Speed and Memory Measures, Study 1

| Measure | Young | | Old | | Old as % of Young | Old in Young (SD) | Correlation with Age |
|---|---|---|---|---|---|---|---|
| Digit Symbol | 71.7 | (11.4)[a] | 45.2 | (8.6) | 63.0 | −2.32 | −.82 |
| Finding A's | 35.0 | (11.4) | 27.5 | (7.3) | 78.6 | −0.66 | −.40 |
| Number Comparison | 27.9 | (5.3) | 21.1 | (3.5) | 75.6 | −1.28 | −.65 |
| Identical Pictures | 37.6 | (5.3) | 21.7 | (2.7) | 57.7 | −3.00 | −.90 |
| Backwards Digit Span | 6.20 | (1.45) | 5.23 | (1.87) | 84.4 | −0.67 | −.31 |
| Subtract Two Span | 5.88 | (1.10) | 4.93 | (1.31) | 83.8 | −0.86 | −.38 |
| Missing Digit Span | 7.35 | (1.81) | 7.13 | (1.31) | 97.0 | −0.12 | −.08 |
| Comp. Span | 3.63 | (1.18) | 2.00 | (1.01) | 55.1 | −1.38 | −.59 |

[a]Values in parentheses are standard deviations.

of performance. (Note that because these correlations are based upon only two extreme age groups they are inflated relative to that expected from a complete distribution of ages.)

Correlations among the eight performance variables are displayed in Table 7.3, with entries above the diagonal based upon data from the young subjects and entries below the diagonal based upon data from older subjects. Values in parentheses along the diagonal are estimated reliabilities obtained by using the Spearman–Brown formula to boost the correlation between the scores on the two administrations of each test to predict the reliability of the average score. Note that although the reliabilities pertain to the average score, they reflect some degree of stability as well as consistency because in each case they are derived from two temporally spaced assessments.

The data in Tables 7.2 and 7.3 can be used to evaluate the eight variables with respect to their suitability as indices of their respective processing resources. Table 7.3 indicates that most of the measures had respectable reliability in at least one of the two age groups. The speed measure with the highest average reliability across young and old groups was Digit Symbol score, with a mean of 0.91, and the memory measure with the highest average reliability was Backwards Digit Span, with a mean of 0.82.

Also evident in Table 7.3 is that the speed and memory measures had the desired pattern of convergent and discriminant validity, in that the correlations among measures indexing the same construct were generally larger than those reflecting different constructs. For the young adults the median correlation among speed measures was .41 and that among memory mea-

TABLE 7.3. Correlation Matrix for Speed and Memory Variables for 20 Young Adults (above diagonal) and 20 Older Adults (below diagonal), Study 1[a]

| | DigSym | FindAs | NumCom | IdPict | BckSpn | SubSpn | MisSpn | CmpSpn |
|---|---|---|---|---|---|---|---|---|
| DigSym | (.92/.90) | .37 | .65** | .45* | .47* | .24 | .28 | −.08 |
| FindAs | .41 | (.89/.89) | .60** | .17 | .11 | .05 | .27 | −.36 |
| NumCom | .43 | .55* | (.85/.81) | .11 | .37 | .12 | .21 | −.32 |
| IdPict | .49* | .54* | .63** | (.84/.56) | −.00 | −.13 | .19 | .14 |
| BckSpn | .14 | .06 | .43 | .11 | (.69/.94) | .64** | .51* | .25 |
| SubSpn | .12 | .26 | .47* | .20 | .84** | (.49/.83) | .37 | .59* |
| MisSpn | .27 | .49* | .33 | .16 | .18 | .43 | (.82/.12) | .13 |
| CmpSpn | .42 | .23 | .00 | .27 | .39 | .53* | .46* | (.65/.57) |

[a]DigSym = digit symbol substitution;
FindAs = finding as;
NumCom = number comparison;
IdPict = identical pictures;
BckSpn = backwards digit span;
SubSpn = subtract two span;
MisSpn = missing digit span;
CmpSpn = computational span;
* = $p < .05$;
** = $p < .01$.

sures was .44, compared to a median across-construct correlation of .17. Results were similar for the older adults in that the medians were .52 for speed-speed correlations and .45 for memory-memory correlations, but only .25 for correlations between speed measures and memory measures.

The data in Table 7.2 indicate that only the Missing Digit Span measure failed to clearly differentiate between young and old subjects. However, additional considerations serve to further limit the measures that might be suitable as indices of processing resources. One is that perceptual factors probably contributed to some of the age differences with the Identical Pictures measure because many of the response alternatives were visually very similar to the target item, and rather poor reproduction quality of the test forms added to the difficulty of discrimination. A second consideration in evaluating the age sensitivity of the various measures as resource indices is that many of the scores in the Computational Span procedure were very near the minimum value. In fact, 45% of the scores of the older subjects consisted of a value of 1, with an additional 28% of the scores consisting of a value of 2. Because very few of the young subjects had scores this low, the sensitivity of the measure to increased age is not in dispute. However, the existence of such a large number of scores near the minimum value is an undesirable measurement characteristic because it makes the true range of scores impossible to determine.

Based upon the information reported here, two reasonable indices of the speed and working-memory resource constructs appear to be Digit Symbol score as a reflection of speed of processing, and Backwards Digit Span as a reflection of working-memory capacity. (See Salthouse, 1985a, for further discussion of the Digit Symbol score as an index of processing speed.) Other measures are certainly possible, but these two possess the desired mix of high reliability and high age sensitivity, and have the additional advantage of having been widely used as subtests in the popular WAIS battery. They were therefore used to index the speed and memory conceptualizations of processing resources in the next study.

## Study 2

Study 2 had three major goals. The first was to determine whether a complexity effect phenomenon would be produced by systematically manipulating the number of repetitions of the same type of processing operation. As discussed earlier, a resource interpretation of age differences in cognition would receive considerable support if it could be demonstrated that the complexity effect phenomenon, that is, the tendency for the magnitude of age differences to increase with the complexity of the task, was evident even when complexity was increased without adding any new processing operations. Three different tasks involving four distinct manipulations of complexity were used to investigate the generality of the complexity effect with quantitative rather than qualitative variations in complexity.

The second goal of the study was to use the data from the task complexity manipulations to derive estimates of the relative quantities of the critical processing resource in older and young adults. That is, following the arguments outlined above, slopes will be computed from the functions relating performance to complexity, and then the ratio of these slopes in young and old subjects will be used to make inferences about the ratio of resource quantities in the two groups. Correlations among the slopes will also be examined to assess the construct validity of the processing-resources notion (i.e., moderate-to-high correlations are expected if the slopes of each function are determined by the quantity of the same type of processing resource).

The third major goal of Study 2 was to examine the correlations among the variables indexing age, cognitive performance, and the speed and memory conceptualizations of processing resources to allow inferences about the nature of the processing resource involved in the age differences in cognition.

Three different types of tasks from the domains of spatial ability and reasoning were employed to provide measures of cognitive performance. Selection of the cognitive tasks was somewhat arbitrary, but guided by two considerations. The first was a desire to assess performance in at least two ability areas seemingly unrelated to the proposed resources of speed and memory. The second consideration in selecting tasks was that the tasks must have been amenable to quantitative variations in complexity by increasing the number of repetitions of some critical processing operation. Tasks that met these qualifications were a Visual Synthesis task involving the integration of spatially distinct figural segments, a Paper Folding task requiring spatial manipulations of a two-dimensional object, and a Geometric Analogies task in which subjects had to decide whether the two terms on each side of an equation had equivalent transformations of their respective elements. Relatively large sample sizes (i.e., $n = 100$ in each age group) were employed to maximize precision in the determination of resource quantity, and to increase confidence in the results of the correlational analyses. In view of the statistical power of the tests with these large samples, a rather conservative .01 level of statistical significance was established.

## Method

*Subjects.* Sixty-two women and 38 men aged between 18 and 25 years (mean, 19.1), and 63 women and 37 men aged between 57 and 67 years (mean, 62.4), participated in a single experimental session of approximately 1.5 hours. Self-reported health status (1 = Excellent, 5 = Poor) averaged 1.2 for the young adults and 2.0 for the older adults; 96% of the former and 94% of the latter reported themselves to be in average or better-than-average health. The range of education in the young group was 12 to 15 years (mean, 12.4), and that in the older group 8 to 20 (mean, 14.2).

*Procedure.* All subjects were tested individually and performed eight tasks in an identical sequence. The first two tasks, which were also administered at the end of the session as the seventh and eighth tasks, were the Digit Symbol Substitution and Backwards Digit Span tasks from the WAIS.

The remaining four tasks were presented in a paper-and-pencil format, with the subject providing oral YES/NO responses. Each task consisted of 16 pages with four problems of the same level of complexity per page. Half of the problems should have been answered YES because they involved similar configurations on the left and right sides of the problem, and half should have been answered NO because they consisted of mismatching configurations on the two sides of an equal sign. The four complexity conditions within each task were distributed across the 16 pages in a counterbalanced order, starting with the least complex problems and then increasing, decreasing, increasing, and finally decreasing again. The subjects were instructed to respond accurately, and as soon as they knew the answer to the problem, but they were allowed as much time as necessary to respond. A stopwatch was used to record the time to answer all four problems on a given page, and this value then divided by four to obtain a measure of average time per problem on that page.

The Visual Synthesis task involved the subject attempting to integrate spatially separated line segments of a 12-segment pattern into a composite figure, and then determine whether it matched a comparison figure. In the least complex condition no integration was required because a single 12-segment figure was presented on both the lett and right sides of the problem. As complexity increased the number of frames needing to be integrated also increased, starting with two frames of 6 segments each, to three frames of 4 segments each, and finally to four frames of 3 segments each.

The Paper Folding test was based on a test of the same name in the ETS Cognitive Reference Battery (French et al., 1963), and consisted of illustrations of zero to three folds of a piece of paper before a hole was punched in the folded paper. The subject in this task was instructed to determine whether, when unfolded, the paper would match the pattern of holes illustrated in a comparison figure. In the least complex condition no spatial manipulation was required because the left and right sides of the problem both contained unfolded pages with patterns of holes. Complexity was increased by adding successively more folds (i.e., one, two, or three) before the indicated punching of the hole.

The remaining two tasks consisted of slightly different versions of a geometric analogies test patterned after a task employed by Mulholland, Pellegrino, and Glaser (1980). Each version consisted of problems of the A:B::C:D form, with the goal of deciding whether the D term was correct for the rest of the analogy. Letters were used as the elements in the problem, with transformations between the two terms on each side of the equation consisting of alterations in size, completeness, rotation, or black/white reversal. One version of the task involved three elements per term with complexity varied by the presence of one, two, three or four elements per term.

## Results and Discussion

The first aspect of the results to be discussed concern those relevant to the complexity effect phenomenon. Figures 7.3, 7.4, 7.5, and 7.6 display the mean time per problem and the mean percentage of errors for the young and older adults at each of four levels of complexity for each task. These data were analyzed with separate two-factor (Age and Complexity Level) analyses of variance on each dependent measure. Both main effects were significant ($F > 10.97, p < .01$) with each variable, with the F values for the Age × Complexity interactions ($df = 3, 594$) ranging from 5.49 (for Paper Folding errors) to 50.13 (for Analogies-Elements time). These interactions, in conjunction with the trends illustrated in Figures 7. 3 through 7.6, indicate that the complexity effect pattern was evident with both time and error measures in all four cognitive tasks.

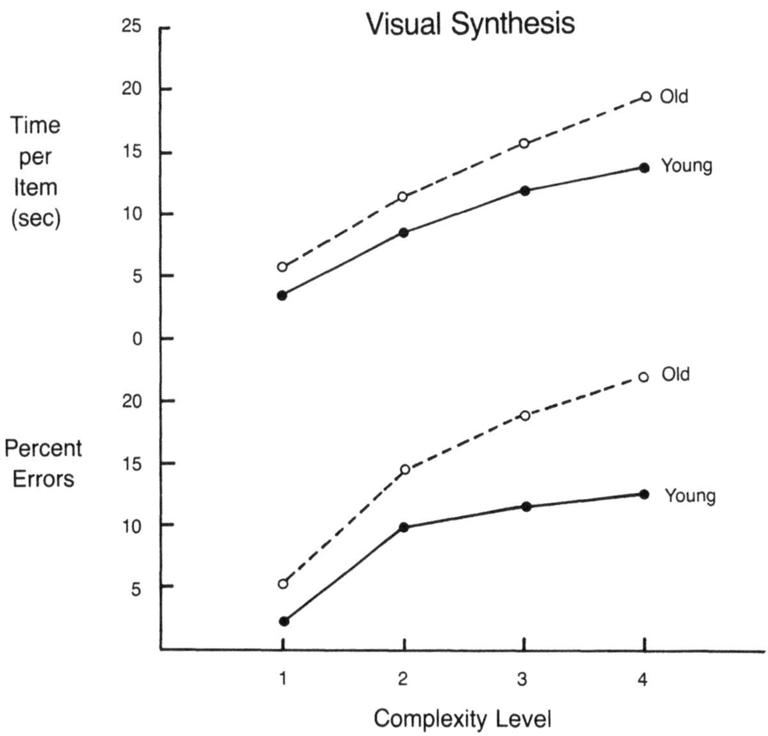


FIGURE 7.3. Mean time per item and percentage of errors at each complexity level for young and old adults in the Visual Synthesis task, Study 2.

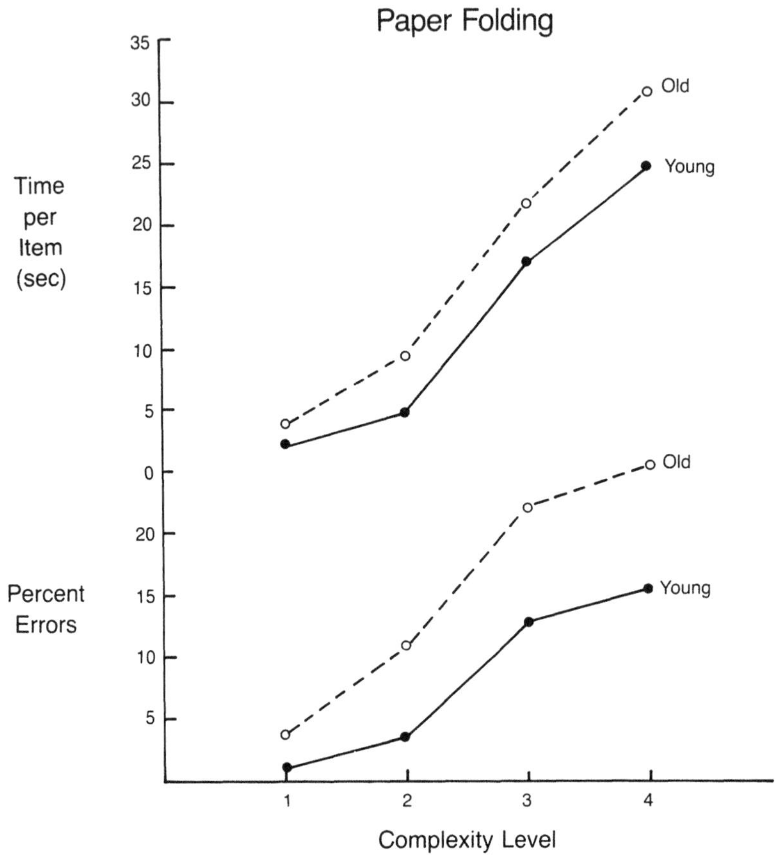


FIGURE 7.4. Mean time per item and percentage of errors at each complexity level for young and old adults in the Paper Folding task, Study 2.

It would have been desirable to summarize performance in each task in terms of a single variable, but the results that age and complexity effects were evident on both time per item and percentage of errors, together with the realization that these variables can exhibit a speed–accuracy tradeoff, precluded that possibility. Subsequent analyses were therefore performed independently on both time and error variables, with the hope that the possible attentuation in magnitude of the phenomena and the loss in quantitative precision associated with an effect being manifested in two variables that might be reciprocally related would be balanced by the gain in generality associated with an increase in the number of variables available for examination.

The existence of the complexity effect with quantitative rather than qualitative manipulations of complexity is consistent with some general-

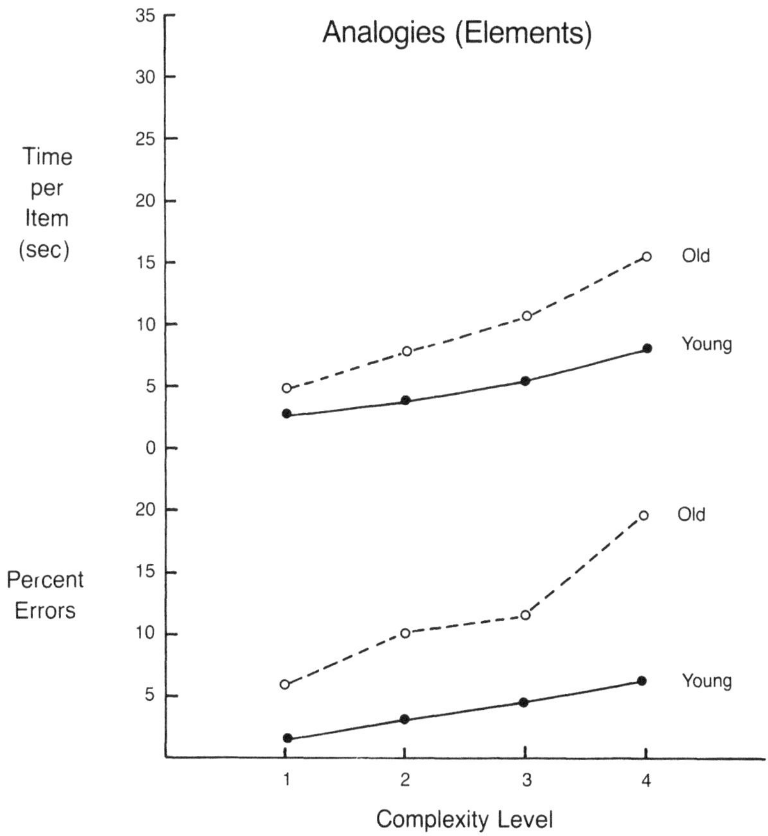


FIGURE 7.5 Mean time per item and percentage of errors at each complexity level for young and old adults in the Analogies task with a variable number of elements, Study 2.

purpose processing resource being involved in the cognitive age differences. These data were therefore used to estimate how much this resource declined from young to old adulthood. Following the reasoning outlined earlier, the slopes of the functions relating mean performance to ordinal complexity level (i.e., 1 for least complex up to 4 for most complex) were computed to serve as resource-dependent indices of performance. The ratio of these slopes in old and young adults was then determined, and its reciprocal used as an estimate of the quantity of resources available to older adults relative to that available to young adults. Relevant data for these computations are summarized in Table 7.4.

The $r^2$ values in Table 7.4 indicate that all of the data except that from the Analogies (Transformations) task were well fit by a linear equation. Figure 7.6 indicates that variations in the number of transformations imposed on

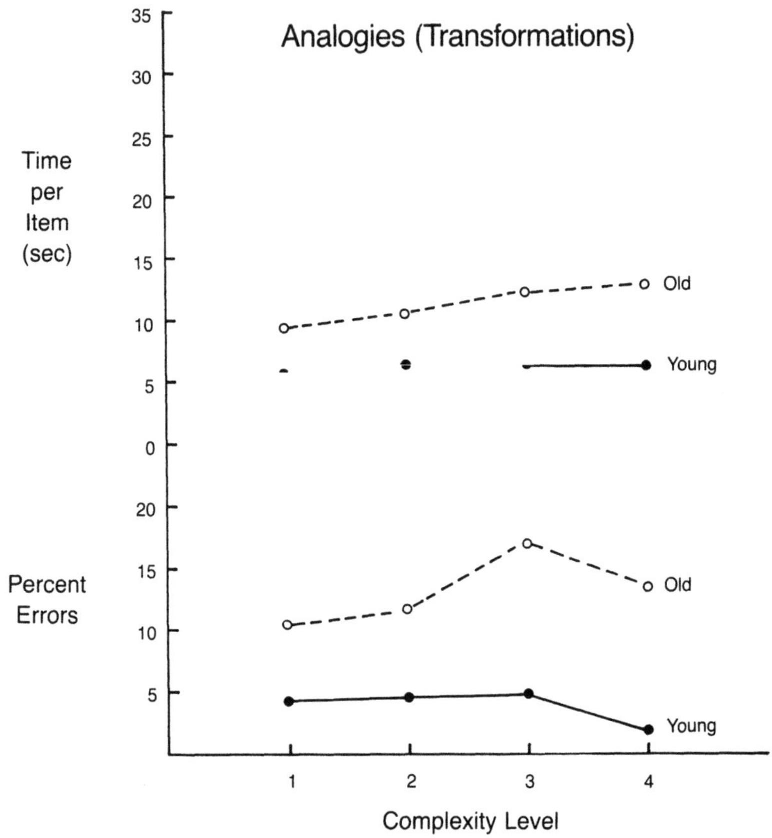


FIGURE 7.6. Mean time per item and percentage of errors at each complexity level for young and old adults in the Analogies task with a variable number of transformations, Study 2.

the elements between terms in these problems had virtually no effect on the performance of the young subjects. The reason this manipulation was ineffective is not clear, particularly because it did result in sizeable effects in the Mulholland et al. (1980) study, but the absence of a substantial linear trend precludes a meaningful interpretation of the quantity of resources from these data. Ratios of old slopes to young slopes with the time and error measures for the remaining tasks ranged from 1.18 to 2.76, which yield estimates that the older adults had between 36.2% and 84.5% as many processing resources available as in the young adults. There is considerable variability in these values, and thus it is probably prudent to view each as only an approximation and to rely on a measure of the central tendency of the values for determining the relative amount of resources in the two groups. The mean ratio for the time measures was 1.48, corresponding to a resource estimate of

TABLE 7.4. Parameters of the Complexity–Performance Functions, Study 2

| Task Measure | Young | | Old | | Old (Slope)/ Young (Slope) |
|---|---|---|---|---|---|
| | Slope | $r^2$ | Slope | $r^2$ | |
| Visual synthesis | | | | | |
| Time per item | 3.51 | .960 | 4.50 | .989 | 1.28 |
| Error percentage | 3.29 | .811 | 5.48 | .935 | 1.67 |
| Paper folding | | | | | |
| Time per item | 7.91 | .953 | 9.34 | .981 | 1.18 |
| Error percentage | 5.27 | .940 | 7.60 | .960 | 1.44 |
| Analogies (elements) | | | | | |
| Time per item | 1.78 | .959 | 3.50 | .972 | 1.97 |
| Error percentage | 1.60 | .995 | 4.41 | .898 | 2.76 |
| Analogies (transformations) | | | | | |
| Time per item | 0.13 | .398 | 1.19 | .981 | 9.15 |
| Error percentage | −0.70 | .424 | 1.44 | .422 | −2.06 |

67.6%, and that for the error measures was 1.96, which yields a resource estimate of 51.0%. The overall mean ratio was 1.72, leading to an estimate that the quantity of resources in older adults was 58.1% the quantity of that in young adults.

Slopes of the functions relating performance to ordinal complexity were also computed on the data from each individual subject with the time-per-item and error percentage data in each task. As expected from the significant Age × Complexity interactions, older adults had significantly ($t > 2.63$, $p < .01$) greater slopes than young adults with each measure. Correlations among these slope parameters are presented in Table 7.5, with values above the diagonal based upon data from young adults and values below the diagonal based upon data from older adults.

Table 7.5 indicates that two of six correlations between slopes with time measures were significantly different from zero for young adults, and four of six were significant for older adults. Both groups had only two significant correlations between slopes with error measures of performance, and none of the correlations between slopes from time measures and slopes from error measures were significant for either age group.

It is difficult to reach a definitive conclusion about the resources construct on the basis of the data summarized in Table 7.5. On the one hand, the significant correlations between the amount of complexity-related increase in time for tasks as distinct as Paper Folding and Geometric Analogies is consistent with the view that a common processing resource is responsible for the complexity effects. On the other hand, the majority of the correlations were quite small, particularly those involving slopes based upon the error measures. The low correlations could have originated because of a true lack

TABLE 7.5. Correlations Among Slopes of the Complexity-Performance Functions for 100 Young Adults (above diagonal) and 100 Older Adults (below diagonal), Study 2

| | SynT | FolT | A-ET | A-TT | SynE | FolE | A-EE | A-TE |
|---|---|---|---|---|---|---|---|---|
| SynT | X | .05 | .01 | .50* | −.17 | .07 | −.04 | −.09 |
| FolT | .47* | X | .26* | −.20 | .08 | .13 | .01 | .12 |
| A-ET | .50* | .38* | X | −.14 | .20 | .11 | .10 | .01 |
| A-TT | .21 | .04 | .39* | X | .04 | −.01 | −.03 | .09 |
| SynE | .23 | .23 | .24 | .18 | X | .30* | .14 | .04 |
| FolE | −.02 | −.06 | −.07 | −.04 | .28* | X | .48* | −.05 |
| A-EE | −.05 | −.03 | .04 | −.10 | .24 | .41* | X | −.16 |
| A-TE | .09 | .17 | .25 | .21 | .15 | .04 | −.02 | X |

SynT = Synthesis Time;
FolT = Folding Time;
A-ET = Analogies (El) Time;
A-TT = Analogies (Tr) Time;
SynE = Synthesis Errors;
FolE = Folding Errors;
A-EE = Analogies (EL) Errors;
A-TE = Analogies (Tr) Errors;
*$p < .01$.

of a relation among the variables, or because of low amounts of systematic variance available for association with other variables (i.e., low reliability of measurement). Unfortunately, these alternatives cannot be distinguished with the present data because there was no means of assessing the reliability of the slope parameters.

Data relevant to the resource predictions outlined in Table 1 are summarized in Table 7.6. For the purposes of this analysis, data were collapsed across complexity conditions and cognitive performance represented by the mean across the four levels of complexity. The mean of the scores from the first and second administrations of the Digit Symbol and Backwards Digit Span tests served as the indices of resource quantity. Reliability coefficients for the mean values estimated from the Spearman–Brown formula were .88 and .96 for young and old adults, respectively, with the Digit Symbol measure, and .74 and .81 for the two groups, respectively, with the Backwards Digit Span measure. Entries in Table 7.6 correspond to the square of the relevant correlation multiplied by 100, indicating the percentage of variance common to the two variables with and without control of the third variable. Statistical significance of the partial correlations was evaluated with the conventional procedure (Edwards, 1976), and the significance of the amount of reduction introduced by the partialing procedure was evaluated by means of the formula presented in Horn (1980).

TABLE 7.6. Percentage of Common Variance Among Age, Resources, and Performance, Study 2[a]

| Resource Index / Cognitive Performance Measure | Age–Perf. | | Age–Perf. (Res.) | Res–Perf. | | Res.–Perf. (Age) |
|---|---|---|---|---|---|---|
| Digit Symbol | | | | | | |
| Synth. Time | 18.5 | > | 2.6 | 19.4 | > | 3.6 |
| Synth. Errors | 16.0 | > | 9.0 | 7.8 | > | 0.3 |
| Fold. Time | 16.8 | > | 7.3 | 10.2 | > | 0.0 |
| Fold Errors | 17.6 | > | 9.6 | 9.0 | > | 0.2 |
| Anal. (El) Time | 41.0 | > | 10.2 | 38.4 | > | 6.8 |
| Anal. (El) Errors | 22.1 | > | 7.8 | 16.0 | > | 0.5 |
| Anal. (Tr) Time | 41.0 | > | 12.2 | 36.0 | > | 4.8 |
| Anal. (Tr) Errors | 27.0 | > | 10.9 | 18.5 | > | 0.3 |
| Mean | 25.0 | > | 8.7 | 19.4 | > | 2.1 |
| Backwards Digit Span | | | | | | |
| Synth. Time | 18.5 | | 16.8 | 2.0 | | 0.0 |
| Synth. Errors | 16.0 | > | 10.2 | 10.2 | > | 4.4 |
| Fold Time | 16.8 | | 14.4 | 2.6 | | 0.0 |
| Fold Errors | 17.6 | > | 12.2 | 9.6 | > | 3.6 |
| Anal. (El) Time | 41.0 | > | 34.8 | 11.6 | > | 2.6 |
| Anal. (El) Errors | 22.1 | > | 16.0 | 12.2 | > | 4.8 |
| Anal. (Tr) Time | 41.0 | > | 34.8 | 10.9 | > | 2.3 |
| Anal. (Tr) Errors | 27.0 | > | 21.2 | 11.6 | > | 4.0 |
| Mean | 25.0 | > | 20.1 | 8.8 | > | 2.7 |

[a]Entries greater than 3.2 ($r = .18$) are significantly ($p < .01$) different from zero. A greater than (>) symbol indicates that the first value is significantly ($p < .01$) greater than the second value.

Two aspects of these results are particularly noteworthy. The first is that the data appear most consistent with Model 2 of Table 7.1. That is, controlling the resource index reduced but did not completely eliminate the degree of association between age and performance, and controlling age reduced but did not completely eliminate the resource–performance association.

The second important result evident in Table 7.6 is that the speed resource index produced greater resemblance to the predictions of the strong resource model (Model 1) than did the working-memory index. In particular, statistical control of the speed measure greatly reduced the degree of age association (from a mean of 25.0% to a mean of 8.7% common variance for the eight cognitive measures), while comparable control of the memory measure resulted in a much smaller attenuation of the age association (from a mean of 25.0% to a mean of 20.1% common variance).

This same pattern of results was obtained when the slopes of the complexity functions served as the cognitive performance measures. Controlling for Digit Symbol score reduced the degree of association between age and performance from a mean of 10.2% common variance to a mean of 3.7% common variance, and controlling for age reduced the Digit Symbol-performance association from a mean of 7.7% common variance to a mean of 1.1% common variance. Effects with the Backwards Digit Span resource index were much smaller, with a reduction of the age-performance association from a mean of 10.2% to a mean of 8.2% after control of the memory measure, and a reduction of the resource-performance association from a mean of 3.1% to a mean of 0.8% after statistical control of age.

A further indication of the relative importance of the two resource indices is available in two additional correlational analyses. First, simultaneously controlling both the speed and memory indices resulted in about the same amount of attenuation of the age-performance association as only controlling speed (i.e., from 25.0% common variance to 8.7% common variance after control of speed and to 8.4% common variance after controlling both speed and memory). This suggests that the memory index is not responsible for much variance not already associated with the speed index. Second, statistical control of the speed index virtually eliminated the age effect with the memory variable (i.e., from 12.2% to 0.6% common variance), while control of the memory index resulted in only a slight reduction in the degree of age association with the speed variable (i.e, from 59.3% common variance to 53.3% common variance). One interpretation of this result is that the age differences in Backwards Digit Span are largely mediated by age differences in speed of information processing, but that age differences in Digit Symbol performance are largely independent of any age differences that might exist in working-memory capacity, at least when the latter is indexed by Backwards Digit Span.

## Study 3

The third study was designed with four goals in mind. The first goal was to attempt to replicate the major results of Study 2. In particular, it was considered desirable to verify three findings: (a) the complexity effect pattern with complexity manipulated by variations in the number, rather than the identity, of the processing operations; (b) the results leading to the inference that adults with an average age in the sixties have approximately 58% as much of a relevant processing resource as adults with an average age of about 20 years; and (c) the configuration of correlations suggesting that processing resources related to speed and working-memory capacity cannot account for all age differences in performance of fluid cognitive tasks, but of the two, speed appears to be more important than working-memory capacity.

A second goal of the study was to administer two of the cognitive tasks twice to allow an assessment of the reliability of the complexity-performance slope parameters, and also to provide additional practice on the tasks in order to determine whether the same pattern would be evident with greater amounts of experience.

The third goal of the present study was to examine new variables as indices of the space or working-memory conceptualization of processing resources. It is possible that despite the attempts to obtain an optimal index of working-memory capacity, the workspace conceptualization of processing resources may not have been adequately indexed by the Backwards Digit Span measure. In particular, because the stimuli in the present cognitive tasks were all visual-spatial in nature, it could be argued that the memory involved in these tasks was more concerned with spatial information than with verbal information. Because the Backwards Digit Span involved auditorily presented alphanumeric material, lack of congruency in the nature of the processing and/or the storage of the material may have contributed to the weak effects with the memory index in Study 2. The present investigated this possibility by including measures of both verbal and spatial memory.

Examination of new speed measures to eliminate the possibility that the earlier results were specific to the Digit Symbol speed measure was the fourth goal of the study. The Number Comparison test was therefore administered to all subjects as well as the Digit Symbol test. An attempt was also made to minimize the contribution of the motor time associated with writing symbols from the Digit Symbol score by measuring the time required to copy symbols without any substitution requirement, and then subtracting this copying time from the Digit Symbol time to obtain a measure of coding time.

## Method

*Subjects.* Fifty women and 50 men aged between 17 and 26 years (mean, 18.9), and 20 women and 20 men aged between 55 and 75 years (mean, 63.6), participated individually in a single experimental session of approximately 1.5 hours. Self-reported health status (1 = Excellent, 5 = Poor) averaged 1.4 for the young adults and 1.9 for the older adults, with 98% of the former and 95% of the latter reporting themselves to be in average or better-than-average health. The range of education in the young group was 11 to 17 years (mean, 12.4), and that in the older group 6 to 20 (mean, 13.3).

*Procedure.* All subjects performed seven tasks in an identical sequence. Five tasks were each administered twice, once at the beginning of the session and once at the end of the session. These consisted of the Digit Symbol Substitution task from the WAIS, a Symbol Copying task, the Number Comparison task from the ETS battery (French et al., 1963), a Verbal Memory task, and a Spatial Memory task.

The Symbol Copying task was based on a procedure introduced by Storandt (1976), and simply required the subject to copy symbols (identical to those in the Digit Symbol Substitution Test) from the top of two vertically aligned boxes in the empty box below. Sixty seconds were allowed to complete as many symbols as possible, but because a large number of the young subjects finished the 100 symbols in less than 60 seconds, all scores were transformed to a sec-per-symbol metric.

The two memory tasks were similar to those described by Salthouse (1974, 1975), and consisted of a 5 × 5 matrix of 25 letters with seven targets printed in inverse (i.e., white on black background instead of black on white background). The task for the subject was to view the matrix for 3 seconds and then attempt to recall the identities of the target letters in the Verbal Memory task, or attempt to recall the locations of the target elements in the Spatial Memory task. Locations were recalled by marking cells in a blank 5 × 5 matrix, while letters were recalled by writing them in any order on a sheet of paper. In both cases the subject was instructed to guess if necessary to produce seven responses on each trial. Four trials were presented in each task at the first administration, with the initial trial serving as practice and not scored, and three trials were presented at the second administration of each task.

The remaining two tasks performed in the session were the Visual Synthesis task and the Geometric Analogies task (with a variable number of elements) from the previous study. There were, however, two modifications in procedure from Study 2. One change was that accuracy was emphasized to a greater extent, and subjects received accuracy feedback and detailed explanations of trials in which an error occurred during the first 4 pages in each task. The second modification from the earlier procedure was that twice as many trials were administered in each task. The additional trials were similar but not identical to the initial set, and resulted in a total of 32 timed pages (with four problems per page) in each task.

## Results and Discussion

The data relevant to the complexity effect phenomenon are displayed in Figure 7.7 (for the Visual Synthesis Task) and Figure 7.8 (for the Geometric Analogies Task). Three-factor (Age, Complexity, and Practice) analyses of variance were conducted on the time and error data in each task. Age, Complexity, and the interaction of Age × Complexity were all statistically significant ($F > 5.27, p < .01$) for each variable, and Practice had a significant ($F > 27.68$, $p < .01$) effect on Synthesis errors, Analogies time, and Analogies errors. The interactions of Age × Practice ($F < 1.75$) and Age × Practice × Complexity ($F < 3.08$) were not significant for any variables. The $F$ values for the interactions of Age × Complexity ($df = 3, 414$) ranged from 5.27 (for Synthesis errors) to 21.30 (for Analogies time). These results and the trends evident in Figures 7.7 and 7.8 again confirm that the magnitude of the age dif-

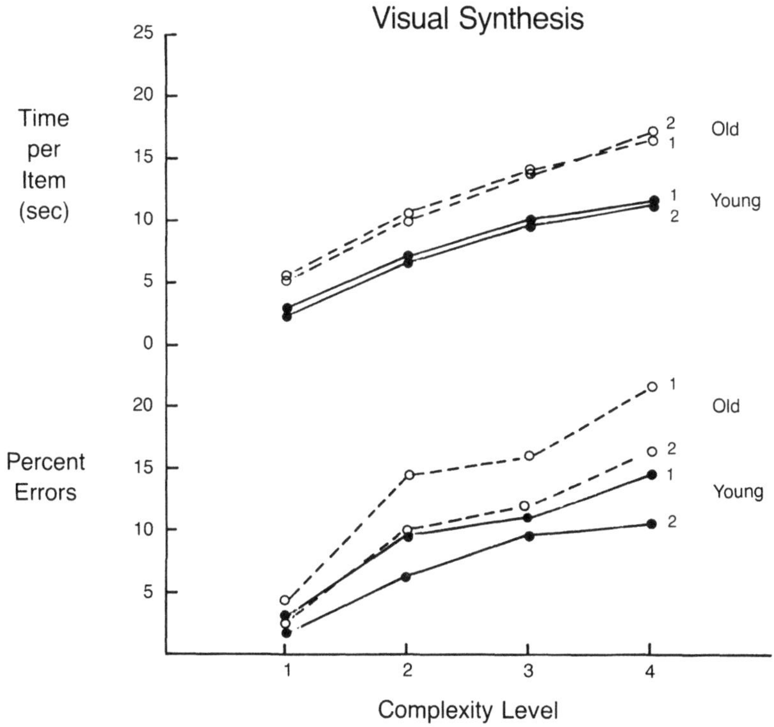


FIGURE 7.7 Mean time per item and percentage of errors at each complexity level and early (1) and late (2) in practice for young and old adults in the Visual Synthesis task, Study 3.

ferences in both time and error measures increases as the complexity of the task increases.

Data relevant to the derivation of estimates concerning the quantity of processing resources available to older adults relative to that available to young adults are summarized in Table 7.7. The $r^2$ values indicate that linear regression equations between ordinal complexity and performance fit the mean time and error data quite well in each task, and for both age groups. Ratios of the slopes of these equations in old and young adults ranged from 1.24 to 2.38, with means of 1.33 and 1.77 for the time and error measures, respectively. The reciprocals of these values yield estimates of older adults having 75.2% and 56.5% the amount of resources available to young adults. The overall mean ratio was 1.55, which is equivalent to a resource estimate of older adults having 64.5% the quantity possessed by young adults.

Slopes of the functions relating performance to ordinal complexity were computed on the data from each individual subject with the time and error measures in each task. The age difference in the slopes was significant ($t >$ 2.82) at $p < .01$ for all slopes except that with the error measure in the second

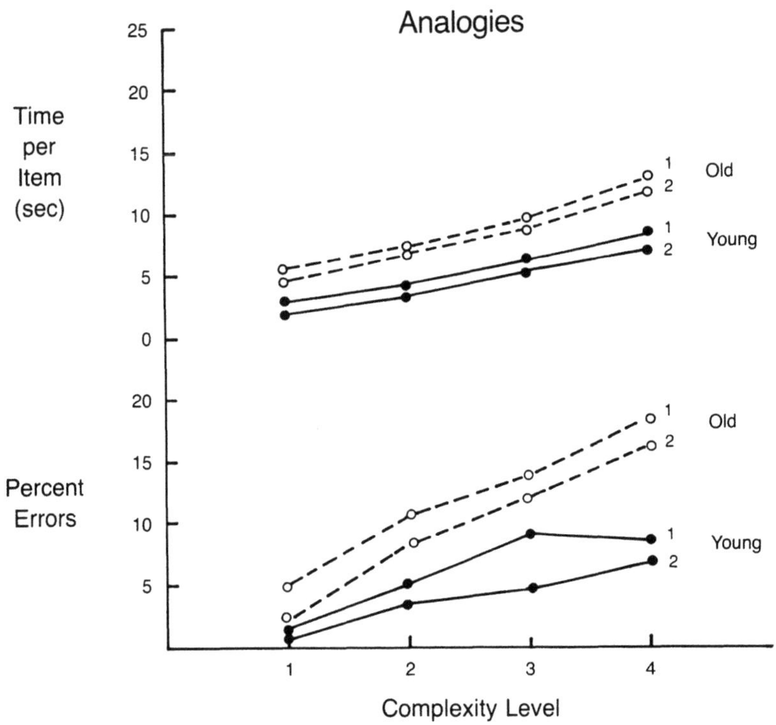


FIGURE 7.8. Mean time per item and percentage of errors at each complexity level and early (1) and late (2) in practice for young and old adults in the Analogies task, Study 3.

TABLE 7.7. Parameters of the Complexity-Performance Functions, Study 3

| Task Measure | Young Slope | Young $r^2$ | Old Slope | Old $r^2$ | Old (Slope)/ Young (Slope) |
|---|---|---|---|---|---|
| Visual synthesis—1 | | | | | |
| Time per item | 2.99 | .957 | 3.72 | .979 | 1.24 |
| Error percentage | 3.69 | .921 | 5.49 | .918 | 1.49 |
| Visual synthesis—2 | | | | | |
| Time per item | 3.01 | .953 | 4.06 | .992 | 1.35 |
| Error percentage | 3.01 | .917 | 4.53 | .960 | 1.50 |
| Analogies—1 | | | | | |
| Time per item | 1.79 | .998 | 2.40 | .983 | 1.34 |
| Error percentage | 2.47 | .838 | 4.25 | .985 | 1.72 |
| Analogies—2 | | | | | |
| Time per item | 1.72 | .991 | 2.37 | .990 | 1.38 |
| Error percentage | 1.99 | .961 | 4.74 | .983 | 2.38 |

administration of the Synthesis task, which was significant ($t$ = 2.38) at $p <$ .05. Correlations among the slope parameters are presented in Table 7.8, with values above the diagonal based upon data from older adults.

The first item to note in Table 7.8 is that the reliabilities of the slope parameters (represented by values in parentheses) were much greater for the slopes based upon time measures than for those based upon error measures. The low reliabilities with the error variables clearly places limits on the maximum between-variable correlation one could expect with these measures because the low within-variable correlation indicates that there is very little systematic variance available for association with other measures. Reliabilities of the slopes with the time measures of performance were adequate, however, and it is noteworthy that all the correlations between different slopes with the time measures were significantly ($p <$ .01) greater than zero for both young and old adults. The finding that the amount of increase in time associated with additional integration operations in the Synthesis task is positively related to the amount of increase in time associated with additional to-be-evaluated elements in the Analogies task is clearly consistent with the view that a common processing resource is involved in the operations in both tasks.

The results of the correlational analyses pertinent to evaluating the predictions from the three models outlined in Table 7.1 are summarized in Table 7.9. Performance in the cognitive tasks was represented by the mean of the

TABLE 7.8. Correlations Among Slopes of the Complexity–Performance Functions for 100 Young Adults (above diagonal) and 40 Older Adults (below diagonal), Study 3[a]

| | S1T | S2T | A1T | A2T | S1E | S2E | A1E | A2E |
|---|---|---|---|---|---|---|---|---|
| S1T | X | (.77*) | .38* | .54* | −.07 | −.13 | −.03 | .17 |
| S2T | (.87*) | X | .47* | .54* | .14 | −.08 | −.08 | .02 |
| A1T | .47* | .44* | X | (.63*) | −.02 | .02 | .01 | −.08 |
| A2T | .45* | .44* | (.64*) | X | .00 | .00 | .01 | .05 |
| S1E | −.15 | −.21 | −.09 | −.00 | X | (.34*) | .26* | −.05 |
| S2E | −.04 | .06 | −.02 | .05 | (.51*) | X | .19 | .09 |
| A1E | .36 | .15 | .36 | .29 | .16 | .03 | X | (.05) |
| A2E | .20 | .12 | −.15 | −.02 | .40 | .37 | (.34) | X |

[a]S1T = Synth. (First) Time;
S2T = Synth. (Second) Time;
S1E = Synth. (First) Errors;
S2E = Synth. (Second) Errors;
A1T = Analog. (First) Time;
A2T = Analog. (Second) Time;
A1E = Analog. (First) Errors;
A2E = Analog. (Second) Errors;
*$p <$ .01.

values across levels of complexity and practice, and the averages of the two scores served as the indices of resource quantity for the speed and memory measures. Spearman-Brown estimated reliabilities, with the value of young adults first and the value of older adults second, were Digit Symbol .92, .93; Number Comparison .88, .90; Coding Time .86, .88; Verbal Memory .65, .58; and Spatial Memory .63, .37.

Table 7.9 indicates that the results with Digit Symbol score as the resource index were very similar to those of Study 2. As before, the age-associated variance was greatly reduced but not eliminated by statistically controlling the Digit Symbol variable, and the variance common to the Digit Symbol score and the cognitive performance measures was reduced but not eliminated by statistically controlling age.

The pattern with the Verbal Memory score serving as the index of a memory processing resource was also like that found with the Backwards Digit Span memory measure in the previous study. The results were more similar to the predictions from Model 2 than to those from Models 1 or 3, but the amount of reduction in age-associated variance by controlling the resource was much less than that obtained with the Digit Symbol score serving as the resource index.

The Number Comparison, Coding Time, and Spatial Memory measures exhibited patterns intermediate to those with the Digit Symbol and Verbal Memory scores. As hypothesized, the Spatial Memory measure resulted in a greater reduction in the age-performance variance when it was controlled, and had larger amounts of resource-performance variance, than did the Verbal Memory measure. However, it was still inferior to the Digit Symbol measure in the amount of reduction in the age association produced by its statistical control, and in the magnitude of the resource-performance association.

As was found in the previous study, analyses of the interrelations of age, Digit Symbol score, and the memory measures revealed that the largest amount of variance was associated with the Digit Symbol score. Statistical control of the Digit Symbol score reduced the percentage of common variance between age and Verbal Memory score from 14.4% to 0.0%, and reduced the percentage of common variance between age and Spatial Memory score from 27.0% to 3.2%. However, partialling out Verbal Memory score only reduced the amount of age-associated variance common to the Digit Symbol score from 57.8% to 50.4%, and partialling out Spatial Memory score only reduced it from 57.8% to 43.6%. Furthermore, simultaneous control of Digit Symbol score and either Verbal Memory score or Spatial Memory score resulted in nearly the same amount of residual age-performance association as that remaining after control of only the Digit Symbol score (i.e., 4.8% common variance after control of Digit Symbol, 4.8% common variance after control of Digit Symbol and Verbal Memory, and 3.8% common variance after control of Digit Symbol and Spatial Memory).

TABLE 7.9. Percentage of Common Variance Among Age, Resources, and Performance, Study 3[a]

| Resource Index / Cognitive Performance Measure | Age–Perf. | | Age–Perf. (Res.) | Res–Perf. | | Res.–Perf. (Age) |
|---|---|---|---|---|---|---|
| Digit Symbol | | | | | | |
| Synth. Time | 33.6 | > | 5.3 | 37.2 | > | 10.2 |
| Synth. Errors | 9.0 | > | 0.3 | 18.5 | > | 10.9 |
| Anal. Time | 51.8 | > | 12.3 | 56.3 | > | 20.3 |
| Anal. Errors | 20.3 | > | 1.4 | 25.0 | > | 7.3 |
| Mean | 28.7 | > | 4.8 | 34.3 | > | 12.2 |
| Number Comparison | | | | | | |
| Synth. Time | 33.6 | > | 21.2 | 26.0 | > | 12.3 |
| Synth. Errors | 9.0 | > | 3.6 | 10.2 | > | 4.8 |
| Anal. Time | 51.8 | > | 41.0 | 32.5 | > | 17.6 |
| Anal. Errors | 20.3 | > | 13.0 | 11.6 | > | 3.2 |
| Mean | 28.7 | > | 19.7 | 20.1 | > | 9.5 |
| Coding Time | | | | | | |
| Synth. Time | 33.6 | > | 18.5 | 24.0 | > | 6.8 |
| Synth. Errors | 9.0 | > | 0.0 | 36.0 | > | 30.3 |
| Anal. Time | 51.8 | > | 34.8 | 37.2 | > | 15.2 |
| Anal. Errors | 20.3 | > | 2.6 | 42.3 | > | 29.2 |
| Mean | 28.7 | > | 14.0 | 34.9 | > | 20.4 |
| Verbal Memory | | | | | | |
| Synth. Time | 33.6 | > | 28.1 | 9.0 | > | 1.2 |
| Synth. Errors | 9.0 | > | 4.0 | 11.6 | > | 6.8 |
| Anal. Time | 51.8 | > | 44.9 | 16.0 | > | 4.0 |
| Anal. Errors | 20.3 | > | 14.4 | 9.6 | > | 2.9 |
| Mean | 28.7 | > | 22.9 | 11.6 | > | 3.7 |
| Spatial Memory | | | | | | |
| Synth. Time | 33.6 | > | 16.8 | 30.3 | > | 13.0 |
| Synth. Errors | 9.0 | > | 1.0 | 18.5 | > | 11.6 |
| Anal. Time | 51.8 | > | 36.0 | 34.8 | > | 13.0 |
| Anal. Errors | 20.3 | > | 9.6 | 16.0 | > | 4.8 |
| Mean | 28.7 | > | 15.9 | 24.9 | > | 10.6 |

[a]Entries greater than 4.6 ($r = .215$) are significantly ($p < .01$) different from zero. A greater than symbol (>) indicates that the first value is significantly ($p < .01$) greater than the second value.

Also consistent with the earlier results was the finding that the same correlational pattern was evident when the slopes of the complexity functions served as the measures of cognitive performance. Statistical control of Digit Symbol score reduced the variance common to age and performance from a mean of 11.7% to a mean of 1.5%, and statistical control of age reduced the variance common to the Digit Symbol resource index and the performance measures from a mean of 13.1% to a mean of 3.1%. Corresponding values with the Verbal Memory resource index were a reduction in the age-performance association from 11.7% to 9.8% after control of the memory resource, and a reduction in the resource–performance association from 2.7% to 0.6% after control of age.

## General Discussion

The studies just described were designed to provide information relevant to three issues concerning the role of processing resources in cognitive aging. These were (a) whether there is evidence that some type of general-purpose processing resource could be involved in the age differences in fluid ability types of cognition; (b) the approximate amount by which the quantity or availability of the hypothesized resource decreased from about age 20 to about age 65; and (c) the specific nature of that processing resource.

Examination of the complexity-effect phenomenon under conditions in which complexity was varied with quantitative rather than qualitative manipulations was the primary analytical strategy employed to investigate the involvement of processing resources in cognitive aging. Because alterations in performance produced by increasing the number of repetitions of the same operation are not easily attributed to the introduction of a new age-sensitive operation or strategy, one plausible interpretation is that they result from a general entity like processing resources. Nonresource interpretations might also be proposed to account for this phenomenon, and thus it cannot be considered a definitive test of the necessity of the resources construct to account for cognitive aging phenomena, but the existence of a quantitatively induced complexity-effect phenomenon is certainly consistent with the resources perspective and is inconsistent with at least some nonresource interpretations.

The slopes of the functions relating task complexity to performance were hypothesized to be inversely proportional to the amount of available resources because more resources should lead to smaller variations in performance as a function of resource demands. That is, if $P = R/D$, and $P = D/R$ when performance is scaled in errors or time, then the slope of the function relating performance to complexity or resource demands should be inversely related to the quantity of available resources; that is, $1/R = P/D$.

As expected from the resource interpretation, older adults had significantly greater slopes than young adults for both speed and accuracy measures of performance in each of four tasks in Study 2, and across the two levels of practice in the two tasks employed in Study 3. Also consistent with the resource interpretation is the finding that the slopes of these complexity functions with the time-based measures of performance were positively correlated with one another. The correlations with the slopes derived from the error measures were not consistently correlated with one another, nor with the slopes from the time measures, but those values were found not to be very reliable and thus there was little systematic variance available for association with other variables.

By assuming that the task demands for resources were comparable in young and old adults, it was possible to use Eq. (6) to estimate the quantity of resources available to older adults relative to that available to young adults. These estimates, which should be considered quite tentative because the necessary assumptions concerning the comparability of the resource-performance functions across age groups have not yet been tested, ranged from 36.2% to 84.5%, with averages of 58.1% in Study 2 and 64.5% in Study 3, respectively. Although the amount of processing resources is postulated to be only one determinant of cognitive performance, the values of 58% to 65% appear plausible because they are similar to the percentages by which the performance of 65-year-olds is of the performance of 20-year-olds in a variety of tests of fluid intellectual ability (cf. Salthouse, 1982).

Results from other studies in which slopes of complexity functions with quantitative manipulations of complexity have been computed for young and old adults are also quite consistent with the present findings. For example, a number of studies have been conducted with the Sternberg memory-scanning procedure in which time to decide whether a probe item was in a previously presented memory set is the primary dependent variable. Salthouse (1982) reviewed seven aging studies of this type and concluded that the slopes of the set size-reaction time functions for adults in their sixties were between 1.6 and 2.0 times greater than those for adults in their early twenties. Reciprocals of these ratios yield estimates that the older adults had between 50% and 62.5% the quantity of resources as young adults.

Several studies have also been reported in which adults of different ages have been administered the Shepard mental-rotation task in which subjects have to make rapid decisions about visual stimuli in varying orientations. The predominant result has been that the functions relating decision time to amount of angular deviation of the stimulus from a vertical orientation had steeper slopes in older adults than in young adults (see Salthouse, 1982, for a review), thus leading to the inference that the latter have more resources than the former. These similarities are impressive because the Sternberg and Shepard tasks are very simple and stress speeded responding, while the tasks in the current studies more closely resemble those from intelligence test batteries and emphasize accuracy much more than speed.

To summarize, the results of the reported studies are consistent with the existence of some type of general-purpose processing resource involved in cognitive functioning that declines by approximately 30% to 40% from the early twenties to the mid-sixties. Because the processing resources concept is more compatible with a holistic rather than a compartmentalized view of the information-processing system, one would not expect an altered quantity of resources to result in discrete and isolated deficits in only certain cognitve components. Instead, "the deficits are likely to be widespread and permeate the whole system—although they may show up more clearly in some circumstances than in others" (Craik & Simon, 1980, p. 95). Because this seems to characterize the observed pattern of age-related cognitive deficits, the quantity of processing resources available for allocation to cognitive tasks may be an important factor contributing to the existence of the age differences in performance in fluid ability cognitive tasks documented in the introduction.

The current data do, however, indicate some limitations of the resource perspective. One weakness is that for none of the combinations of resource indices or performance variables was the pattern of correlations consistent with the expectations from the strong resource model (i.e., Model 1 of Table 7.1). The data were also inconsistent with Model 3, and since this model postulates that the performance variables and the resource indices are independent consequences of aging, it can be inferred that there are some common factors involved in the age differences in different types of cognitive tasks. However, the best-fitting model, Model 2 of Table 7.1, explicitly acknowledges the contribution of nonresource determinants of the age differences in performance and thus it can be considered a relatively weak exemplar of the resource perspective.

Although not elaborated earlier, the processing resource interpretation was only moderately successful when examined at the level of individual subjects within each age group. Two sets of data are relevant in this connection. One is the pattern of positive correlations, across subjects within each age group, among the slopes of the complexity functions for the time variables. This finding is consistent with the view that the complexity functions result from reliance upon a common processing resource rather than being determined by independent task-specific processes.

The other set of data is derived from the resource–performance correlations across levels of complexity. If it is postulated that variations in the quantity of processing resources contribute to the individual differences in performance within, as well as between, age groups, then the correlations between the index of resource quantity and performance should increase as the resource demands increase with greater task complexity. Means of the absolute value of the correlations across eight performance variables in each study (i.e., time and accuracy for each of four tasks in Study 2, and time and accuracy for each of two tasks at two levels of practice in Study 3) are summarized in Table 7.10. It is clear from these results that the relations between the resource indices and the performance variables do not increase systematically with increased task complexity, and thus they provide no support for a contribution of processing resources to variations in performance among individuals within groups homogeneous with respect to age. A restricted range of resource quantity within relatively homogeneous groups may contribute to this failure, but the apparent inability to account for complexity-influenced performance variations within comparably aged individuals is nevertheless an embarrassment for the processing resource perspective.

TABLE 7.10. Mean Absolute Correlations Between Resource Indices and Performance Measure Across Levels of Complexity

| | | | Complexity Level | | | |
|---|---|---|---|---|---|---|
| Resource Index | Study | Age | 1 | 2 | 3 | 4 |
| Digit Symbol | 2 | Young | .14 | .14 | .10 | .09 |
| | | Old | .17 | .13 | .14 | .14 |
| Backwards Digit Span | 2 | Young | .12 | .12 | .17 | .15 |
| | | Old | .15 | .17 | .12 | .14 |
| Digit Symbol | 3 | Young | .26 | .23 | .20 | .21 |
| | | Old | .40 | .43 | .41 | .45 |
| Verbal Memory | 3 | Young | .28 | .22 | .19 | .09 |
| | | Old | .32 | .28 | .27 | .24 |

Also unresolved in the present studies is the exact nature of the hypothesized processing resource. As mentioned above, none of the indices of different types of processing resources produced results congruent with a strong version of the resource interpretation, although the measures did appear to vary in their degree of correspondence to the predictions from that perspective. Of the six measures examined in Studies 2 and 3, score on the Digit Symbol Substitution test resulted in a pattern of correlations most consistent with the view that age differences in cognition are mediated by age differences in a type of processing resource indexed by that variable. But because the similarity to the predictions was lower with two other speed measures, including the Coding Time measure that presumably incorporates all of the cognitive components from the Digit Symbol measure, it is premature to conclude that the processing resource involved in age differences in cognition is analogous to rate of processing information. A resource related to speed does appear to have been more important than a resource related to working-memory capacity with the tasks employed in these studies. However, the variability in the results with different speed measures suggests that the conceptualization of processing resources in terms of time or rate of processing is not yet sufficiently well understood to function as a single or all-inclusive explanatory mechanism.

## Reappraisal of the Resources Construct

While the results of the present studies are consistent with the view that age-related reductions in the quantity or efficiency of processing resources mediate age differences in fluid cognition, they are probably also consistent with certain interpretations that do not rely upon the concept of processing resources. Alternative nonresource interpretations that can account for a large variety of cognitive aging phenomena have apparently not yet been formulated, but it is still appropriate to question the usefulness of the processing resources concept. Specifically, it is worth considering three objections to the notion of processing resources as an explanatory factor in age-related differences in cognitive functioning.

Perhaps the most pessimistic perspective is that processing resources simply do not exist, and consequently all efforts to assess their quantity or to determine their nature are doomed to failure. While this view cannot be dismissed outright, it is not very compelling without an explanation for the evidence that seems to support the existence of processing resources. In the area of cognitive aging, this entails an interpretation of why age-related performance differences are observed in so many diverse tasks, why the magnitude of those age differences increases when the number of postulated operations, or task complexity, increases, why the slopes of these complexity functions are positively correlated with one another, and why statistical control of variables thought to index processing resources greatly attenuates the effects of age on other variables. Until parsimonious alternative accounts of these phenomena are available, therefore, the concept of general-purpose processing resources seems to serve a useful explanatory and integrative function.

A second perspecitve on processing resources is that while they may exist, they are in principle not measurable. In other words, there might be something that functions like processing resources, but no single variable or collection of variables (latent or manifest) may ever be adequate to capture its essence. This argument can also be challenged because it violates the familiar dictum that if something exists, it exists in some amount and therefore should ultimately be measurable. Furthermore, while it may not be necessary to have a precise operational definition of every construct employed in a theoretical system, the resources construct plays such a fundamental role in the resource perspective of cognitive aging that this view is in danger of being considered mere speculative fantasy without at least some evidence for its existence independent of the phenomena for which it is intended to explain.

A related but much less serious objection is that the classification of resources into three categories is misleading because the different conceptualizations are all interrelated. This possibility was briefly discussed in the introduction, and it is clearly conceivable that resources viewed in terms of space, energy, and time are interchangeable, and perhaps merely reflect different facets of the same mechanism or phenomenon. To the extent that this is the case, a correlational approach to determine the exact nature of the processing resource involved in cognitive aging is unlikely to be successful because different resource indices may simply consist of alternative manifestations of the same resource.

While the idea that what appear to be different types of resources are actually interrelated complicates analyses of the processing resources construct, it is still possible to investigate the role of processing resources in cognitive aging under this perspective. What is necessary is to explore many more potential measures of processing resources, both in isolation and in combination, and to seek evidence from as great a variety of research strategies as possible. As a means of progressing toward this latter goal, the next section consists of a discussion of advantages and disadvantages of six different research strategies that might be used to investigate the nature of the processing resources hypothesized to contribute to age differences in cognition.

## New Approaches to Identifying Age-Related Processing Resources

One research strategy is essentially a multivariate extension of the correlational analyses employed in the current studies. That is, several different indices or markers of each resource construct might be obtained in addition to performance measures from a variety of different cognitive tasks. The existence of multiple measures of each hypothesized resource should allow each construct to be defined and assessed more precisely, perhaps by relying on factors identified from factor analytic techniques or latent variables derived from latent variable causal modeling to serve as the indices of the various resources. Horn (1980, 1982; Horn, Donaldson, & Engstrom, 1981) has employed an approach of this type with factors derived from the fluid-crystallized theory of intelligence serving as the predictor (resource) and criterion (cognitive performance) variables. Despite considerable differences in the procedures and variables employed, there were some interesting similarities between Horn's results and those of the present studies. In particular, Horn et al. (1981) found that the amount of age-related decline was greater for a speed (CPS, or Clerical-Perceptual Speed) factor than for a factor (SAR, or Short-Term Acquisition and Retrieval) claimed to be comparable to the concept of working memory. Computations from the values contained in the correlation matrices of that report also reveal that the amount of attenuation in the association between age and fluid ability was greater after control of the speed factor than after control of the memory factor.

One disadvantage of the multivariate approach is that unless the number of predictor variables used to define the resource is small, the investigator runs the risk of, in effect, examining age differences in cognition after statistically controlling for cognition. In other words, when the number of variables contributing to the controlled factor increases, so also does the probability increase that the factor being controlled and the variable or factor being explained are no longer conceptually independent. Another complication with the use of factor-analytically defined resource indices is that the addition of multiple measures of the resource makes it much more cumbersome to establish the stability aspect of reliability because the entire ensemble of measurements must be replicated. That is, because internal consistency assessments of reliability are inadequate if one is concerned that performance could be affected by strategies that vary across time, some type of test-retest procedure is the more desirable means of determining reliability (cf. Salthouse, 1985a), and the time needed for these repeated measurements obviously increases in direct proportion to the number of relevant measures.

A second possible strategy for investigating the type of processing resources presumed to be involved in cognitive aging is to rely on physiological measures as the indices of different types of processing resources. This approach would also be similar to that employed in the current studies, but with physiological measures substituting for the behavioral measures as the resource indices in examining the predictions outlined in Table 7.1. This reductionistic approach offers the potential of leading to more immediate insights about the relations between physiology and cognition, as well as contributing to greater understanding about the exact nature of the hypothesized processing resource.

An additional advantage of focusing on physiological variables is that they may provide the most suitable indices of the conceptualization of processing resources in terms of energy or attentional capacity. Many candidate measures could be identified (e.g., cerebral blood flow, rate of glucose metabolism, magnitude of pupil dilation, components of the evoked response potential in the EEG, various indices of arousal, etc.), but it is important that whatever measure is employed satisfies the criteria for a suitable resource index enumerated earlier. In particular, the measure should be reliable, positively correlated with cognitive effectiveness, and negatively correlated with adult age. Reliability in the sense of temporal stability is essential because if the behavioral differences one is attempting to explain are stable then the processes presumed to be responsible for those differences should exhibit comparable stability. It is also necessary that the variable exhibit a positive association with measures of cognition and a negative association with age if the negative relation between age and performance is to be explained in terms of a reduction in the resource indexed by that variable.

Another conceivable approach to investigating processing resources involves comparing the patterns of deficit associated with increased age with the patterns of deficit observed under conditions known to be affected by altered quantities of a specified type of resource. A discovery of parallel patterns of impairment relative to a normative group such as healthy young adults could be interpreted as indicating that the previously identified resource may contribute to the age differences in cognition. However, this strategy is unlikely to be fruitful if the other condition is not so well understood that the impairments can be unambiguously attributed to a diminished quantity of a particular type of resource. Because this degree of understanding is characteristic of few, if any, of the conditions (e.g., alcoholic intoxication, brain damage, childhood, division of attention among two or more concurrent tasks, fatigue, hypoxia, schizophrenia, etc.) in which parallels have been drawn, successful application of this strategy may be delayed until appropriate advances have been made in the knowledge about causes of other types of cognitive impairment.

Investigation of tasks or processes postulated to make no demands on certain types of processing resources is a fourth possible strategy for investigating the involvement of different types of processing resources in cognitive aging. For example, if it is hypothesized that a particular task can be performed with no demands on working-memory capacity, then examination of age differences on that task could elucidate the involvement of the processing resource related to working-memory capacity in cognitive age differences. A finding that young and old adults performed equivalently on the task would be consistent with the view that an age-related reduction in working-memory capacity is responsible for many age differences in cognition. On the other hand, a discovery that older adults performed more poorly on the task than young adults might be interpreted as contradicting the hypothesis that resources related to working-memory capacity are responsible for age differences in cognitive functioning.

Unfortunately, there are several weaknesses with this line of argument, and it is not yet clear whether this approach would really be informative about the type of processing resource involved in cognitive aging. It is very difficult to establish that hypothesized task processes are truly independent of a particular type of processing resource. To illustrate, a popular manipulation to examine the degree of resource independence involves contrasting performance in the task under incidental and intentional instructional conditions, because it has been proposed that a defining characteristic of automatic or resource-independent processing is that it is unaffected by voluntary control. However, intentionality may be a weak manipulation for this purpose because it is not clear exactly what, or how much, it does. For example, intention may be necessary for the allocation of resources, or it may only be sufficient in which case resources could also be allocated without intention. And if resources can be allocated without intention, it is then meaningful to ask if intention adds more resources, channels the same amount of resources more effectively, or has effects unrelated to resource quantity such as utilization of a more optimal strategy of task performance.

A second difficulty with the approach of focusing on resource-independent tasks or processes is that the requisite knowledge about the specific resources of which a task is independent is simply not available for any currently used cognitive task. If one is not certain about the identity of the resource that is presumably not required for successful performance of the task, then this procedure will be of little help in identifying the nature of the age-affected resource.

Still another problem with the resource-independent procedure is that both the absence and the presence of age differences in task performance could be explained by factors unrelated to processing resources. For example, the absence of significant age differences might be attributable to low statistical power or to insensitive or unreliable measurement rather than to the task not requiring processing resources, and the presence of age differences might result from a variety of factors unrelated to the quantity of relevant resources because the amount of processing resources is hypothesized to be only one possible determinant of cognitive performance.

Experimental manipulation of the quantity of a particular type of processing resource is another possible strategy for determining the kind of processing resources involved in the age differences in cognition. If some means could be devised for altering the amount of a particular type of processing resource available to an individual, and if it is the quantity of that resource that is responsible for much of the cognitive aging phenomena, then it should be possible to mimic aging effects by reducing the quantity in young adults. Even more interesting is the potential for reversing age-related decline by increasing the quantity available to older adults.

Although if successful this strategy might well be the most convincing of those discussed, as well as the one with the greatest practical importance, it is only a matter of conjecture at the present time because knowledge about how it might be implemented is almost completely lacking. Ultimately resource quantity might be alterable with certain drug or surgical interventions, but this does not appear feasible with currently available information and procedures. What is clear, however, is that the amount of these internal resources is unlikely to be affected by simple external manipulations. For example, the quantity of resources related to working-memory capacity will probably not be affected by the presence or absence of memory aids such as a tape recorder or note pad, and the quantity of resources related to time will probably not be affected by increasing or decreasing the duration of stimulus presentation or the time allowed for a response. Manipulations such as these may alter the influence of the resource quantity in certain situations, but it is unrealistic to assume that they will completely eliminate the consequences of different amounts of an internal resource. As an illustration, manipulating the rate of stimulus presentation may influence the quality of stimulus encoding, but there is no reason to believe that it will also influence the efficiency of forming associations to the encoded representation, establishing relations among associations, determining higher level abstractions, etc. Because a general-purpose processing resource is presumed to influence the efficiency of a great many internal processes such as these, manipulations of the durations available for registering or responding to external events is unlikely to mimic all effects of time or speed when it is viewed as a resource involved in information processing.

The sixth and final strategy for investigating the nature of the processing resources hypothesized to be involved in the age differences in cognition is exploring the consequences of different types of resource limitations in formal and explicit models of the processing involved in particular cognitive tasks. The viability of different types of processing resources can then be examined by using the results from the models to serve as predictions in actual empirical studies.

An initial such step was described by Salthouse (1985a), who constructed a computer program designed to simulate the activity of a simple hierarchical network. The different conceptualizations of resources were implemented by manipulating the maximum number of nodes that could be active at one time as a reflection of the space resource, manipulating the total amount of activation in the network to correspond to the energy resource, and manipulating the number of time cycles between propagation of activation from one node to the next as a reflection of the time resource. All consequences of these manipulations have not yet been thoroughly explored, but preliminary results suggest that manipulations of the number of time cycles between propagation of activation produces particularly robust complexity effects of the type interpreted as supporting the existence of an influence of processing resources in cognitive aging. Much weaker (and sometimes absolutely no) complexity effects were apparent with the particular parameters examined thus far by manipulating the variables hypothesized to correspond to the space and energy conceptualizations of processing resources.

This model-based approach is obviously hampered by limited knowledge about the specific processes involved in any cognitive task, but it may offer one of the most promising techniques for understanding the consequences of specified resource limitations in a highly complex and interrelated system such as that responsible for human cognition. A major factor contributing to the lack of progress in understanding the role of processing resources in cognitive functioning has been inadequate, often naive, conceptualizations of the nature of, and consequences of limitations in, different types of processing resources. Implementation of alternative interpretations of resource limitations in mathematical or computer simulation models of cognition is one means of alleviating this problem by forcing the theorist to be explicit about the nature of the resource, and allowing detailed examination of the effects of restricting its quantity.

# Conclusion

This chapter examined the viability of a processing resource interpretation of cognitive age differences. Past usages of the processing resources concept have been too vague and imprecise to allow empirical examination; thus, several assumptions were made explicit and indices of different types of processing resources were identified to provide a means of investigating the validity of this perspective.

The results were moderately supportive of the view that age-related reductions in some type of processing resource contribute to age differences in cognitive functioning; less evidence supports a role of processing resources as a determinant of individual differences in performance within age groups. Although many of the individual results could probably be interpreted without invoking the resources concept, there is a need for a parsimonious explanation of the reductions of nearly 40% in the efficiency of processes involved in reasoning, spatial, and memory abilities between the twenties and the sixties. The proposal that age-related reductions in some type of general-purpose processing resources are responsible for at least some of these effects is still plausible, and therefore serves a useful integrative function. However, the processing resources notion should not be considered truly explanatory until the nature and role of these resources are better understood, and until detailed process analyses of individual tasks can specify when and how cognitive performance is affected by resource quantity.

*Acknowledgments.* This research was supported by grants from the National Institute on Aging (R01 AG04226) and Research Career Development Award (K04 AG00146). I thank K. Berry, S. Lawrence, S. Saults, and D. Smittle for assistance in collecting data, and Don Kausler for comments on an earlier draft of this manuscript.

## References

Arbuckle, T.Y., & Harsany, M. (1985). Adult age differences in recall of a moral dilemma under intentional, incidental, and dual task instructions. *Experimental Aging Research, 11,* 175–177.

Arenberg, D., & Robertson-Tchabo, E.A. (1985). Adult age differences in memory and linguistic integration revisited. *Experimental Aging Research, 11,* 187–191.

Attig, M., & Hasher, L. (1980). The processing of frequency of occurrence information by adults. *Journal of Gerontology, 35,* 66–69.

Baddeley, A. 1981. The concept of working memory: A view of its current state and probable future development. *Cognition, 10,* 17–23.

Birren, J.E., & Renner, V.J. (1977). Research on the psychology of aging: Principles and experimentation. In J.E. Birren & K.W. Schaie (Eds.), *Handbook of the psychology of aging* (pp. 3–38). New York: Van Nostrand Reinhold.

Botwinick, J. (1978). *Aging and behavior.* New York: Springer-Verlag.

Brainerd, C.J., & Kingma, J. (1985). On the independence of short-term memory and working memory in cognitive development. *Cognitive Psychology, 17,* 210–247.

Bromley, D.B. (1958). Some effects of age on short-term learning and remembering. *Journal of Gerontology, 13,* 398–406.

Byrd, M. (1985). Age differences in the ability to recall and summarize textual information. *Experimental Aging and Research, 11,* 87–91.

Carroll, J.B. (1976). Psychometric tests as cognitive tasks: A new "structure of intellect." In L.B. Resnick (Ed.), *The nature of intelligence* (pp. 27–56). Hillsdale, NJ: Erlbaum.

Cerella, J., Poon, L.W., & Williams, D.M. (1980). Age and the complexity hypothesis. In L.W. Poon (Ed.), *Aging in the 1980s* (pp. 332–340). Washington, DC: American Psychological Association.

Charness, N. (1985). Aging and problem solving. In N. Charness (Ed.), *Aging and human performance* (pp. 225–259). Chichester, England: Wiley.

Cohen, G. (1979). Language comprehension in old age. *Cognitive Psychology, 11,* 412–429.

Cohen, G. (1981). Inferential reasoning in old age. *Cognition, 9,* 59–72.
Craik, F.I.M., & Byrd, M. (1982). Aging and cognitive deficits: The role of attentional resources. In F.I.M. Craik & S.E. Trehub (Eds.), *Aging and cognitive processes* (pp. 191–211). New York: Plenum Press.
Craik, F.I.M., & Rabinowitz, J.C. (1984). Age differences in the acquisition and use of verbal information: A tutorial review. In H. Bouma & D.G. Bouwhuis (Eds.), *Attention and performance, 10,* (pp. 471–499). Hillsdale, NJ: Erlbaum.
Craik, F.I.M., & Simon, E. (1980). Age differences in memory: The roles of attention and depth of processing. In L.W. Poon, J.L. Fozard, L.S. Cermak, D. Arenberg, & L.W. Thompson (Eds.), *New directions in memory and aging* (pp. 95–112). Hillsdale, NJ: Erlbaum.
Crowder, R.G. (1980). Echoic memory and the study of aging memory systems. In L.W. Poon, J.L. Fozard, L.S. Cermak, D. Arenberg, & L.W. Thompson (Eds.), *New directions in memory and aging* (pp. 181–204). Hillsdale, NJ: Erlbaum.
Daneman, M., & Carpenter, P.A. (1980). Individual differences in working memory and reading. *Journal of Verbal Learning and Verbal Behavior, 19,* 450–466.
Duchek, J.M. (1984). Encoding and retrieval differences between young and old: The impact of attentional capacity usage. *Developmental Psychology, 20,* 1173–1180.
Edwards, A.L. (1976). *An introduction to linear regression and correlation.* San Francisco: Freeman.
Eysenck, H.J. (1967). Intelligence assessment: A theoretical and experimental approach. *British Journal of Psychology, 37,* 81–98.
French, J.W., Ekstrom, R.B., & Price, R.B. (1963). *Manual for kit of reference tests for cognitive factors.* Princeton, NJ: Educational Testing Service.
Hartley, A.A., & Anderson, J.W. (1983). Task complexity and problem-solving performance in younger and older adults. *Journal of Gerontology, 38,* 72–77.
Hartley, J.T. (1986). Reader and text variables as determinants of discourse memory in adulthood. *Psychology and Aging, 1,* 150–158.
Hasher, L., & Zacks, R.T. (1979). Automatic and effortful processes in memory. *Journal of Experimental Psychology: General, 108,* 356–388.
Hess, T.M. (1982). Visual abstraction processes in young and old adults. *Developmental Psychology, 18,* 473–484.
Hess, T.M. (1985). Aging and context influences on recognition memory for typical and atypical script actions. *Developmental Psychology, 21,* 1139–1151.
Hess, T.M., & Slaughter, S.J. (1986). Aging effects on prototype abstraction and concept identification. *Journal of Gerontology, 41,* 214–221.
Horn, J.L. (1978). Human ability systems. In P.B. Baltes (Ed.), *Life-span development and behavior* (Vol. 1, pp. 211–256). New York: Academic Press.
Horn, J.L. (1980). Concepts of intellect in relation to learning and adult development. *Intelligence, 4,* 285–317.
Horn, J.L. (1982). The theory of fluid and crystallized intelligence in relation to concepts of cognitive psychology and aging in adulthood. In F.I.M. Craik & S. Trehub (Eds.), *Aging and cognitive processes* (pp. 237–278). New York: Plenum Press.
Horn, J.L., & Cattell, R.B. (1967). Age differences in fluid and crystallized intelligence. *Acta Psychologica, 26,* 107–129.
Horn, J.L., Donaldson, G., & Engstrom, R. (1981). Apprehension, memory, and fluid intelligence decline in adulthood. *Research on Aging, 3,* 33–84.
Hoyer, W.J., & Plude, D.J. (1980). Attentional and perceptual processes in the study of

cognitive aging. In L.W. Poon (Ed.), *Aging in the 1980s* (pp. 227–238). Washington, DC: American Psychological Association.
Hoyer, W.J., & Plude, D.J. (1982). Aging and the allocation of attentional resources in visual information processing. In R. Sekuler, D. Kline, & K. Dismukes (Eds.), *Aging and human visual function* (pp. 245–263). New York: Alan R. Liss.
Inman, V.W., & Parkinson, S.R. (1983). Differences in Brown-Peterson recall as a function of age and retention interval. *Journal of Gerontology, 38,* 58–64.
Jensen, A.R. (1982). Reaction time and psychometric g. In H.J. Eysenck (Ed.), *A model for intelligence* (pp. 93–132). New York: Springer-Verlag.
Kahneman, D. (1973). *Attention and Effort.* Englewood Cliffs, NJ: Prentice-Hall.
Kausler, D.H., & Hakami, M.K. (1983). Memory for activities: Adult age differences and intentionality. *Developmental Psychology, 19,* 889–894.
Kausler, D.H., Hakami, M.K., & Wright, R.E. (1982). Adult age differences in frequency judgments of categorical representations. *Journal of Gerontology, 37,* 365–371.
Kausler, D.H., Lichty, W., & Davis, R.T. (1985). Temporal memory for performed activities: Intentionality and adult age differences. *Developmental Psychology, 21,* 1132–1138.
Kausler, D.H., & Puckett, J.M. (1980). Frequency judgments and correlated cognitive abilities in young and elderly adults. *Journal of Gerontology, 35,* 376–382.
Kausler, D.H., & Puckett, J.M. (1981). Adult age differences in memory for sex of voice. *Journal of Gerontology, 36,* 44–50.
Light, L.L., & Anderson, P.A. (1983). Memory for scripts in young and older adults. *Memory & Cognition, 11,* 435–444.
Light, L.L., & Anderson, P.A. (1985). Working-memory capacity, age, and memory for discourse. *Journal of Gerontology, 40,* 737–747.
Light, L.L., Zelinski, E.M., & Moore, M. (1982). Adult age differences in reasoning from new information. *Journal of Experimental Psychology: Learning, Memory and Cognition, 8,* 435–447.
Macht, M.L., & Buschke, H. (1983). Age differences in cognitive effort in recall. *Journal of Gerontology, 38,* 695–700.
Mulholland, T.M., Pellegrino, J.W., & Glaser, R. (1980). Components of geometric analogy solution. *Cognitive Psychology, 12,* 252–284.
Navon, D. (1984). Resources: A theoretical soup stone? *Psychological Review, 91,* 216–234.
Navon, D., & Gopher, D. (1979). On the economy of the human processing system. *Psychological Review, 86,* 214–255.
Newell, A., & Simon, H.A. (1972). *Human problem solving.* Englewood Cliffs, NJ: Prentice-Hall.
Norman, D.A., & Bobrow, D.G. (1975). On data limited and resource limited processes. *Cognitive Psychology, 7,* 44–64.
Parkinson, S.R., Inman, V.W., & Dannenbaum, S.E. (1985). Adult age differences in short-term forgetting. *Acta Psychologica, 60,* 83–101.
Parkinson, S.R., Lindholm, J.M., & Urell, T. (1980). Aging, dichotic memory and digit span. *Journal of Gerontology, 35,* 87–95.
Petros, T., Tabor, L., Cooney, T., & Chabot, R.J. (1983). Adult age differences in sensitivity to semantic structure of prose. *Developmental Psychology, 19,* 907–914.
Plude, D.J., & Hoyer, W.J. (1985). Attention and performance: Identifying and localiz-

ing age deficits. In N. Charness (Ed.), *Aging and human performance* (pp. 47–99). Chichester, England: Wiley.
Plude, D.J., & Hoyer, W.J. (1986). Age and the selectivity of visual information processing. *Psychology and Aging, 1,* 4–10.
Plude, D.J., Hoyer, W.J., & Lazar, J. (1982). Age, response complexity, and target consistency in visual search. *Experimental Aging Research, 8,* 99–102.
Puglisi, J.T. (1986). Age-related slowing in memory search for three-dimensional objects. *Journal of Gerontology, 41,* 72–78.
Rabinowitz, J.C., & Ackerman, B.P. (1982). General encoding of episodic events by elderly adults. In F.I.M. Craik & S. Trehub (Eds.), *Aging and cognitive processes* (pp. 145–154). New York: Plenum Press.
Rabinowitz, J.C., Ackerman, B.P., Craik, F.I.M., & Hinchley, J.L. (1982). Aging and metamemory: The roles of relatedness and imagery. *Journal of Gerontology, 37,* 688–695.
Rabinowitz, J.C., Craik, F.I.M., & Ackerman, B.P. (1982). A processing resource account of age differences in recall. *Canadian Journal of Psychology, 36,* 325–344.
Reisberg, D., Rappaport, I., & O'Shaughnessy, M. (1984). Limits of working memory: The digit-digit span. *Journal of Experimental Psychology: Learning, Memory and Cognition, 10,* 203–221.
Rose, A.M. (1980). Information-processing abilities. In R.E. Snow, P. Federico, & W.E. Montague (Eds.), *Aptitude, learning, and instruction* (Vol. 1, pp. 65–86). Hillsdale, NJ: Erlbaum.
Salthouse, T.A. (1974). Using selective interference to investigate spatial memory representations. *Memory & Cognition, 2,* 749–757.
Salthouse, T.A. (1975). Simultaneous processing of verbal and spatial information. *Memory & Cognition, 3,* 221–225.
Salthouse, T.A. (1982). *Adult cognition: An experimental psychology of human aging.* New York: Springer-Verlag.
Salthouse, T.A. (1985a). *A theory of cognitive aging.* Amsterdam: North-Holland.
Salthouse, T.A. (1985b). Speed of behavior and its implications for cognition. In J.E. Birren & K.W. Schaie (Eds.), *Handbook of the psychology of aging* (2nd ed., pp. 400–426). New York: Van Nostrand Reinhold.
Spearman, C. (1927). *The abilities of man.* New York: Macmillan.
Spilich, G.J. (1983). Life-span components of text processing: Structural and procedural differences. *Journal of Verbal Learning and Verbal Behavior, 22,* 231–244.
Spilich, G.J. (1985). Discourse comprehension across the span of life. In N. Charness (Ed.), *Aging and human performance* (pp. 143–190). Chichester, England: Wiley.
Storandt, M. (1976). Speed and coding effects in relation to age and ability level. *Developmental Psychology, 12,* 177–178.
Wickens, C.D. (1980). The structure of attentional resources. In R.S. Nickerson (Ed.), *Attention and performance, VIII* (pp. 239–257). Hillsdale, NJ: Erlbaum.
Wright, R.E. (1981). Aging, divided attention, and processing capacity. *Journal of Gerontology, 36,* 605–614.

# 8. Internal Validity Threats in Studies of Adult Cognitive Development

*K. Warner Schaie*

## Introduction

If development is viewed as a process that implicitly requires time to elapse to observe quantitative change or qualitative transformations, it then follows that age-comparative studies or other experimental manipulations can at best simulate development. It is obviously impossible to assign experimental subjects at random to different ages or different measurement occasions. The formal investigation of developmental processes, therefore, typically involves quasi-experiments in which carefully selected population samples are followed over time to observe whether or not hypothesized transformations can indeed be observed.

The concept of the quasi-experiment was popularized by the classical Campbell and Stanley (1967) research design monograph. These authors collectively denote as quasi-experiments "many natural social settings in which the research person can introduce something like experimental design . . . even though he lacks the full control over the scheduling of experimental stimuli . . . which make a true experiment possible" (p. 34). One example of a quasi-experiment for the study of cognitive aging, is the typical cross-sectional study in which aging effects are modeled by comparing subsamples that differ in age but which are assumed to be matched in all other aspects (Salthouse, 1982). A more complex example of a quasi-experiment in this substantive field would be a longitudinal study in which subjects are tested at specified ages, and re-examined at regular time intervals, where amount of practice is controlled for by adding matched controls groups at successive measurement points (Schaie, 1983a).

Because of the fact that quasi-experiments do not permit random assignment of study participants to different conditions with respect to which hypotheses are to be examined, the issue of the validity of such studies looms large. Campbell and Stanley (1967) distinguish between internal and external validity threats. The former refer to alternative interpretations which arise as a consequence of design flaws, the latter reflect the degree to which findings from internally valid studies can be generalized to other populations. Both of these classes of validity threats have substantial effects on the interpretability of studies of adult cognitive development (cf. Schaie, 1977). Specifically, these validity threats force us to examine the possibility that design flaws may be equally or more parsimonious in explaining results than the experimenter's stated hypothesis. Interestingly enough, at least some studies of adult cognitive aging have collected data that allow the investigator either to control for or to assess the validity threats inherent in their study designs. It is the unusual research report, however, that provides adequate documentation to show whether or not the reported findings might be more parsimoniously attributable to a detectable design flaw.

In this chapter I call attention to those threats to the internal validity of quasi-experiments that should be of concern to developmentalists at all stages of the life span, but that have been most directly addressed thus far in studies of adult cognitive development. All of the validity threats discussed here are directly amenable to experimental control or empirical assessment, given appropriate design strategies (cf. Schaie, 1973, 1977). Explicit designs derived from the longitudinal-sequential approach (Schaie, 1965) are examined to show how internal validity threats can be effectively handled in longitudinal studies. Finally, some empirical data are provided that show applications of these designs to the assessment of the significance of internal validity threats for data on adult cognitive behavior.

## Threats to the Internal Validity of Developmental Studies

Eight different threats to the internal validity of quasi-experiments have been described by Campbell and Stanley (1967). One of these, maturation, represents no threat to the validity of developmental studies, if their intent is to test hypotheses about effects of aging. The remaining seven threats to be considered in order represent rival hypotheses to the effect of aging (i.e., maturational or age-specific changes). They involve the rival hypotheses of the effects of history, testing (reactivity), instrumentation, statistical regression, experimental mortality (attrition), selection, and certain interactions thereof. I briefly review the implications of these threats as they apply to the interpretability of findings in aging studies. A representative paradigm in such studies would be the natural experiment format of the typical pretest-treatment-posttest variety, in which the "treatment" is assumed to be the aging of the organism under study. In this design I compare the behavior of a sample of individuals at two points in time ($T_1$ and $T_2$) and infer that a change observed in the dependent variable has occurred as a function of the treatment; that is, the lapse of time during which the organism has matured. I now examine specific potential flaws to this inference.

## History

With the exception of well-controlled animal studies, it is inevitable that events may occur in the environment between $T_1$ and $T_2$ that could account for the observed behavioral change, whether or not a maturationally determined change had occurred. We have no assurance that the unknown environmental event that resulted in behavioral change will recur with similar impact if we were to replicate our study over another time interval (Schaie, 1982). For example, age differences in life satisfaction for black and while elderly have been shown to exhibit different temporal patterns as a consequence of environmental changes that had more dramatic effects on the black than the white elderly (Schaie, Orshowsky, & Parham, 1982). We must conclude then that the single-cohort longitudinal study fails to control for history. This flaw might not be unduly bothersome in studies of physiological development during childhood, except during periods of intense political turbulence that create special hazards (e.g., malnutrition, exposure to excess radiation). In adults, however, changing conditions of health care and or stress may quite readily suppress or exacerbate maturational phenomena. In behavioral studies, there are so many possible sources of events at all age levels that can affect the dependent variable differentially across time that the single-cohert longitudinal study will rarely be useful to detect reliably generalizable behavioral changes (cf. Schaie, 1972; Nesselroade & Baltes, 1974).

## Reactivity (Testing or Practice Effects)

Administering a test or survey instrument or introducing an observer into a behavioral situation may also result in effects that might erroneously be interpreted to be maturational. In the cognitive literature in particular, practice effects may be particularly serious over short periods of time but long-term reactivity effects may also prevail (cf. Schaie & Parham, 1974). For example, it is not clear whether differential aging patterns in fluid and crystallized intelligence (Horn, 1982) may not be attributable to the fact that greater practice opportunities are available for crystallized abilities. The reactivity threat to the validity of a longitudinal study can be controlled for by carrying a randomly assigned untested control group to be examined at $T_2$ only. However, this simple approach is also flawed because reactivity will be confounded with effects of experimental mortality that in this design cannot be assessed for the control group.

## Instrumentation

Changes in measurement instruments, experimenters, or protocol between $T_1$ and $T_2$ are the most obvious sources of artifactual changes that could be caused by instrumentation effects. Other more subtle sources reflect changes in the projection of observed (measured) variables on the latent constructs of interest (unmeasured variables), changes that may well be substantial if comparisons are made over different developmental stages or extensive time periods (cf. Schaie & Hertzog, 1982, 1985). The latter effects can, of course, be examined only if a study contains multiple markers of the constructs at all measurement points (an empirical example testing the construct equivalence for a cognitive data set in adults is provided in Schaie, Willis, Hertzog, & Schulenberg, 1987). Instrumentation effects for single variables can be untangled from practice effect, but will remain confounded with the effect of history.

## Statistical Regression

The concept of statistical regression implies that when the position of an individual at $T_2$ is predicted from that person's score at $T_1$, the best prediction would be that the score at $T_2$ will be closer to the mean of the group. The degree of such movement will be directly influenced by the reliability of the measurement operations; the lower the reliability, the greater the regression to the mean. It should be noted, however, that the concept of statistical regression is a function of the system of linear predictions (cf. Hays, 1963, pp. 500–501). In the typical research situation, regression to the mean may occur for empirical as well as statistical reasons. For example, it has been argued that age may be more kind to the more able, but empirical studies do not necessarily support this argument (Baltes et al., 1972).

If the regression effect results from unreliability of the measures, then one would expect the variance at $T_2$ to be lower than that at $T_1$, but such reduction in variance is not guaranteed when regression to the mean occurs as a consequence of interventions that have differential effects at different portions of the range of talent. In any event, it is likely that mean scores above the population average at $T_1$ will be lower at $T_2$ while low means will increase. Such regression effects would serve to enhance or obscure true maturational effects (Furby, 1973). There have been some arguments to support the contention that regression effects should not be cumulative across successive occasions (Nesselroade, Stigler, & Baltes, 1980). Regression effects must, nevertheless, be taken seriously in any longitudinal two-point comparisons. Examples of intuitive methods using a time-reversal paradigm that will differentiate maturational and regression effects have been described elsewhere

(Baltes et al., 1972; Campbell & Stanley, 1967; Schaie and Willis, 1986b), but will not be considered further in this chapter.

## Experimental Mortality (Attrition)

A major threat to the internal validity of a pretest-treatment-posttest design occurs when all subjects tested at $T_1$ are not available for retest at $T_2$. In studies of cognitive aging, experimental mortality would include death, disability, disappearance, and simple failure to cooperate for the second test. There is a substantial literature that reports differences in base performance between those who appear and those who fail to appear for the second or subsequent tests. Typically the dropouts at base score lower on ability variables and describe themselves as possessing less socially desirable traits than to the retest survivors (e.g., Baltes, Schaie, & Nardi, 1971; Cooney, Schaie, & Willis, 1988; Riegel, Riegel, & Meyer, 1967; Schaie, Labouvie, & Barrett, 1973). As a consequence it has been argued that longitudinal studies may represent successively more elite groups, and may no longer be sufficiently generalizable. This proposition can be tested, however, and suitable adjustments for attrition are readily available.

## Selection

Differential selection per se is not a problem in single-cohort longitudinal studies. However, it becomes the major internal validity threat in cross-sectional and other nonequivalent control group designs. It has long been known that it is virtually impossible to rule out the likelihood that differences observed across groups selected at different ages may well be a function of differential recruitment, particularly when snowball or other voluntary panels of subjects are utilized (Schaie, 1959). Selections effects in developmentally oriented studies have typically been considered under the rubric of cohort effects (cf. Baltes, Cornelius, & Nesselroade, 1979; Schaie, 1965, 1977, 1986). More complex designs are required to control for or assess these effects (see following).

## Interactions

A number of interactions of the threats discussed may also be problematic for the design of studies of adult cognitive development.

### Maturation by History

This interaction is of particular concern in cross-sectional studies in which one must consider the possibility that effects of environmental impact could have differential import depending on the life stage of the individual when the impact occurred. For example, the effects of the Vietnam era made a much greater impact on the cohort then liable to be drafted than on younger or older persons. In longitudinal studies, the possibility of differential maturation by history effects must also be considered when individuals are followed over several measurement points.

## Maturation by Experimental Mortality

Drop-out effects do not necessarily occur in a symmetrical fashion. In particular, drop out due to death or disability may be systematically related to the age of the sample studied. For example, among the young-old, drop-out effects are greatest for individuals lost by illness, while for the old-old the effects are greatest for those lost due to death (Cooney et al., 1988). Experimental mortality by age effects can be estimated only when more than one cohort is followed longitudinally.

## Maturation by Reactivity

Again, practice or other reactivity effects may well differ by age. This interaction may reflect prior differential exposure to the measurement operations at different ages. For example, college students are likely to have attained an asymptotic level with respect to many ability measures because of similar recent experiences during the educational process. Older individuals, by contrast, may not have taken educational tests for several decades. Assessment of the significance of this interaction requires the assessment of practice effects at two or more age levels.

## Maturation by Selection

Maturational effects can have differential magnitudes depending on the selection conditions prevailing when sampling occurs. For example, changes in rate of cognitive decline will lead to differential representation of well-functioning older persons for successive generations. The disaggregation of aging and selection (cohort) effects requires the study of two or more cohorts at two or more ages.

Controlling for any of these complex validity threats or disaggregating the effects attributable to maturation from the various confounded sources of variance typically requires multiple test occasions and replications of cross-sectional or longitudinal studies or their combination in a single design. We next examine appropriate design complications that have been proposed for use in the study of adult cognitive development. Later, empirical examples of an application of each of these designs are presented.

# The Longitudinal-Sequential Approach As a Method for the Control or Assessment of Internal Validity Threats

In this section, I discuss a number of designs that can be utilized to control or assess most of the internal validity threats discussed above. To begin, a number of rather simple design variations that control for a single rival hypothesis are described. Designs that control for multiple threats are then presented. The reader should note that the most carefully controlled or complex design is not necessarily the best. In fact, the first step in design selection must be to reason out whether or not a given threat has a high probability of occurrence for the dependent variable of interest. All controls are expensive in experimenter effort and resources, and controls should therefore be imposed only when absolutey required to protect the integrity of a given study. Good research paradigms are therefore always driven by meta-theoretical context (cf. Costa & McCrae, 1982; Hultsch & Hickey, 1978; Labouvie, 1982; Nesselroade & Labouvie, 1985; Schaie & Hertzog, 1982). The following designs have been developed in a dialectic process that involved conducting studies that were discovered to have design flaws, designing paradigms that would remedy these flaws, and then discovering that the new designs required acquisition of further data sets (cf. also Schaie, 1959; 1973; 1977; 1986; Schaie & Willis, 1986, pp. 23–34).

## Direct Assessment of Attrition Effects

Attrition effects can be assessed directly in a pretest-treatment-posttest design by testing the null hypothesis for the dependent variable at $T_1$, comparing participants who have returned for the $T_2$ measurement with those who have not (cf. Baltes, Schaie, & Nardi, 1971; Schaie et al., 1973). Because of the cross-sectional nature of the comparison, however, this most direct analysis will only provide information on the changing nature of our longitudinal sample; it will not provide an estimate of the effects of attrition on the measurement of age changes. Nor can this level of attrition analysis account for the possible confounding of attrition with practice, or the interaction with maturation, and selection. More complex analyses, as are described later in this chapter are required to resolve these confounds.

## Direct Assessment of Practice Effects

The most direct assessment of practice (reactivity) effects is accomplished either by carrying a control group that has not been examined at $T_1$, or by drawing a new random sample from the cohort tested at $T_1$ for assessment at $T_2$. Since experimental and control groups differ at $T_2$ only in that the control has not received previous practice, differences in performance at $T_2$ can then be treated as a reasonable estimate of the magnitude of practice effects. An important caveat for this design, however, must be that attrition effects are equivalent for the experimental and control groups. But attrition effect estimates require that $T_1$ scores be available for both experimental and control groups. We obviously do not have this information for the control group, and must conclude that the most direct estimate will necessarily be confounded with attrition effects. Nevertheless, if attrition is relatively limited, the direct assessment of practice as suggested here may be the most viable approach. Moreover, if we are willing to assume that attrition effects in the experimental and control group are comparable, it is then possible to adjust estimates of practice effects by the differentials between dropouts and controls at the $T_1$ assessment (see examples described later in this chapter).

It has been shown that nonrandom effects of experimental mortality are most pronounced from $T_1$ to $T_2$; thereafter, attrition continues but tends to become somewhat more random with respect to the dependent variable until advanced ages are reached (cf. Gribbin & Schaie, 1979). An alternative, somewhat more complex, design for estimating practice effects (that would also control for nonpractice-related reactivity to the first measurement) would require carrying both experimental and control groups for one more measurement occasion. The estimate of practice would then be the difference between groups of equivalent maturational level at $T_3$, at which time we would be testing for the effect of one additional unit of practice. In this case it would, incidentially, be possible to assess the equivalence of attrition effects from $T_2$ to $T_3$ across experimental and control groups (see above).

## Designs That Combine Controls for the Effects of History or Selection With the Assessment of Attrition Effects and/or Practice

The more complex designs required to handle more than one internal validity threat or those involving interactions are derived from what has been called "a general model for the study of developmental problems" (Schaie, 1965, 1977, 1986) and typically involve a further complication of one of the longitudinal-sequential strategies. These strategies allow three basic options: The first approach crosses maturational and selection effects (cohort-sequential design) by sampling two or more cohorts over the same age range, thus conducting a multicohort longitudinal study. The second option crosses maturational and history effects (time-sequential design) by sampling two or more age levels at two or more measurement points; this is a replicated cross-sectional study. The third approach crosses maturational and selection effects (cross-sequential design) by sampling two cohorts across the same time interval—a mixed cross-sectional and longitudinal approach.

### History by Attrition Designs

We can assess the effects of history and attrition by considering two longitudinal samples carried over the same age range: that is, sample 1 is followed from $T_1$ to $T_2$ and sample 2 from $T_2$ to $T_3$. Because only the first measurement points are considered for either sample, this design is cross-sectional and thus controls for testing and reactivity. This design can be analyzed by a two-way ANOVA that crosses attrition and time of measurement. Note, however, that this approach does not control for selection effects.

The time-sequential strategy allows a more general (and interesting) format for this design in that it allows estimating the components of variance associated with maturation, history, and attrition. The sampling plan and ANOVA model for this general approach have previously been described (Schaie, 1977, p. 53, Table 10; also see following example). This design requires a minimum of two age levels from two samples initially assessed at $T_1$ or $T_2$. The attrition information is obtained by assessing sample 1 also at $T_2$ and sample 2 at $T_3$. The last assessment point does not enter the analysis.

### Selection by Attrition Designs

A more complex approach is required to cross maturational, selection and attrition effects. This can be accomplished by extending the standard cohort-sequential design (Schaie, 1977, p. 44, Table 2). Two cohorts are followed over a minimum of two ages. The first cohort is assessed at $T_1$, $T_2$, and $T_3$, while the second cohort is assessed at $T_2$, $T_3$, and $T_4$. In each case the final assessment is for the purpose of identifying dropouts and does not enter the analysis. Note that this design does not control for testing and reactivity. That is, attrition and practice effects must necessarily be confounded. However, it is possible to include the necessary controls by utilizing the cohort-sequential design with independent measurements (Schaie, 1977, p. 45, Table 3). In this instance, we would need to carry a minimum of two samples from each of two cohorts at two age levels. Again four assessment points are required: $C_1A_1S_1$ is tested at $T_1$ and $T_2$; $C_1A_2S_2$ and $C_2A_1S_1$ are tested at $T_2$ and $T_3$; and $C_2A_2S_2$ is tested at $T_3$ and $T_4$. Only data at first time of test are included in this analysis to control for testing and reactivity.

### History by Selection by Attrition Designs

During those periods of adulthood when maturational change is minimal, it is also possible to specify designs that allow crossing attrition effects, with both history and selection. These designs involve extensions of the cross-sequential approach (Schaie, 1977, p. 49, Tables 7 and 8). These designs follow a minimum of two cohorts over at least two times of measurement, with an additional measurement point at $T_3$ to determine dropouts following the $T_2$ assessment. The repeated measures design requires classification into dropouts and survivors after the first and second assessment. Experimental mortality at $T_2$ consequently is confounded with practice effects. In the independent measurement variant, practice is controlled for, but separate samples must be assessed twice for each level of the design.

### History by Practice Designs

Crossing history and practice for a particular age level requires a minimum of four samples and three measurement occasions. Data are compared at $T_2$ and $T_3$ for samples of equivalent age that were either previously assessed at $T_1$ and $T_2$, or that are assessed at $T_2$ and $T_3$ for the first time. A more general format of this design, which balances ages at pretest, is an extension of the time-sequential design that crosses maturation, history and practice (see Schaie, 1977, p. 47, Table 6). This design requires four samples at each of two age levels, half of which are pretested at an earlier occasion before generating the data that enter this analysis. Note that this design confounds practice with attrition.

### Selection by Practice Designs

The cohort-sequential design with independent measurements can be expanded to permit crossing of maturation, selection, and practice. A minimum of two samples are required at each age level for each cohort, half of whom have received practice at a previous data point that does not enter analysis. As a consequence, a minimum of four assessment points will be required for this design, which also confounds practice with attrition (see Schaie, 1977, p. 46, Table 4).

### History by Selection by Practice Designs

Once again, for those adult age levels when maturation can be assumed to be trivial, it would be possible to cross history, selection, and practice by an extended version of the cross-sequential design with independent measurements. The minimum design here requires three assessment points. That is, each of the four possible cohort/time of measurement combinations (at $T_2$ and $T_3$) would require two samples, one of which received practice at $T_1$ or $T_2$ respectively (see Schaie, 1977, p. 50, Table 9).

### Designs Crossing Practice and Attrition

Using the independent measurement designs allows assessing the effects of experimental mortality while controlling for practice. The converse approach (assessing effects of practice while controlling for experimental mortality) is not feasible because study participants returning for a second assessment represent, by definition, only the group of retest survivors. It is possible, however, to cross attrition and practice, if rather than comparing only survivors and dropouts after $T_1$, we also consider survivors and dropouts after $T_2$. In this case a prior occasion not entering analysis is required for half of our groups, and all individuals must be followed to the occasion beyond the last analysis point, to determine dropouts and survivors for each subset. All the designs described can be treated in this manner, but an additional assessment occasion is required. Thus designs crossing practice, attrition, maturation, and history, or those crossing practice, attrition, selection, and history will require four assessment occasions. The design that crosses practice, attrition, selection, and history requires a minimum of five occasions (see Schaie, 1977, pp. 54–55, Table 11).

# Empirical Data on the Significance of Internal Validity Threats for Data on Adult Cognitive Development

## Description of the Data Base

The data to be discussed come from the Seattle Longitudinal Study (SLS), a multiwave panel study that uses as its population frame the membership of a metropolitan health maintenance organization (cf. Schaie, 1983b). All 3442 participants were, at first test, community-dwelling adults who were randomly selected from each 7-year age stratum included in each panel. These data were collected in 1956 ($N$ = 500; ages 22–70 years), 1963 ($N$ = 997; ages 22–77), 1970 ($N$ = 705; ages 22–84); 1977 ($N$ = 612; ages 22–84), and 1984 ($N$ = 628; ages 22–84 years). At each successive data point as many survivors of the previous wave as possible were reexamined. Thus we have 1357 participants for whom 7-year longitudinal data at $T_2$ are available for four data sets: 1963 ($N$ = 303; ages 29–77), 1970 ($N$ = 420; ages 29–84), 1977 ($N$ = 340; ages 29–91), and 1984 ($N$ = 294; ages 29-91). Fourteen-year longitudinal data at $T_3$ are available for 723 participants in three data sets: 1970 ($N$ = 162; ages 36–84), 1977 ($N$ = 337; ages 36–91), and 1984 ($N$ = 224; ages 36–94). Twenty-one-year longitudinal data at $T_4$ exist for 355 participants in two data sets: 1977 ($N$ = 130; ages 43–91), and 1984 ($N$ = 225; ages 43–94). Finally, there is one 28-year longitudinal data set in 1984 at $T_5$ ($N$ = 97; ages 50–94 years).

All participants were in good health when tested, and were representative of the upper 75% of the socioeconomic stratum. For the total data base educational levels averaged 13.27 years (range, 4–20 years), and occupational status averaged 6.25 on a 10-point scale using census classifications ranging from unskilled labor to professional.

Throughout the study, subjects were assessed with the first five primary mental abilities (Schaie, 1985; Thurstone & Thurstone, 1941), the Test of Behavioral Rigidity (Schaie & Parham, 1975), and a demographic information form. All subjects were tested in small groups in sessions, which for the first three waves lasted about 2 hours, for the fourth wave about 3 hours, and for the fifth wave in two sessions of 2.5 hours each (necessary because multiple markers of the abilities and other additional measures were added). For the examples in this chapter we will limit our discussion to the five primary abilities: Verbal Meaning, the ability to comprehend words, a measure of recognition vocabulary; Spatial Orientation, the ability to mentally rotate objects in two-dimensional space; Inductive Reasoning, the ability to infer rules from examples that contain regular progressions of information; Number, the ability to manipulate number concepts, as measured by checking simple addition problems; and Word Fluency, a measure of recall vocabulary.

## Some Basic Findings

The foregoing data base by now contains sufficient information to allow us to conduct virtually all of the analyses that I have described, allowing either controls for or assessment of the magnitude of effects of the internal validity threats described previously. I begin my discussion by presenting some basic data and then proceeding through some further analyses investigating the effects of the internal validity threats. For ease of comparison across the different measurement variables, all raw scores have been scaled to T-score form ($M = 50, SD = 10$) on the basis of the total sample of 3442 individuals at first test across all five test occasions. All data have been organized in subsets with equal interval boundaries; that is, all age and cohort groupings are expressed in 7-year intervals to conform to the 7-year intervals between assessment occasions.

### The Cross-Sectional Sequence

The initial test data can be conceptualized as a sequence of five cross-sectional studies. Table 8.1 provides the scaled means for each separate sample for all available age groups. Weighted means across the five data sets are also provided, and the significance level (from one-way ANOVAs) is indicated for those age levels at which the means for the separate samples differ in a nonchance manner. Significant findings here provide evidence for the presence of selection by history effects. Significant variation across time (time lags) are characteristic for most age levels of all the Primary Mental Ability (PMA) variables, with the exception of Spatial Orientation.

These data of course do not allow direct inferences on age change in cognitive behavior within individuals. They are, however, relevant for a description of age differences among groups of individuals, as well as the identification of peak performance ages, at particular points in time. Over the age range from 25 to 67 years (data available for all five test occasions), for example, peak performance ages for Verbal Meaning have shifted upwards from age 32 in 1956 to age 46 in 1984, and the range of mean age differences has

TABLE 8.1. Scaled Means for the Primary Mental Abilities for Five Cross-Sectional Samples Assessed at 7-Year Intervals

| Mean Age | 1956 | 1963 | 1970 | 1977 | 1984 | Average |
|---|---|---|---|---|---|---|
| Verbal Meaning | | | | | | |
| 25 | 52.64 | 53.30 | 53.84 | 54.68 | 55.46 | 53.94 |
| 32 | 54.87 | 54.05 | 53.80 | 56.22 | 54.83 | 54.64 |
| 39 | 51.90 | 54.20 | 53.95 | 54.96 | 56.86 | 54.83** |
| 46 | 53.36 | 51.73 | 54.86 | 52.49 | 57.36 | 53.54*** |
| 53 | 49.10 | 48.35 | 54.45 | 52.87 | 54.79 | 51.43*** |
| 60 | 44.45 | 46.84 | 52.30 | 50.64 | 52.46 | 49.16*** |
| 67 | 42.56 | 42.57 | 45.26 | 46.44 | 48.68 | 44.86*** |
| 74 | — | 39.66 | 39.85 | 40.88 | 44.32 | 41.11** |
| 81 | — | — | 37.92 | 35.72 | 40.60 | 37.92** |
| Spatial Orientation | | | | | | |
| 25 | 54.00 | 53.30 | 53.84 | 54.68 | 55.46 | 53.94* |
| 32 | 54.95 | 54.16 | 57.28 | 55.98 | 54.02 | 55.14 |
| 39 | 51.96 | 53.16 | 53.84 | 54.78 | 53.10 | 53.38 |
| 46 | 51.12 | 51.76 | 54.73 | 52.72 | 53.82 | 52.71 |
| 53 | 47.28 | 48.99 | 50.82 | 51.00 | 49.51 | 49.52 |
| 60 | 46.16 | 48.14 | 48.85 | 47.65 | 48.08 | 47.87 |
| 67 | 44.10 | 44.22 | 43.77 | 46.98 | 43.97 | 44.55 |
| 74 | — | 41.97 | 42.16 | 41.68 | 41.72 | 41.88 |
| 81 | — | — | 40.70 | 39.44 | 39.82 | 39.92 |
| Inductive Reasoning | | | | | | |
| 25 | 55.19 | 58.60 | 59.84 | 59.02 | 60.01 | 58.23*** |
| 32 | 55.67 | 56.02 | 58.14 | 57.72 | 58.86 | 56.91* |
| 39 | 51.07 | 53.84 | 54.13 | 56.60 | 57.83 | 54.53*** |
| 46 | 51.68 | 50.07 | 53.56 | 52.61 | 56.18 | 52.29*** |
| 53 | 48.41 | 46.45 | 51.09 | 51.55 | 53.72 | 49.56*** |
| 60 | 42.63 | 44.83 | 49.52 | 48.31 | 50.97 | 47.10*** |
| 67 | 42.04 | 40.53 | 42.80 | 45.02 | 46.83 | 43.13*** |
| 74 | — | 39.86 | 39.51 | 40.82 | 44.16 | 41.03*** |
| 81 | — | — | 38.81 | 38.91 | 38.86 | 38.86 |
| Number | | | | | | |
| 25 | 48.79 | 50.73 | 51.29 | 49.25 | 48.22 | 49.69 |
| 32 | 51.67 | 53.78 | 53.49 | 50.72 | 50.55 | 52.35 |
| 39 | 51.25 | 54.31 | 52.37 | 51.17 | 48.83 | 52.10** |
| 46 | 53.58 | 53.01 | 55.46 | 48.07 | 51.52 | 52.57*** |
| 53 | 52.80 | 50.66 | 54.74 | 51.80 | 48.99 | 51.77** |
| 60 | 47.58 | 49.64 | 55.20 | 50.42 | 49.50 | 50.45*** |
| 67 | 47.67 | 46.55 | 48.24 | 49.94 | 48.79 | 48.06* |
| 74 | — | 44.33 | 44.90 | 44.64 | 46.91 | 45.19 |
| 81 | — | — | 41.35 | 42.07 | 41.73 | 41.74 |

TABLE 8.1 *Continued*

| Mean Age | 1956 | 1963 | 1970 | 1977 | 1984 | Average |
|---|---|---|---|---|---|---|
| Word Fluency | | | | | | |
| 25 | 53.96 | 52.34 | 53.36 | 53.50 | 55.19 | 53.63 |
| 32 | 56.65 | 52.54 | 50.78 | 54.71 | 54.90 | 53.71** |
| 39 | 54.30 | 51.91 | 50.36 | 52.00 | 54.71 | 52.45* |
| 46 | 56.49 | 50.80 | 52.66 | 49.55 | 53.47 | 52.20*** |
| 53 | 55.63 | 47.68 | 52.82 | 50.91 | 51.98 | 51.15*** |
| 60 | 50.00 | 49.15 | 50.42 | 50.09 | 47.70 | 49.43 |
| 67 | 47.95 | 44.64 | 44.12 | 47.68 | 46.95 | 46.01* |
| 74 | — | 44.66 | 41.54 | 43.07 | 44.78 | 43.45* |
| 81 | — | — | 42.46 | 41.82 | 41.24 | 41.84 |

*$p < .05$; **$p < .01$; ***$p < .001$.

been reduced from approximately 1 *SD* to 0.6 *SD*. For Inductive Reasoning, the range of age differences has remained the same, but the peak performance age has shifted upwards from age 32 to age 46. For Word Fluency the range of age difference has increased slightly, and the peak performance age has shifted downward from 32 to 25. Age difference patterns have remained fairly stable for Spatial Orientation, while substantial nonsystematic fluctuation occurred for Number skill.

It should be evident that any particular set of age differences will be confounded with cohort (selection) differences, and that an assessment of reasonably stable age differences will require aggregation of data for several cross-sectional studies covering the same age ranges. Such average data are given in the last column of Table 8.1.

## THE LONGITUDINAL SEQUENCES

The estimates of mean level obtained at various ages from the longitudinal studies are not directly interpretable since they reflect data from attrited samples. Direct estimates of within-individual change over time are consequently more informative. Table 8.2 provides data on longitudinal change for the PMA variables over a 7-year period aggregated across the four longitudinal sequences described. The last column in this table aggregates 7-year changes regardless of level of prior practice to obtain the largest possible sample sizes. It will be noticed that on average small gains are experienced into the thirties, and that decremental age changes are quite small and only reach Cohen's (1977) criterion of a minimally interesting effect size (0.2 *SD*) for some variables by age 67. Such changes, increasing in magnitude, are then seen for successive 7-year intervals.

It is of interest further to note the cumulative effect of longitudinal age changes as derived from the overall estimates in the last column of Table 8.2.

TABLE 8.2. Magnitude of Longitudinal Age Changes for the Primary Mental Abilities Across a 7-Year Interval[a]

| | $T_1$ to $T_2$ | | $T_2$ to $T_3$ | | $T_3$ to $T_4$ | | $T_4$ to $T_5$ | | Average | |
|---|---|---|---|---|---|---|---|---|---|---|
| Mean Ages | *N* | *d* | *N* | *d* | *N* | *d* | *N* | *d* | *N* | *d* |
| **Verbal Meaning** | | | | | | | | | | |
| 25–32 | 135 | +1.42 | | — | | — | | — | 135 | +1.42 |
| 32–39 | 169 | +1.70 | 69 | +0.08 | | — | | — | 238 | +1.23 |
| 39–46 | 213 | +1.06 | 96 | +0.02 | 34 | −2.26 | | — | 343 | +0.45 |
| 46–53 | 204 | +0.54 | 108 | −0.56 | 52 | −0.95 | 13 | −0.73 | 377 | −0.03 |
| 53–60 | 223 | −0.28 | 126 | −0.55 | 56 | −1.60 | 17 | −1.67 | 422 | −0.68 |
| 60–67 | 170 | −1.59 | 117 | −2.24 | 70 | −2.82 | 17 | −0.65 | 374 | −2.03 |
| 67–74 | 163 | −2.12 | 66 | −3.17 | 55 | −3.00 | 22 | −3.28 | 306 | −2.59 |
| 74–81 | 60 | −1.79 | 49 | −4.05 | 21 | −2.61 | 14 | −5.93 | 144 | −3.43 |
| 81–88 | 18 | −4.68 | 8 | −9.70 | 10 | −9.25 | 3 | −8.67 | 39 | −7.36 |
| **Spatial Orientation** | | | | | | | | | | |
| 25–32 | 135 | +0.99 | | — | | — | | — | 135 | +0.99 |
| 32–39 | 169 | +0.27 | 69 | +0.24 | | — | | — | 238 | +0.26 |
| 39–46 | 212 | +0.03 | 96 | −0.45 | 34 | +0.96 | | — | 342 | −0.02 |
| 46–53 | 204 | +0.13 | 108 | −0.73 | 52 | −1.57 | 13 | −2.89 | 377 | −0.45 |
| 53–60 | 222 | −0.26 | 126 | −1.14 | 56 | −0.40 | 17 | −3.03 | 421 | −0.66 |
| 60–67 | 168 | −2.05 | 117 | −1.41 | 69 | −3.16 | 17 | +0.41 | 371 | −1.94 |
| 67–74 | 162 | −2.81 | 64 | −1.49 | 54 | −2.91 | 21 | +0.04 | 301 | −2.35 |
| 74–81 | 59 | −4.10 | 49 | −2.15 | 21 | −1.53 | 14 | −5.47 | 143 | −3.19 |
| 81–88 | 18 | −4.68 | 7 | −4.06 | 8 | −4.96 | 3 | −6.97 | 36 | −4.81 |
| **Inductive Reasoning** | | | | | | | | | | |
| 25–32 | 135 | +0.48 | | — | | — | | — | 135 | +0.48 |
| 32–39 | 169 | +0.68 | 69 | −0.24 | | — | | — | 238 | +0.42 |
| 39–46 | 213 | +0.08 | 96 | −0.34 | 34 | −0.48 | | — | 343 | −0.09 |
| 46–53 | 204 | −0.31 | 108 | +0.30 | 52 | −0.29 | 13 | +0.72 | 377 | −0.10 |
| 53–60 | 223 | +0.19 | 126 | −0.20 | 56 | −1.75 | 17 | −1.77 | 422 | −0.26 |
| 60–67 | 170 | −2.28 | 117 | −1.49 | 70 | −2.51 | 17 | −2.28 | 374 | −2.07 |
| 67–74 | 163 | −2.07 | 66 | −2.88 | 55 | −3.60 | 22 | −3.53 | 306 | −2.63 |
| 74–81 | 60 | −2.28 | 48 | −2.59 | 21 | −0.92 | 14 | −2.68 | 143 | −2.22 |
| 81–88 | 17 | −2.54 | 8 | −8.34 | 10 | −3.44 | 3 | −2.24 | 38 | −3.97 |
| **Number** | | | | | | | | | | |
| 25–32 | 135 | +1.32 | | — | | — | | — | 135 | +1.32 |
| 32–39 | 169 | + .14 | 69 | −1.36 | | — | | — | 238 | −0.29 |
| 39–46 | 213 | −0.10 | 96 | −0.85 | 34 | −1.14 | | — | 343 | −0.41 |
| 46–53 | 204 | −0.48 | 108 | −2.50 | 52 | −0.95 | 13 | −0.86 | 377 | −1.14 |
| 53–60 | 222 | −0.22 | 126 | −1.40 | 56 | −1.43 | 17 | −1.43 | 421 | −0.78 |
| 60–67 | 171 | −1.56 | 117 | −2.47 | 70 | −3.09 | 17 | −0.76 | 375 | −2.13 |
| 67–74 | 163 | −2.24 | 66 | −2.34 | 55 | −3.00 | 22 | +1.03 | 306 | −2.17 |
| 74–81 | 60 | −4.41 | 49 | −5.01 | 21 | +0.91 | 14 | −3.47 | 144 | −3.75 |
| 81–88 | 18 | −5.08 | 8 | −7.03 | 10 | −4.80 | 3 | −7.80 | 39 | −5.61 |

Table 8.2 *Continued*

| Mean Ages | $T_1$ to $T_2$ N | $T_1$ to $T_2$ d | $T_2$ to $T_3$ N | $T_2$ to $T_3$ d | $T_3$ to $T_4$ N | $T_3$ to $T_4$ d | $T_4$ to $T_5$ N | $T_4$ to $T_5$ d | Average N | Average d |
|---|---|---|---|---|---|---|---|---|---|---|
| Word Fluency | | | | | | | | | | |
| 25–32 | 135 | +0.89 | | — | | — | | — | 135 | +0.89 |
| 32–39 | 169 | −0.55 | 69 | +0.75 | | — | | — | 238 | −0.17 |
| 39–46 | 213 | −0.12 | 96 | +0.69 | 34 | −1.24 | | — | 343 | +0.01 |
| 46–53 | 204 | −0.79 | 108 | −0.90 | 52 | −0.79 | 13 | −0.77 | 377 | −0.82 |
| 53–60 | 223 | −1.25 | 126 | −1.31 | 56 | −0.74 | 17 | −0.40 | 422 | −1.17 |
| 60–67 | 171 | −2.48 | 117 | −1.07 | 70 | −1.17 | 17 | −2.73 | 375 | −1.81 |
| 67–74 | 163 | −2.49 | 66 | −2.08 | 55 | −2.84 | 22 | −2.88 | 306 | −2.56 |
| 74–81 | 60 | −4.07 | 49 | −2.70 | 21 | −2.88 | 14 | −4.25 | 144 | −3.44 |
| 81–88 | 18 | −4.19 | 8 | −1.73 | 10 | −2.96 | 3 | +2.29 | 39 | −2.57 |

[a]Data in T-score points.

The magnitudes of these cumulative changes are given in Table 8.3. For Verbal Meaning, the most crystallized of our measures, cumulative gain remains significantly above the base age until age 60. Early cumulative gains do not reach levels of statistical significance.

In terms of Cohen's criteria, cumulative decrement reaches a small but significant level for Number and Word Fluency by age 67 and for all other variables by age 74. The effects of cumulative decrement become moderately severe (0.5 *SD*) by age 74 for Number and Word Fluency, and by age 81 for

Table 8.3. Cumulative Magnitude of Longitudinal Age Changes for the Primary Mental Abilities From Base Age 25 to Ages 32–88[a]

| Mean Age | Verbal Meaning | Spatial Orientation | Inductive Reasoning | Number | Word Fluency |
|---|---|---|---|---|---|
| 32 | +1.42 | +0.99 | +0.48 | +1.32 | +0.89 |
| 39 | +2.65* | +1.25 | +0.90 | +1.03 | +0.72 |
| 46 | +3.10** | +1.23 | +0.81 | +0.62 | +0.73 |
| 53 | +3.03** | +0.78 | +0.71 | −0.52 | −0.09 |
| 60 | +2.35* | +0.12 | +0.45 | −1.30 | −1.26 |
| 67 | +0.32 | −1.82 | −1.62 | −3.43** | −3.07** |
| 74 | −2.27* | −4.17** | −4.25** | −5.60** | −5.63** |
| 81 | −6.00** | −7.36** | −6.47** | −9.35** | −9.07** |
| 88 | −13.36** | −12.17** | −10.44** | −14.96** | −11.64** |

[a]Data in T-score points.
*Significant at or beyond the 5% level of confidence.
**Significant at ar beyond the 1% level of confidence.

the other variables. However, substantial effect sizes (>1 *SD*) are reached only by age 88 for all variables.

The first four columns of Table 8.2 disaggregate the longitudinal data into separate estimates for those subjects who had no prior practice before the initial point of the 7-year interval, and for those who had either one, two, or three earlier experiences with the test material. With few exceptions, the groups with no prior experience show either greater gain or less decline than those with greater prior experience. One might infer from these data that the estimates for the first longitudinal interval could be inflated by favorable practice effects. It should be noted, however, that this conclusion can be preliminary only, since different levels of practice are confounded with experimental mortality (drop-out) effects. Moreover, the disaggregated data in Table 8.2 may also be disparately affected by history; that is, given the cumulative nature of the data, $T_1/T_2$ data are cumulated over four 7-year periods, $T_2/T_3$ data over three periods, and $T_3/T_4$ data over two periods; $T_4/T_5$ data are available only for a single period. These differences are of course also reflected in disparate sample sizes as shown for each estimate in Table 8.2. Some of these problems can be directly or indirectly addressed utilizing the analytic strategies mentioned for which examples utilizing our data base are now provided.

## The Estimation of Attrition and Practice Effects in Longitudinal Data

I first report complete data on well-replicated direct estimates of attrition, practice, and practice adjusted for attrition effects based on large samples covering the entire age ranges represented in the Seattle Longitudinal Study. I examine how these effects have differential impact on estimates of longitudinal change at different age levels. Finally, more limited examples controlling for the interaction of attrition and practice with other validity threats are examined.

### Direct Estimates of Attrition

I begin by investigating the magnitude of attrition effects, using the direct estimates described on page 247. These effects can be examined for several longitudinal sequences to contrast the base performance of individuals for whom longitudinal data are available and those who dropped out after the initial assessment, and it is also possible to consider shifts in direction and magnitude of attrition effects that may occur after multiple assessment occasions. Because the overall means are affected by slightly different age compositions, I report attrition data as the difference in average performance between dropouts and returnees (Table 8.4). Attrition effects vary across samples originally assessed at different points in time, but after the first test generally range from 0.3 to 0.5 *SD*, and must therefore be characterized as

TABLE 8.4. Difference in Average Performance at Base Assessment Between Dropouts and Returnees[a]

| | Sample 1 $N = 500$ | Sample 2 $N = 997$ | Sample 3 $N = 705$ | Sample 4 $N = 612$ |
|---|---|---|---|---|
| After Test 1 | | | | |
| Verbal meaning | 4.07** | 6.38** | 6.27** | 6.12** |
| Spatial orientation | 2.52** | 4.00** | 4.08** | 4.25** |
| Inductive reasoning | 3.06** | 5.28** | 5.70** | 6.70** |
| Number | 1.97* | 3.95** | 5.16** | 4.45** |
| Word fluency | 3.06** | 3.66** | 4.84** | 3.68** |
| After Test 2 | | | | |
| Verbal meaning | 3.51** | 1.97* | 3.71** | |
| Spatial orientation | 2.16** | 1.35 | 5.09** | |
| Inductive reasoning | 5.14** | 2.54** | 5.81** | |
| Number | 2.13* | 1.65* | 2.87** | |
| Word fluency | 2.41* | 1.01 | 2.67** | |
| After Test 3 | | | | |
| Verbal meaning | 4.10* | 2.30* | | |
| Spatial orientation | 4.85** | 0.48 | | |
| Inductive reasoning | 4.35** | 4.73** | | |
| Number | 0.58 | 1.89 | | |
| Word fluency | 3.96* | 1.16 | | |
| After Test 4 | | | | |
| Verbal meaning | 4.72** | | | |
| Spatial orientation | 3.45* | | | |
| Inductive reasoning | 4.45* | | | |
| Number | 1.35 | | | |
| World fluency | 4.25* | | | |

[a]Data in T-score points.
*$p < .05$; **$p < .01$. Note: All differences are in favor of the returnees.

being of at least moderate effect size. Attrition effects after the second test and beyond are somewhat less pronounced, but remain of significant magnitude.

Before being overly impressed by the substantial differences between dropouts and returnees, we must note that the extent to which these differences will bias our projections based on the survivors only will depend on the proportion of dropouts; that is, if attrition is modest the effects will be small, or vice versa. Table 8.5 presents the net attrition effects (in T-score points) for our samples, showing different attrition patterns. As can be seen the effect is largest for those occasions when the greatest proportion of dropouts occur, and becomes smaller as the panels stabilize and remaining loss occurs primarily through death or disabilities.

The attrition data clearly indicate that parameter estimates of levels of cognitive function from longitudinal data, in the presence of significant attri-

TABLE 8.5. Attrition Effects Calculated as Difference Between Base Means for Total Sample and Returnees[a]

| | Sample 1 $N = 500$ | Sample 2 $N = 997$ | Sample 3 $N = 705$ | Sample 4 $N = 612$ |
|---|---|---|---|---|
| Attrition after $T_1$ | 38.2% | 53.5% | 51.9% | 52.3% |
| Verbal meaning | 1.52* | 3.41** | 2.97** | 3.20** |
| Spatial orientation | 0.96 | 2.14** | 2.12** | 1.40* |
| Inductive reasoning | 1.17 | 2.82** | 2.96** | 2.22** |
| Number | 0.76 | 2.11** | 2.68** | 2.46** |
| Word fluency | 1.17 | 1.95** | 2.51** | 2.33** |
| Attrition after $T_2$ | 25.0% | 16.0% | 16.5% | |
| Verbal meaning | 1.59 | 0.70 | 1.54 | |
| Spatial orientation | 1.02 | 0.48 | 1.40 | |
| Inductive reasoning | 2.33** | 0.91 | 1.99 | |
| Number | 0.93 | 0.59 | 0.98 | |
| Word fluency | 1.09 | 0.36 | 0.74 | |
| Attrition after $T_3$ | 8.0% | 7.4% | | |
| Verbal meaning | 0.97 | 0.57 | | |
| Spatial orientation | 1.12 | 0.12 | | |
| Inductive reasoning | 1.03 | 1.14 | | |
| Number | 0.16 | 0.47 | | |
| Word fluency | .94 | 0.29 | | |
| Attrition after $T_4$ | 6.6% | | | |
| Verbal meaning | 1.21 | | | |
| Spatial orientation | 0.86 | | | |
| Inductive reasoning | 1.14 | | | |
| Number | 0.35 | | | |
| Word fluency | 1.09 | | | |

[a]Data in T-score points.
*$p < .05$; **$p < .01$. Note: All differences are in favor of the returnees.

tion, will be substantially higher in most instances than would be the case if an entire population sample could be followed over time. It does not necessarily follow, however, that rates of change will be overestimated unless it can be shown that there is a substantial positive correlation between base level performance and age change. On the basis of the favorable attrition, we would expect modest negative correlations due to regression effects, even though the stability of the PMA variables is quite high. The relevant correlations are reported in Table 8.6, and suggest that there is no evidence for a more favorable rate of change for the higher scoring members of the panel. In fact, some of the larger negative correlations may reflect greater age changes on some variables (e.g., Number and Word Fluency) for the more able, implying that the longitudinal panel data might in some instances be overestimating the extent of age-related decline in the general population.

TABLE 8.6. Correlations of Gain Scores With Base Scores

| | Sample 1 | Sample 2 | Sample 3 | Sample 4 |
|---|---|---|---|---|
| At Test 1 | | | | |
| Verbal meaning | −.24 | −.26 | −.15 | −.23 |
| Spatial orientation | −.33 | −.27 | −.24 | −.23 |
| Inductive reasoning | −.18 | −.26 | −.20 | −.17 |
| Number | −.25 | −.28 | −.37 | −.19 |
| Word fluency | −.28 | −.43 | −.27 | −.18 |
| At Test 2 | | | | |
| Verbal meaning | −.17 | −.10 | −.15 | |
| Spatial orientation | −.18 | −.33 | −.19 | |
| Inductive reasoning | −.16 | −.02 | −.20 | |
| Number | −.25 | −.19 | −.21 | |
| Word fluency | −.23 | −.36 | −.17 | |
| At Test 3 | | | | |
| Verbal meaning | −.10 | −.20 | | |
| Spatial orientation | −.23 | −.25 | | |
| Inductive reasoning | −.25 | −.22 | | |
| Number | −.22 | −.26 | | |
| Word fluency | −.08 | −.22 | | |
| At Test 4 | | | | |
| Verbal meaning | −.08 | | | |
| Spatial orientation | −.37 | | | |
| Inductive reasoning | −.14 | | | |
| Number | −.40 | | | |
| Word fluency | −.29 | | | |

## DIRECT ASSESSMENT OF PRACTICE EFFECTS

The possible inflation of longitudinal change estimates because of practice effects can be studied by comparing individuals at the same age who are retest returnees with the performance of individuals assessed for the first time at $T_2$. It will be seen from Table 8.7 that the apparent practice effects estimated in this manner, at first glance, appear to be impressively large. However, these comparisons involve the comparisons of attrited and random samples. The mean values for the longitudinal group must therefore be adjusted for attrition to permit a valid comparison. The appropriate values for this adjustment are not those from Table 8.4 (the differences between the survivors and returnees), but rather the mean differences between the returnees and the entire sample at base as shown in Table 8.5. Data for the raw and adjusted practice effects are provided in Table 8.7. Because we expect practice effects to be positive, all significance tests used in this instance are one-tailed. The raw practice effects appear to be statistically significant for virtually all variables and samples, but none of adjusted effects reach significance except for Verbal Meaning in sample 1.

TABLE 8.7. Raw and Attrition-Adjusted Effects of Practice by Sample and Test Occasion[a]

| | Sample 1 | | Sample 2 | | Sample 3 | | Sample 4 | |
|---|---|---|---|---|---|---|---|---|
| | Raw | Adj. | Raw | Adj. | Raw | Adj. | Raw | Adj. |
| From Test 1 to Test 2 | | | | | | | | |
| Verbal | 2.83** | 1.31* | 4.02** | 0.61 | 3.25** | 0.28 | 1.21* | −1.99 |
| Spatial | 1.02 | 0.06 | 3.00** | 0.86 | 2.28** | 0.28 | 2.06** | 0.14 |
| Reasoning | 2.03** | 0.86 | 3.43** | 0.61 | 2.77** | −0.19 | 1.33* | −0.69 |
| Number | 1.02 | 0.26 | 1.29* | −0.82 | 3.09** | 0.41 | 1.60* | −0.86 |
| Word fluency | 1.71* | 0.54 | 2.94** | 0.99 | 2.97** | 0.87 | 1.10 | −1.23 |
| From Test 2 to Test 3 | | | | | | | | |
| Verbal | −3.07 | −2.77 | 3.11** | 1.97* | −3.15 | −4.46 | | |
| Spatial | −0.03 | 0.13 | 2.05** | 0.65 | 1.68* | −0.06 | | |
| Reasoning | 1.16 | 0.48 | 2.71** | 1.34 | 1.93* | −0.80 | | |
| Number | −0.50 | −0.08 | 1.84* | 1.82* | 1.13 | −0.07 | | |
| Word fluency | 0.22 | −0.09 | 0.41 | 0.61 | 2.15** | 1.23 | | |
| From Test 3 to Test 4 | | | | | | | | |
| Verbal | 0.20 | 0.20 | −0.78 | 0.79 | | | | |
| Spatial | 0.14 | −0.34 | 0.30 | 0.63 | | | | |
| Reasoning | −0.17 | −0.97 | 0.04 | 0.09 | | | | |
| Number | −1.03 | −0.18 | 0.10 | 0.59 | | | | |
| Word fluency | 0.10 | −0.80 | −0.99 | −0.34 | | | | |
| From Test 4 to Test 5 | | | | | | | | |
| Verbal | 0.90 | 0.29 | | | | | | |
| Spatial | 0.81 | −0.41 | | | | | | |
| Reasoning | −0.09 | −0.86 | | | | | | |
| Number | −1.83 | −1.66 | | | | | | |
| Word fluency | 1.74 | 0.05 | | | | | | |

[a]Data in T-score points.
*$p < .05$; **$p < .01$.

Similar analyses can be conducted to assess the continuing effects of practice at additional assessment points in the study. Data are provided up to the fifth assessment occasion. It will be seen that a few raw effect estimates are significant for practice from $T_2$ to $T_3$, but attrition-adjusted effects remain significant only for Verbal Meaning and Number in sample 2. Neither raw nor adjusted effects reach significant levels for practice from $T_3$ to $T_4$ or from $T_4$ to $T_5$.

## Effects of Adjustments for Practice and Attrition on Findings of Longitudinal Age Changes

The estimates for attrition-adjusted practice effects can, of course, be derived also for the age changes described in Table 8.2. To obtain maximum cell sizes, we have computed these estimates aggregated for all our subjects at each age for which all of the required 7-year longitudinal data were available. Because the primary concern here is empirical examples of the methods advocated for dealing with internal validity threats, I present data for this and the following analyses only for the variable of Verbal Meaning over the age range from 25 to 81 years. The attrition effects are obtained by finding the differences between dropouts and returnees at $T_1$. Raw practice effects are obtained by obtaining differences between means for returnees at $T_2$ and samples of the same age tested for the first time at $T_2$.

Again, small attrition effects are observed that reach statistical significance for the mean ages 39 to 60. Raw practice effects are statistically significant at all ages, but do not reach significance at any age when adjusted for attrition effects. Virtually all effects, however, are in a positive direction. When these values are used to adjust the raw longitudinal age changes, early increments (from 25 to 46) are no longer statistically significant, while significant decline is found to occur earlier, by age 60. I therefore plotted a comparison of data obtained from the cross-sectional averages (from Table 8.1), the unadjusted longitudinal changes estimated on the basis of all $T_1/T_2$ data (from Table 8.2), and longitudinal changes adjusted for practice and attrition effects (from Table 8.8). These adjusted values still represent within-individual change that is considerably less than would be suggested by the cross-sectional data, but do show steeper decline than the unadjusted longitudinal estimates.

The adjustments to the longitudinal age changes for practice and attrition shown are rather straightforward. As noted earlier, however, they used data aggregated across several samples studied over the same age range but at different time periods. The resultant adjustments consequently would be excessive if average secular trends had been negative or insufficient if such trends were positive. Likewise, positive selection (cohort) effects could result in overestimating the raw practice effects, whereas negative selection effects would result in underestimates. Data are now presented for analyses that ex-

TABLE 8.8. Adjustment of 7-Year Longitudinal Age Changes for Practice and Attrition Effects for Verbal Meaning[a]

| Mean Age | N | Attrition Effect | Practice Effect Raw | Practice Effect Adjusted | Raw Age Change | Adjusted Age Change |
|---|---|---|---|---|---|---|
| 25–32 | 135 | +1.41 | +1.96 | +0.55 | +1.42* | +0.87 |
| 32–39 | 169 | +1.09 | +2.39** | +1.30 | +1.70** | +0.40 |
| 39–46 | 213 | +1.77* | +2.27** | +0.50 | +1.06* | +0.56 |
| 46–53 | 204 | +3.81** | +3.61** | −0.20 | +0.54 | +0.74 |
| 53–60 | 223 | +1.84* | +2.74** | +0.90 | −0.28 | −1.18** |
| 60–67 | 170 | +2.65** | +3.31** | +0.66 | −1.59** | −2.25** |
| 67–74 | 163 | +1.48 | +2.69** | +1.21 | −2.12** | −3.33** |
| 74–81 | 60 | +3.11 | +3.68** | +0.57 | −1.79** | −2.36** |

[a]Data in T-score points.
*$p < .05$; **$p < .01$.

emplify how practice and/or mortality effects can be disentangled when suitably crossed with the effects of history and selection.

## ESTIMATING HISTORY BY ATTRITION EFFECTS

Using ANOVA, overall attrition and history effects can be estimated, controlled for maturation, and estimates of history-specific and age-specific attrition effects can be provided. The 2 (attrition) × 3 (times-of-measurement) × 8 (age levels) time-sequential ANOVA employs 2205 subjects over the age

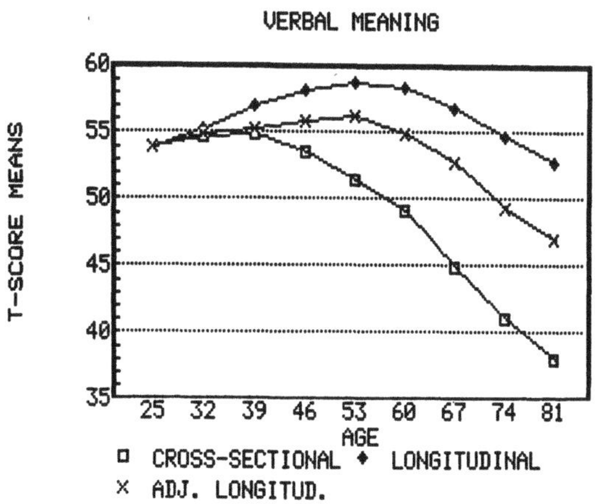


FIGURE 8.1. Comparison of cross-sectional age differences, raw longitudinal age changes, and longitudinal age changes adjusted for practice and attrition.

range from 25 to 74 years who were first tested either in 1963, 1970, or 1977; attrition information was obtained from the second assessment of each sample 7 years later (1970, 1977, or 1984, respectively). Results of this analysis are reported in Table 8.9. All main effects are statistically significant, as is the age by history interaction. However, the age by attrition interaction is not significant, suggesting that attrition effects are randomly distributed with respect to age. The history by attrition interaction approaches statistical significance. While the overall attrition effect amounts to 3.60 *T*-score points, history-specific attrition effects were found to be 4.79, 2.84, and 3.14 points, respectively, for 1963, 1970, and 1977. I did not report age-specific attrition effects in this instance, because the age by attrition interaction failed to reach statistical significance.

## Estimating Selection by Attrition Effects

Age-specific attrition effects can also be estimated, while controlling for the effects of maturation and selection effects, by a series of ANOVAs that cross any two adjacent ages and cohorts. The current example represents data for two 2 (attrition) × 2 (cohort) × 2 (age levels) cohort-sequential analyses with independent samples of 385 subjects for ages 53 and 60 and 366 subjects for ages 60 and 67. Data for the first cohort in each analysis come from the 1963 and 1970 data collections; the second cohort was assessed in 1970 and 1977. Attrition information on each of the four samples entering these analyses was obtained at the assessment that occurred 7 years beyond the data point entering the analysis. Results are shown in Table 8.10. The comparison at ages 53 and 60 yields significant selection and attrition effects, but no significant age effects. However, there is a significant age by selection interaction, revealing stability across age in the earlier born cohort but negative age differences in the later born cohort. In the comparison of samples at ages 60 and 67, main effects are significant for all three factors. The significant age by

TABLE 8.9. Time-Sequential Analysis of Variance Partitioning Effects Attributable to Age, History, and Attrition

| Effect | *df* | Mean Square | *F* Ratio | *p* | Omega$^2$ |
|---|---|---|---|---|---|
| Age | 7 | 6534.87 | 67.89 | < .001 | .168 |
| History | 2 | 1097.83 | 11.41 | > .001 | .006 |
| Attrition | 1 | 8260.99 | 85.82 | < .001 | .054 |
| Age × history | 14 | 248.10 | 2.58 | < .001 | .014 |
| Age × attrition | 7 | 88.56 | .92 | ns[a] | — |
| History × attrition | 2 | 264.45 | 2.75 | < .06 | .004 |
| Age × history × attrition | 14 | 79.80 | .83 | ns | — |
| Error | 2157 | 96.26 | — | — | — |

[a]ns, not significant.

TABLE 8.10. Cohort-Sequential Analysis of Variance Partitioning Effects Attributable to Age, Selection, and Attrition

| Effect | *df* | Mean Square | *F* Ratio | *p* | Omega$^2$ |
|---|---|---|---|---|---|
| Comparison at Ages 53 and 60 | | | | | |
| Age | 1 | 5.47 | .05 | ns[a] | |
| Selection | 1 | 622.82 | 6.11 | <.01 | .011 |
| Attrition | 1 | 2695.60 | 26.46 | <.001 | .087 |
| Age × selection | 1 | 2092.01 | 20.54 | <.001 | .134 |
| Age × attrition | 1 | 29.26 | .29 | ns | — |
| Selection × attrition | 1 | 22.90 | .22 | ns | — |
| Age × selection × attrition | 1 | 284.26 | 2.79 | ns | — |
| Error | 377 | 101.86 | — | — | — |
| Comparison at Ages 60 and 67 | | | | | |
| Age | 1 | 1652.46 | 15.21 | <.001 | .048 |
| Selection | 1 | 788.34 | 7.26 | <.01 | .010 |
| Attrition | 1 | 1056.35 | 9.72 | <.01 | .034 |
| Age × selection | 1 | 400.96 | 3.69 | <.05 | .034 |
| Age × attrition | 1 | 116.58 | 1.07 | ns | — |
| Selection × attrition | 1 | 146.46 | 1.35 | ns | — |
| Age × selection × attrition | 1 | 7.27 | .07 | ns | — |
| Error | 358 | 108.64 | — | — | — |

[a]ns, not significant.

selection interaction, again favors the earlier born over the later born cohort. Attrition effects in both analyses appear to be random with respect to age and selection. The magnitude of the attrition effects, however varies substantially across sets (4.77 and 3.01 *T*-score points, respectively).

### ESTIMATING HISTORY BY PRACTICE EFFECTS

We can disaggregate history and practice effects while controlling for maturation by means of a time-sequential ANOVA that includes four samples per age level, two of which are assessed at first assessment and two that would have previously experienced the same measures. Data are presented for 2 (levels of practice) × 2 (times of measurement) × 7 (age levels) time-sequential analysis involving 1764 subjects aged 32 to 74 with assessments of independent random samples occurring in 1970 and 1977. Note that half of the subsamples were assessed 7 years earlier, in 1963 or 1970; the earlier data do not enter this analysis. This analysis (Table 8.11) is *not* controlled for effects of attrition, which, in this design, remain confounded with the practice effects. As seen in the earlier history by attrition analysis, no significant history effects are found between 1970 and 1977. As expected the age effect is highly significant, as is the practice effect. The magnitude of the latter (average raw practice effect) amounts to 2.61 *T*-score points. No significant in-

TABLE 8.11. Time-Sequential Analysis of Variance Partitioning Effects Attributable to Age, History, and Practice

| Effect | *df* | Mean Square | *F* Ratio | *p* | Omega² |
|---|---|---|---|---|---|
| Age | 6 | 7390.17 | 81.73 | <.001 | .218 |
| History | 1 | 4.77 | .05 | ns[a] | — |
| Practice | 1 | 3754.57 | 41.52 | <.001 | .031 |
| Age × history | 1 | 158.91 | 1.76 | ns | — |
| Age × practicen | 1 | 128.85 | 1.43 | ns | — |
| History × practice | 1 | 6.36 | .07 | ns | — |
| Age × history × practice | 1 | 1179.46 | 1.98 | <.06 | .023 |
| Error | 1761 | 90.42 | — | — | — |

[a]ns, not significant.

teractions are found between age and practice, but the three-way interaction is marginally significant. Theoretically, this interaction would reflect age-specific practice effects that differ by time of assessment. Magnitudes for these specific effects are not reported; they may occur primarily because of the failure to control for the attrition confound in this design.

## ESTIMATING SELECTION BY PRACTICE EFFECTS

Age-specific practice effects, of course, can also be estimated while controlling for the effects of selection effects. A series of ANOVAs is used to cross any two adjacent ages and cohorts. This example has two 2 (levels of practice) × 2 (cohort) × 2 (age levels) cohort-sequential analyses with independent samples. The first analysis is of 625 subjects aged 53 and 60. The second analysis, with 571 subjects, compares ages 60 and 67. Data for the first cohort in each analysis come from the 1963 and 1970 data collections; the second cohort was assessed in 1970 and 1977. Two samples are involved at each data point. For exmple, one of the samples from cohort 1 tested in 1963 is at first test, while the other sample from this cohort was previously assessed in 1956. Likewise, one sample from cohort 2 tested in 1977 was tested earlier in 1970, and so on. Data from the earlier tests do not enter these analyses, and attrition is not controlled for.

Results of these analyses are shown in Table 8.12. Main effects are statistically significant for both analyses, although the selection effect is only marginally so in the comparison of ages 53 and 60. Of particular interest here are the age by practice and triple interactions. These are clearly significant in the first analysis, and marginally significant in the second. These results suggest that practice effects may indeed not be random with respect to age, particularly under specific selection conditions. Practice effects estimated in these analyses attain magnitudes of 3.16 and 3.75 *T*-score points, respectively.

TABLE 8.12. Cohort-Sequential Analysis of Variance Partitioning Effects Attributable to Age, Selection, and Practice

| Effect | *df* | Mean Square | *F* Ratio | *p* | Omega$^2$ |
|---|---|---|---|---|---|
| Comparison at Ages 53 and 60 | | | | | |
| Age | 1 | 392.11 | 3.89 | <.05 | .010 |
| Selection | 1 | 295.41 | 2.93 | <.08 | .007 |
| Practice | 1 | 1872.14 | 18.56 | <.001 | .053 |
| Age × selection | 1 | 274.27 | 2.72 | ns[a] | — |
| Age × practice | 1 | 433.46 | 4.30 | <.05 | .022 |
| Selection × practice | 1 | 178.30 | 1.77 | ns | — |
| Age × selection × practice | 1 | 1358.81 | 13.47 | <.001 | .129 |
| Error | 617 | 100.84 | | | |
| Comparison at Ages 60 and 67 | | | | | |
| Age | 1 | 916.48 | 8.46 | <.00 | .024 |
| Selection | 1 | 969.84 | 8.95 | <.01 | .026 |
| Practice | 1 | 2392.68 | 22.09 | <.001 | .068 |
| Age × selection | 1 | 82.26 | .76 | ns | — |
| Age × practice | 1 | 341.60 | 3.15 | <.07 | .018 |
| Selection × practice | 1 | 155.58 | 1.44 | ns | — |
| Age × selection × practice | 1 | 359.25 | 3.32 | <.07 | .038 |
| Error | 563 | 108.33 | — | — | — |

[a]ns, not significant.

Note that at specific age and selection levels, practice effects range from a low of −.08 to a high of 8.33 *T*-score points.

It would have been possible in each of the two preceding examples to control for attrition effects by using in the "no practice" cells only those individuals who had been identified as having returned for further assessment of a subsequent test occasion. I do not provide examples for these further controls because data on age-specific attrition-adjusted practice effects have already been reported in the section on direct assessment of practice effects. Instead, the final example provides results of a design that directly crosses attrition and practice effects.

## JOINT ESTIMATES OF HISTORY, SELECTION, ATTRITION, AND PRACTICE

The final example disaggregates the effects of attrition and practice from history and selection effects. This analysis requires subsamples examined at four different assessment points even though only data collected on two of these occasions are used; the other two occasions are required to establish two subsamples within each selection/history/attrition combination. One has been assessed on one more occasion than the other, and a subsample of each has remained in the study for one further assessment. The example represents a 2 (selection levels) × 2 (times of measurement) × 2 (practice levels)

× 2 (attrition levels) cross-sequential ANOVA with independent samples. Data from 606 subjects collected in 1970 and 1977, from two cohorts that were aged 46 and 53 in 1970 and aged 53 and 60 in 1977, respectively, are used. Each of the four history by selection combinations is divided into four further subsets. Two of these have not had prior testing, while two were previously assessed. Further, each is divided into one sample whose members left the study after the assessment included in this analysis; the other subset consists of individuals who returned for at least one other occasion. In this particular example, I am not interested in age-specific estimates, but wish to consider the relative magnitude of the four internal validity threats under study. For this reason, an age interval is selected in which earlier data suggest that maturational (age-related) change will be zero or trivial, and equal time intervals are used for all comparisons (cf. Botwinick & Arenberg, 1976). Results of this analysis are given in Table 8.13.

When we cross all four internal validity threats under these conditions, statistically significant main effects are found for history, practice, and attrition with a marginally significant effect for selection. However, none of the interactions is statistically significant. Over a 7-year interval, it appears that the largest effect is from attrition (2.62 *T*-score points in favor of the returnees), followed by history (2.48 *T*-score points in favor of the groups assessed at the earlier point in time), and practice (2.40 *T*-Score points in favor of the practiced groups). The selection effect amounts to 1.35 *T*-score

TABLE 8.13. Cross-Sequential Analysis of Variance Partitioning Effects Attributable to Time, Selection, Practice, and Attrition

| Effect | *df* | Mean Square | *F* Ratio | *p* | Omega$^2$ |
|---|---|---|---|---|---|
| Time | 1 | 966.25 | 11.22 | <.001 | .021 |
| Selection | 1 | 283.91 | 3.30 | <.07 | .001 |
| Practice | 1 | 905.43 | 10.52 | <.01 | .026 |
| Attrition | 1 | 1082.07 | 12.57 | <.001 | .031 |
| Time × selection | 1 | 74.02 | .85 | ns[a] | — |
| Time × practice | 1 | 77.00 | .89 | ns | — |
| Time × attrition | 1 | 195.53 | 2.27 | ns | — |
| Selection × practice | 1 | 1.12 | .01 | ns | — |
| Selection × attrition | 1 | .33 | .00 | ns | — |
| Practice × attrition | 1 | 151.69 | 1.76 | ns | — |
| Time × selection × practice | 1 | 2.24 | .02 | ns | — |
| Time × selection × attrition | 1 | 10.72 | .12 | ns | — |
| Selection × practice × attrition | 1 | 92.61 | 1.07 | ns | — |
| Time × selection × practice × attrition | 1 | 3.49 | .04 | ns | — |
| Error | 569 | 86.10 | — | — | — |

[a]ns, not significant.

points in favor of the later born cohort. These results might suggest that the validity threats investigated here may indeed be cumulative and, although independent of each other, must all be considered. The reader should be cautioned further that, as illustrated earlier, interactions between maturational level and the other variables considered are likely to be found both in young adulthood and advanced old age, those age levels at which positive or negative age changes are expected to occur for many cognitive variables.

## Some Concluding Remarks

It is well known that cross-sectional studies of cognitive aging tend to paint unduly pessimistic pictures because positive selection (cohort) effects inflate age change estimates when modeled by age comparative studies (also see Willis, 1985, 1987). In reaction to these problems, there have been major efforts in recent years to obtain substantial longitudinal data bases that permit direct estimates of age changes. Much information can be gained from longitudinal data that is simply not available in cross-sectional studies (cf. Schaie, 1983c). What has not been given enough attention, however, is that longitudinal studies are plagued with even more complex internal validity threats.

In this chapter I have outlined the nature of these threats with specific reference to their import for studies of cognitive aging in adulthood. I have examined in detail experimental paradigms that allow the investigator to control for or assess the magnitude of effects for the validity threats of attrition, practice, history, and selection (cohort). As has been pointed out by Campbell and Stanley (1967), there is little that one can do to deal with these issues in "one-shot" studies, which should probably always be considered pilot efforts at best.

I have tried to show, however, that there are relatively simple methods available that can be applied in those situations in which at least two estimates are available for comparable groups, as is the case in many studies reported in the adult cognitive literature. Naturally, such data can only be investigated for a single threat at a time, and the investigator must use theoretical rationales to defend the selected paradigm. As the number of data points across time available to an investigator increase, so do the possibilities of investigating multiple validity threats. Again I have presented a number of alternatives and empirical examples that show why the pursuit of these matters is not esoteric at all, but may have important substantive consequences.

At least for several of the Primary Mental Abilities, attrition effects nearly always lead to an overestimate of performance levels, but not necessarily to an overestimate of rate of change. The matter of practice effects is more equivocal, because the more practiced group will always have experienced greater attrition than the less practiced group. Designs that can disaggregate both practice and attrition from aging effects are complex, however, and require multiple data points. When such disaggregation is actually accomplished, small practice effects tend to remain, suggesting that longitudinal data for some variables and over some age ranges may indeed overestimate gain in early adulthood and slightly underestimate loss in old age. However, selection effects confounding cross-sectional data remain of far greater magnitude in those instances where it has been possible to disaggregate selection and aging effects.

I conclude, then, that longitudinal parameter etimates, particularly when available for multiple data points, remain the preferred sources of our understanding of cognitive aging, if only because longitudinal designs provide the very data that can be used to apply the correctives needed to address the internal validity threats here considered.

*Acknowledgments.* Preparation of this chapter was partially supported by research grant AG04770-03 from the National Institute on Aging. The cooperation of staff and members of the Group Health Cooperative of Puget Sound who participated in this study is gratefully acknowledged.

## References

Baltes, P.B. Cornelius, S.W., & Nesselroade, J.R. (1979). Cohort effects in developmental psychology. In J.R. Nesselroade & P.B. Baltes (Eds.), *Longitudinal research in the study of behavior and development* (pp. 61–88). New York: Academic Press.

Baltes, P.B., Nesselroade, J.R., Schaie, K.W., & Labouvie, E.W. (1972). On the dilemma of regression effects in examining ability level-related differentials in ontogenetic patterns of intelligence. *Developmental Psychology, 6,* 78–84.

Baltes, P.B., Schaie, K.W., & Nardi, A.H. (1971). Age and experimental mortality in a seven-year longitudinal study of cognitive behavior. *Developmental Psychology, 5,* 18–26.

Botwinick, J., & Arenberg, D. (1976). Disparate time spans in sequential studies of aging. *Experimental Aging Research, 2,* 55–61.

Campbell, D.T., & Stanley, J.C. (1967). *Experimental and quasi-experimental designs for research.* Chicago: Rand McNally.

Cohen J. (1977). *Statistical power analysis for the behavioral sciences* (rev. ed.). New York: Academic Press.

Cooney, T.M., Schaie, K.W., & Willis, S.L. (1988). The relationship between prior functioning on cognitive and personality variables and subject attrition in psychological research. *Journal of Gerontology: Psychological Sciences, 43,* 12–17.

Costa, P.T., Jr., & McCrae, R.R. (1982). An approach to the attribution of aging, period, and cohort effects. *Psychological Bulletin, 92,* 238–250.

Furby, L. (1973). Interpreting regression toward the mean in developmental research. *Developmental Psychology, 8,* 172–179.

Gribbin, K., & Schaie, K.W. (1979). Selective attrition in longitudinal studies: A cohort-sequential approach. In H. Orino, K. Shimada, M. Iriki, & D. Maeda (Ed.), *Recent advances in gerontology* (pp. 549–551). Amsterdam: Excerpta Medica.

Hays, W.L. (1963). *Statistics.* New York: Holt, Rinehart & Winston.

Horn, J.L. (1982). The theory of fluid and crystallized intelligence in relation to concepts of cognitive psychology and aging in adulthood. In F.J.M. Craik & S. Trehub (Eds.), *Aging and cognitive processes.* New York: Plenum Press.

Hultsch, D.F., & Hickey, T. (1978). External validity in the study of human development: Methodological considerations. *Human Development, 21,* 76–91.

Labouvie, E.W. (1982). Issues in life-span development. In B.B. Wolman (Ed.), *Handbook of developmental psychology* (pp. 54–62). Englewood Cliffs, NJ: Prentice-Hall.

Nesselroade, J.R., & Baltes, P.B. (1974). Adolescent personality development and historical change: 1970–1972. *Monographs of the Society for Research In Child Development, 39* (1, Whole No. 154), 1–80.

Nesselroade, J.R., & Labouvie, E.W. (1985). Experimental design in research on aging. In J.E. Birren & K.W. Schaie (Eds.), *Handbook of the psychology of aging.* (2nd ed., pp. 35–60). New York: Van Nostrand Reinhold.

Nesselroade, J.R., Stigler, S.M., & Baltes, P.B. (1980). Regression towards the mean and the study of change. *Psychological Bulletin, 88,* 622–637.

Riegel, K.F., Riegel, R.M., & Meyer, G. (1967). A study of the dropout rates of longitudinal research on aging and the prediction of death. *Journal of Personality and Social Psychology, 5,* 342–348.

Salthouse, T.A. (1982). *Adult cognition: An experimental psychology of human aging.* New York: Springer-Verlag.

Schaie, K.W. (1959). Cross-sectional methods in the study of psychological aspects of aging. *Journal of Gerontology, 14,* 208–215.

Schaie, K.W. (1965). A general model for the study of developmental change. *Psychological Bulletin, 64,* 92–107.

Schaie, K.W. (1972). Can the longitudinal method be applied to psychological studies of human development? In F.Z. Moenks, W.W. Hartup, & J. DeWit (Eds.), *Determinants of behavioral development* (pp. 3–22). New York: Academic Press.

Schaie, K.W. (1973). Methodological problems in descriptive developmental research on adulthood and aging. In J.R. Nesselroade & H.W. Reese (Eds.), *Life-span developmental psychology: Developmental issues* (pp. 253–280). New York: Academic Press.

Schaie, K.W. (1977). Quasi-experimental research designs in the psychology of aging. In J.E. Birren and K.W. Schaie (Eds.), *Handbook of the psychology of aging* (pp. 39–58). New York: Van Nostrand Reinhold.

Schaie, K.W. (1982). Longitudinal data sets: Evidence for ontogenetic development or chronicles of cultural change? *Journal of Social Issues, 38,* 65–72.

Schaie, K.W. (1983a). *Longitudinal studies of adult psychological development.* New York: Guilford Press.

Schaie, K.W. (1983b). The Seattle Longitudinal Study: A twenty-one year exploration of psychometric intelligence in adulthood. In K.W. Schaie (Ed.), *Longitudinal studies of adult psychological development* (pp. 64–135). New York: Guilford Press.

Schaie, K.W. (1983c). What can we learn from the longitudinal study of adult psychological development? In K.W. Schaie (Ed.), *Longitudinal studies of adult psychological development* (pp. 1–19). New York: Guilford Press.

Schaie, K.W. (1985). *Manual for the Schaie-Thurstone Test of Adult Mental Abilities (STAMAT).* Palo Alto, CA: Consulting Psychologists Press.

Schaie, K.W. (1986). Beyond calendar definitions of age, time and cohort: The general developmental model revisited. *Developmental Review, 6,* 252–277.

Schaie, K.W., & Hertzog, C. (1982). Longitudinal methods. In B.B. Wolman (Ed.), *Handbook of developmental psychology* (pp. 91–115). Englewood Cliffs, NJ: Prentice-Hall.
Schaie, K.W., & Hertzog, C. (1985). Measurement in the psychology of aging. In J.E. Birren & K.W. Schaie (Eds.), *Handbook of the psychology of aging* (2nd ed., pp. 61–92). New York: Van Nostrand Reinhold.
Schaie, K.W., Labouvie, G.V., & Barrett, T. J. (1973). Selective attrition effects in a fourteen-year study of adult intelligence. *Journal of Gerontology, 28,* 328–334.
Schaie, K.W., Orshowsky, S.J., & Parham, I.A. (1982). Measuring age and sociocultural change: The case of race and life satisfaction. In R.C. Manuel (Ed.), *Minority aging: Sociological and social psychological issues* (pp. 223–230). Westport, CT: Greenwood Press.
Schaie, K.W., & Parham, I.A. (1974). Social responsibility in adulthood: Ontogenetic and sociocultural changes. *Journal of Personality & Social Psychology, 30,* 483–492.
Schaie, K.W., & Parham, I.A. (1975). *Manual for the test of behavioral rigidity.* Palo Alto, CA: Consulting Psychologists Press.
Schaie, K.W., & Willis, S.L. (1986a). *Adult development and aging* (2nd ed.). Boston: Little, Brown.
Schaie, K.W., & Willis, S.L. (1986b). Can decline in adult cognitive functioning be reversed? *Developmental Psychology, 22,* 223–232.
Schaie, K.W., Willis, S.L., Hertzog, C., & Schulenberg, J.E. (1987). Effects of cognitive training upon primary mental ability structure. *Psychology and Aging, 2,* 233–242.
Thurstone, L.L., & Thurstone, T.G. (1941). *Factorial studies of intelligence.* Chicago: University of Chicago Press.
Willis, S.L. (1985). Towards an educational psychology of the older learner: Intellectual and cognitive bases. In J.E. Birren & K.W. Schaie (Eds.), *Handbook of the psychology of aging* (pp. 818–847). New York: Van Nostrand Reinhold.
Willis, S.L. (1987). Cognitive training and everyday competence. In K.W. Schaie (Ed.), *Annual review of gerontology and geriatrics* (Vol. 7, pp. 159–188). New York: Springer.

# 9. Physical Activity, Age, and Cognitive/Motor Performance

*Michael J. Stones and Albert Kozma*

## Introduction

Ways to prevent, postpone, or compensate for the deterioration in cognitive performance with age are of interest to everybody. Our focus in this chapter is on regular physical activity as one such intervention. The attempt to develop models of the impact of physical activity on the functional capability of aging humans has attracted the attention of researchers from several disciplines (e.g., demography, physical education, physiology, psychology, sociology). We are as aware as anyone working at this multidisciplinary interface that the human functional system is composed of a set of physical and psychological attributes that are interrelated. This knowledge colors our orientation toward research and theory. We prefer to ask questions about general systems characteristics first, and only then focus in on particular components of the system. Consequently, space will be devoted in this chapter to a consideration of functional age, a higher order construct that encompasses both physical and cognitive/motor functions. Subsequently, specific effects of physical activity on cognitive/motor functions will be examined.

The chapter contains a number of theoretical innovations intended to advance the field and, in addition, some new findings. A new model of functional age is described and evaluated against previously unpublished data. In subsequent sections, the hypothesis that physical activity impacts on functional age is tested against other models of physical activity effects by reference to published and unpublished findings. Finally, we test, in two new studies, a theoretical model that incorporates both general effects resulting from chronic activity (i.e., effects on functional age) and specific effects associated with overpractice in the cognitive/motor domain.

The initial section of this chapter provides some basic definitions and a historical context. The second section focuses on measurement and methodology. In the third section, three theoretical perspectives on the effects of physical activity on cognitive variables are described, and a new model of functional age is developed. The fourth section contains an evaluation of this functional age model by reference to unpublished analyses from the *Functional Age and Physical Activity (FAPA)* study. The fifth, sixth, and seventh sections evaluate the various models of physical activity effects in relation to findings from intervention studies and studies on undifferentiated and differentiated age trends. In the ninth and tenth sections, an inclusive model on the impact of physical activity on cognitive/motor performance is tested in two new studies. The final section contains our conclusions.

## Definitions

Our main intent is to examine the implications of *chronic physical activity* for *age-dependent psychological functions,* in particular, *speeded* cognitive/motor functions. The two constructs permit a general definition as well as those operational definitions more commonly encountered in research.

Chronic physical activity is understood to mean a life-style that includes regular bouts of prolonged, strenuous physical activity. Such activity often is represented in research by persistent participation in sport or exercise classes (i.e., for durations ranging from months to years in various studies), but it also has been indexed using nonformal leisure time activity (Morris, Chave, Adam, Sirey, & Epstein, 1956) or physical activity in the workplace (Montoye, 1975). As we stated, the focus of this chapter is the relationship of chronic physical activity to levels on psychological functions. We do not examine the literature on the *transient* cognitive changes produced by *acute* exercise (i.e., a single bout), recently surveyed by Tomporowski and Ellis (1986). To date, the latter research has not examined whether the effects of acute exercise differ across age levels.

Age-dependent psychological functions refer to cognitive and cognitive/motor performances that typically show linear or accelerating deterioration with age. Many such functions show cross-sectional stability between ages of 20 and 40 years, and longitudinal stability of even longer duration, but deterioration thereafter. They frequently are indexed in research by tests of reaction time, movement time, "don't hold" subtests on intelligence scales (Wechsler, 1958), and neuropsychological tests. Tests involving movement are particularly sensitive to aging efffects, with the deterioration more from a slowing in the processing, decision, and monitoring phases than peripheral factors associated with the musculature (Erber, 1986; Welford, 1977, 1984).

## Some Historical Antecedents to Contemporary Models

The idea that physical activity promotes physical and psychological vitality has had a long but controversial history. For reasons not entirely clear, opinions as to why exercise is or isn't "good for you" tend toward the extremes. Our suspicion is that the polarized attributions are based on approach or avoidance tendencies, respectively, toward the physical discomfort entailed in strenuous exercise. The overenthusiasm of some protagonists may be a strategy to cope with the self-imposed discomfort they endure, whereas antagonists may simply have a low tolerance for physical strain. Historically, three models have emerged for the reasons regular physical activity reduces the ravages of age on cognitive functions: (1) the promotion of good health, (2) the retention of physical integrity, and (3) an effect on functional age.

### The Health Mediation Model

By the fourth centruy B.C., Xenophon had espoused via Socrates the doctrine that physical exercise helps postpone deterioration in power of thinking by preventing ill health (McIntosh, 1968). Recent formulations compatible with Xenophon's illness-mediation model have specified hypertension and ischaemic heart disease as illnesses that adversely affect cognitive performance (Eisdorfer & Wilkie, 1977) but may be postponed or prevented by regular exercise (Morris et al., 1956; Paffenbarger, Hyde, Wing, & Steinmetz, 1984; Shephard, 1978). Yet some writers were antagonistic to Xenophon's notion that physical exercise promotes health. This antipathy was made apparent to Reverend Charles Wordsworth, who instituted the famous annual boat race between the universities at Oxford and Cambridge in 1829: "we used to be told that no man in a racing boat could expect to live to the age of 30". Forty years later, Mr. Frederick Skey, a noted surgeon of that era, called that race a "national folly." Skey's hypothesis of the life-threatening propensity of strenuous rowing was discredited as early as 1873 by J.E. Morgan (cited in Shephard, 1978), and studies since then have failed to produce convincing evidence that rowers die younger than appropriate controls. In fact, evidence indicates that the life span of other categories of sportsmen (e.g., skiers, track participants) may slightly exceed that of nonsportsmen (Shephard, 1978) and regular participants in nonspecified forms of exercise may live somewhat longer than nonexercisers (Paffenbarger et al., 1984). Yet despite inadequate evidence that regular strenuous exercise increases mortality, passionate rhetoric has continued to plague discussion on exercise and illness: Friedman and Rosenman (1974) on jogging and sport:

> This miserable postcollegiate athletic travesty [jogging] has already killed scores, possibly hundreds, of Americans;
>
> violent sports [such as tennis, handball, and squash] ... rank next to jogging in potential lethality. (pp. 182–184)

Friedman and Rosenman (1974) believe that jogging is "custom made for the Type A person" (p. 183) prone to cardiac disorder. Yet the bulk of evidence is contrary, suggesting that bias may override objectivity even among eminent physicians who should know better.

## The Moderator Variable Model

This model rests on the notion that lifelong exercising postpones or even arrests age change in processes that underlie performance capability; exercise, therefore, may moderate age change. Spirduso (1982) quoted the thirteenth century belief of Cornaro (1225; reprinted in 1979) as an early example. Cornaro claimed that sloth and extravagance, not aging, are responsible for any deterioration in cognitive function. Cornaro's austere life-style, consistent with his beliefs, was such that certain among his contemporaries claimed that he lived miserably in order to die fulfilled (W.A. McKim, personal communication).

Some authors who have proclaimed forms of the moderation model enthusiastically also have been guilty of paying too little attention to the quantity and quality of evidence cited to support their claims. Thus Smith and Gilligan reported to *The Physician and Sportsmedicine,* "Disuse accounts for about half of the functional decline [in physical working capacity] that occurs between ages 30 and 70, and aging the other half" (1983, p. 91), but neglected consideration of the methodology of the two studies cited to support this sweeping inference. Yet the methodology of much of the research on fitness training effects has been criticized. Folkins and Sime (1981) commented on research relating physical fitness training to psychological variables as follows: "Only about 15% of the studies reviewed . . . qualified as true experiments, and most of these were studies on clinical populations" (p. 386). Probably the best known recent statements of this model are provided by Spirduso:

> The hypothesis that has been guiding our research is that chronic physical activity has profound influences on the brain, and that many of these influences result in improved cognitive function. (Spirduso, 1982, p. 208)

> . . . exercise may prevent or postpone a commonly existing cycle: disuse decreases metabolic demands in motor and somatosensory brain tissue, which may decrease the need for circulatory flow, which may result in neuronal destruction, leading to disuse of brain tissue, and so on. (Spirduso, 1980, p. 860)

## The Functional Age Model

A model implicit in everday thinking suggests that chronic exercise has generalized benefit for the organism, but does not assume that the aging process itself is affected by exercise. The effects of chronic exercise therefore can be described as *tonic,* meaning that vigor and vitality are restored to the performance of a range of functions. The general form of this model assumes that chronological age and various life-style factors (e.g., chronic physical activity, smoking, etc.) contribute independently to overall capability to function. In recent history, this type of model has come under the general rubric of functional age.

Functional age has a meaning in everyday language that often is misrepresented in technical discussion. In everyday parlance, the implicit use of the construct is evidenced by statements of the form, "Mr. X acts older [younger] than his years." The meaning simply is that Mr. X's general functioning capability differs from his age peers. This usage is similar in form to that of the IQ in intelligence testing. We believe that the early researchers in the field understood this meaning, and tried to operationalize the construct for the benefit of medical and biological science (Benjamin, 1947; Murray, 1951). Sadly, their efforts went astray. Most of them opted to use empirical test construction methods in which the main (and often sole) criterion used to select measures was an independent relationship either with chronological age (Dirken, 1972; Murray, 1951) or remaining life span (Brown & Forbes, 1976; Nuttall, 1972). Missing from this pursuit of empiricism was serious consideration of the meaning of functional age, with the result that measures included in a functional age index might have no bearing on a person's ability to function (Costa & McCrae, 1980; Stones & Kozma, 1981a) (e.g., greying of hair). Many measurement problems that subsequently arose could have been avoided had the early researchers used a construct validity approach that placed primary emphasis on contruct meaning.

Despite its sometimes problematic history, conceptual advances in functional age models have been proposed (e.g., the "cascade" model of Birren & Cunningham, 1985) and major technical breakthroughs have been reported (Borkan & Norris, 1980a, 1980b). We now know that the average 65-year-old can expect to spend 7.5 years of the anticipated 17 years of life remaining in a state of some functional disability (Wilkins & Adams, 1983), a duration that might be reduced if regular exercise were incorporated into the life-style (Shephard, 1978, 1984a). We also can identify those physiological and cognitive measures that correlate highly both with chronological age and (with age partialled out) remaining life span (Borkan & Norris, 1980a, 1980b). For such reasons, several well-known researchers continue to advocate the development of new and better functional age models in gerontology (Birren & Cunningham, 1985; Schaie & Parr, 1981). In later sections of this chapter, we show how a construct validity approach to functional age aids our understanding of physical activity effects on cognitive/motor performance.

## Measurement and Methodology

### Indexing Physical Fitness and Physical Activity

Any research on the effects of physical activity must provide either some means for differentiating between physically active and inactive people in a cross-sectional design or a means of indexing change in activity and/or fitness if the design contains a longitudinal component. The literature on indexing physical activity and fitness has been reviewed (Andersen, Masironi, Rutenfranz, & Seliger, 1978; Cardus, 1978; Stones & Kozma, 1985a), and only the most recent and pertinent discussion is addressed here.

## Indexes of Physical Fitness

The first issue the researcher must consider is whether the independent variable of primary interest is physical activity or physical fitness. If the focus is on the chronic implications of physical activity for cognitive performance, measures of both activity and fitness are desirable. Physical fitness is not a unitary concept, and measures of several aspects of fitness that can be used with people of all ages are available (Cardus, 1978; Standardized Test of Fitness, 1981). The most commonly cited aspect of fitness is endurance capability that can be indexed by aerobic power under maximal or submaximal workload conditions (Astrand & Rodahl, 1977; Smith & Gilligan, 1983). Other aspects of fitness that have received attention in research with older people are strength (Moritani & deVries, 1980), muscular endurance (Stephens, Craig, & Ferris, 1986b), balance (Overstall, 1980; Stones & Kozma, 1987) and flexibility (Adrian, 1981; Rikli & Busch, 1986; Stones, Kozma, & Stones, 1985). These various aspects of fitness differ with respect to age dependency. Aerobic power, muscular endurance, and balance all exhibit marked deterioration with age, whereas flexibility and grip strength show less deterioration (Potvin, Syndulko, Tourtellotte, Lemon, & Potvin, 1980; Stephens et al., 1985).

## Quantitative Indexes of Activity

The quantitative procedure used in much epidemiological research involves the derivation of an overall index of metabolic cost. This index is obtained by summing the product of intensity and duration for all relevant activities within a given time period. Tables of representative rates of energy expenditure for various activities, which are contained in Andersen et al. (1978), supplement earlier tables prepared by Durin and Passmore (1967). Taylor et al. (1978) provided similar tables for leisure time physical activities. Each value in the tables represents the intensity of an activity that can be expressed alternatively on scales of energy expenditure, oxygen consumption, or as a multiple of basal metabolic rate. The time allocated to each activity within the given period has been appraised in different studies by a standardized retrospective interview (van der Sluiijs, 1972), a retrospective activity questionnaire (Morris et al., 1956), or current time budget diaries (Durin & Passmore, 1967). The general problems with this procedure are fairly obvious: The intensity values pertain to an "average" person rather than being tailored to individuals; faulty recall or deliberate misrepresentation may introduce error into the estimates of time allocation (Sidney & Shepard, 1977); etc. Yet despite these sources of error, Montoye (1975) reported correlations greater than .85 between derived indices and judges' ratings of the habitual activity of respondents.

Other investigators have examined the reliability and validity of a single item measure of leisure time physical activity: How frequently did the respondent exercise vigorously enough to "get sweaty" during a preceding period of specified duration (Godin, Jobin, & Bouillon, 1986; Siconolfi, Tasater, Snow, & Carlton, 1985). Godin et al. (1986) report that this measure has moderate 2-week test-retest reliability ($r = .64$) and correlates between .38 and .54 with such measures of fitness as aerobic power and muscular endurance.

### Qualitative Indexes of Activity

A qualitative procedure common in behavioral research involves classification of persons as high activity or low activity based on occupation or leisure time propensities. Spirduso (1975) and Borkan and Norris (1980b) used this procedure to differentiate between sportsmen and nonsportsmen where the former had shown enduring participation in regularly scheduled and frequent bouts of physical exercise.

### Relationships Between the Fitness and Activity Indexes

The relationship between qualitative indexes of activity (e.g., sportsman/nonsportsman) and endurance fitness tends to be positive (Borkan & Norris, 1980b; Heath, Hagberg, Ehsami, & Holloszy, 1981). However, three other factors may suppress or moderate the extent of this relationship: (1) sportspersons of either sex more frequently are self-selected from the higher socioeconomic strata (McPherson & Kozlik, 1980; Stephens, Craig, & Ferris, 1986a); (2) aerobic power is affected not only by physical activity but also by biological "limiting factors" that probably result from genetic predisposition (Astrand & Rodahl, 1977, pp. 324–325), and (3) relationships between type of physical activity and aspects of fitness are characterized by specificity (e.g., strength training does not benefit aerobic power appreciably).

Quantitative indexes of activity have been found to relate only minimally to endurance fitness (Borkan & Norris, 1980b; Dirken, 1972). Borkan and Norris (1980b) reported that indexes based on metabolic cost relate more strongly to the strength and power aspects of fitness than to endurance.

## Research Design and Methodology

A conceptual distinction between two types of aging often is made by researchers: Primary aging is "normal", disease-free aging, whereas secondary aging is disease related. Birren and Cunningham (1985, pp. 21–23) illustrated this distinction by reference to a "cascade" model wherein secondary aging is purported to have deleterious effects on a broader range of psychological functions than does primary aging. They suggest that while primary aging is central to much research in the psychology of aging, attempts to avoid contamination from secondary aging may be less successful than many researchers believe. Birren and Cunningham also point out the importance of secondary aging if the findings from research are to be generalized to the older population as a whole. The distinction between types of aging is particularly relevant to this chapter, because chronic physical activity has been cited with reference to both primary (Spirduso, 1980, 1982) and secondary aging (Shephard, 1984b).

Three research designs, cross-sectional, longitudinal, and intervention, have been used in gerontology to investigate these issues. These designs are not equally represented in the literature on physical activity and cognitive performance. In this section, the advantages and limitations of the designs are discussed from the perspective of physical activity research.

## The Cross-Sectional Design

Two sampling strategies have been used to gather cross-sectional data. First, the normative strategy requires a representative sample of subjects from whom a wide array of measures is usually obtained. This strategy has been used in many functional age studies (Dirken, 1972; Heron & Chown, 1967). Aside from the confounding of age and cohort effects that Schaie has discussed at length (Schaie, 1977, this volume), this type of design requires multivariate analysis and may be less suitable than other designs for differentiating primary aging effects from secondary aging effects. Findings from the use of this design usually indicate that cognitive performance covaries with indexes of endurance potential such as aerobic power and vital capacity (Dirken, 1972; Heron & Chown, 1967; Jalvisto, 1965).

The second strategy is quasi-experimental: Data from elite groups are contrasted either with normative reference data (Stones & Kozma, 1980; Stones, Stones, & Kozma, 1987) or data from selected contrast groups. Spirduso and Clifford (1978) used the latter approach to compare sportspersons and sedentary persons at each of two age levels. This type of design has the advantage that the group selection criteria can be specified so as to exclude persons with acute or chronic health problems. However, disadvantages arise because subjects are not randomly assigned to groups but instead are self-selected. Being an older athlete implies not only a high level of physical activity but also less tendency to engage in health-detrimental behaviors such as heavy smoking (Stones, Kozma, McNeil, & Stones, 1986) and excessive alcohol consumption.

## The Longitudinal Design

Longitudinal studies usually persist over many years and contain no intervention component. Longitudinal designs that either examined chronic exercisers or contrasted physically active and inactive persons have been used to explore age changes in physiological functions and physical performance, but not changes in psychological functions. A few studies have compared longitudinal trend in athletes who remained active with former athletes who had either retired or become much less active. A problem with this latter design is that many athletes who retire from competition take up smoking and drinking habits to greater excess than persons never participant in sports (Montoye, Van Huss, Olson, Pierson, & Hudec, 1957); consequently, any difference in trends between groups cannot unequivocally be attributed to aging effects. A tentative conclusion from this type of research is that a combination of nonsmoking and chronic fitness training is associated with lower longitudinal deterioration on such indicators of cardiorespiratory function as aerobic power and vital capacity (e.g., Dill, Robinson, & Ross, 1967; Pollock, Foster, Rod, Hall, & Schmidt, 1982).

Among athletes who retain competitive habits or resume competitive practice later in life, deterioration in athletic performance is lower when appraised longitudinally than cross-sectionally (Stones & Kozma, 1982a). The longitudinal trends apparently reflect a combination of performance facilitation effects from accumulated training and deterioration from aging (Stones & Kozma, 1984a). Because training effects may accumulate over several years, cross-sectional trends may provide the more realistic estimate of aging effects on athletic performance. When analyzed by appropriate methods (Stones & Kozma, 1984b, 1986a), cross-sectional change in athletic performance accords well with a model that deterioration is greater on events for which the peak power output taxes the available power more severely (Stones & Kozma, 1980, 1981b, 1982b, 1985a, 1986b).

## The Intervention Design

Ideally, this design should include the random assignment of subjects to either fitness training or appropriate control conditions, and measurement of cognitive/motor performance both before and after the intervention. If random assignment is not possible, acceptable alternative procedures may include a waiting-list control condition. Folkins and Sime (1981) reviewed the gamut of exercise intervention studies aimed at improving cognitive performance and mental health. They concluded that the scientific quality was poor in most instances. They classified nearly half the studies as preexperimental and basically uninterpretable. More than one-third of the studies were quasi-experimental but such that an unsatisfactory control condition rendered the conclusions ambiguous. True experimental designs, characterized by random assignment of persons to conditions, accounted for only 15% of studies they reviewed.

## Theoretical Perspectives

Most models that specify relationships between physical activity and age-dependent cognitive functions can be classified as prediction or process, respectively. Prediction models merely describe the type of relationship(s) among the relevant variables. Process models attempt to explain how physical activity benefits cognitive performance by reference to underlying processes. At the current state of knowledge, we can test between prediction models but differentiation among the various process models has barely begun.

The functional age model lies outside of the preceding classification. This model assumes that chronic exercise has tonic effects that compensate for losses with age over a range of functions. The theoretical assumptions made (i.e., that cognitive functions covary with physiological functions and that both sets can be apprehended as attributes of a general construct) transcend the atheoretical slant of the prediction models. Neither does the functional age model share the reductionist flavor of the process models. We think that the functional age perspective is important because (1) it provides a meaningful higher order construct in which to embed interdependent cognitive and physical functions, (2) chronic physical activity is anticipated to affect both sets of functions, and (3) a compound measurement index may be more sensitive to the effects of chronic activity than any of the component functions taken separately. Later in this section a construct validity approach to functional age measurement is described that subsequently is related to physical activity research.

### Prediction Models

Three prediction models that relate chronic physical activity to age change in cognitive performance are the mediation, moderation, and suppression models, respectively. First, the *mediation* model proposes that physical activity decreases as people age, with the effect that cognitive performance deteriorates. This model encompasses Xenophon's illness-mediation model but is not necessarily restricted to mediation via ill health. The critical assumption of this model is that people become less active with age. Second, the *moderation* model assumes that aging and physical activity interact to determine the level of function. This model differs from the mediation model in that diminishing physical activity is not construed as a universal consequence of aging. Some people become increasingly sedentary with age, whereas others remain lifelong exercisers. Chronic physical *in*activity is assumed to contribute to deterioration over time in cognitive performance, but the latter may be postponed in people who retain an active life-style. Two extreme categories of persons are thereby identified: active people who are predicted to retain their psychological capabilities and inactive people who are predicted to suffer major losses in function (e.g., see Spirduso, 1980, 1982, for one version of this model). Finally, the *suppression* model emphasizes effects caused by self-selection. Chronic exercisers differ from the chronically inactive in ways other than exercise habits. These other dimensions, rather than effects from exercise, may be responsible for any group differences in cognitive performance. An illustration of this model from the field of physiology is provided by Suominen, Heikkinen, Parkatti, Forsberg, and Kiiskinen (1980). Their findings indicate that people self-selected for endurance activity differ from inactive people on the basis of inherited traits relevant to muscle fiber composition.

## Process Models

Two classes of model refer to biological and psychological processes, respectively.

### Biological Processes

Dustman, Ruhling, Russell and Shearer (1984) described a version of a hypoxia-reduction model in the context of fitness training effects. They claimed that chronic aerobic physical activity facilitates cerebral metabolic activity in the following ways: (1) enhanced transportation and utilization of oxygen, (2) an increase in glucose metabolism at the cellular level, and (3) a greater turnover of neurotransmitters. These effects are purported to facilitate cognitive and motor performance. They noted that hypoxia is common among older people in poor health, and cited the following findings as providing further convergent validation for their model: Cognitive performance may be improved after administration of oxygen to geriatric patients with chronic, obstructive, pulmonary disease; and cognitive performance is decreased in a high-altitude, oxygen-diminished environment.

Spirduso (1980, 1982) also proposed that enhanced oxygen transport and neurotransmitter availability might underlie the benefit to psychomotor performance associated with lifelong exercising; however, this version was formulated in the context of the moderation model. Spirduso further suggested that structural deterioration in the motor centers may be postponed by lifelong exercise habits.

### Psychological Processes

Alternative formulations were phrased in terms of arousal and decreased susceptibility to distraction. Welford (1977, p. 471) suggested that physical exercise increases central arousal and thereby facilitates the processing of information. Central arousal usually decreases with age, in contrast to phasic arousal that may increase (Woodruff, 1985). A moderate increase in central arousal may decrease the distractability that can impair performance on cognitive tests.

In an opposite vein, Schwartz, Davidson, and Goleman (1978) proposed that regular exercise may reduce the effects of phasic arousal such that any transitory distraction from anxiety is minimized. Consistent with this notion is a finding by deVries and Adam (1972) that physical exercise lowered muscle tension in older patients.

Because arousal models have had a problematic history in psychology, models using this construct seem unlikely to gain wide acceptance. However, findings that the age impairment in cognitive performance is greater under conditions of high distraction (Erber, 1986), and that older nonexercisers are especially disadvantaged under such conditions (Del Rey, 1982), suggest that meaningful models may yet be developed. A change in theoretical perspective to consider the effects of chronic exercise on attention control (Shute, Fitzgerald, & Haynes, 1986) or inhibitory capacity (Woodruff, 1985) might add direction to the field.

## Functional Age Models

A strong form of the general functional age model suggests that aging is a unitary force that affects both physiological and psychological functions (Dirken, 1972). A weaker version considers different bodily systems to vary in rate of aging across subsamples in the population (Borkan & Norris, 1980a, 1980b). The strong and weak versions differ mainly with regard to the expected magnitude of intercorrelations among the cognitive and physical functions. In this section, we address issues that concern functional age models and measurement before evaluating the construct validity of a specific model against new data. Later in the chapter the impact of physical activity on functional age is appraised. The hypothesis derived from the model is that chronic exercise has tonic effects that compensate for aging effects on performance.

### The Meaning of Functional Age

The first issue concerns what functional age scores are supposed to represent. Costa and McCrae (1980) argued that functional age denotes *rate* of aging. They correctly pointed out that functional age scores are misleading if interpreted in this way (i.e., that a person is aging at a slow, fast, or expected rate). Clearly, any scores obtained are influenced also by early established individual differences (e.g., differences from inheritance or of childhood origin) and later life-style effects on the functions. Consequently, they argued that the construct is flawed because measures of functional age reflect multiple sources of causation.

We are unconvinced that most pioneer investigators concur that functional age denotes rate of aging. Dirken (1972) was interested in measuring a person's capability to function in an industrial setting. Murray (1951) was concerned with the implications for medicine. Both investigators intended to measure *relative functional capability* (i.e., relative to age peers) on variables that are age dependent. Costa and McCrae (1980) misinterpreted this intent, probably because it was realized inadequately and/or inappropriately in the early functional age studies. If the meaning of functional age has to do with relative functional capability, it is not very important that functional age indexes reflect multiple causation (e.g., effects from inherited dispositions, lifestyle, aging, etc.). What matters more is ecological validity: Does a person with a favorable (or unfavorable) functional age score have the capability to function more (or less) adequately than age peers in a representative environment?

## Interrelationships Among Measures

A neglected issue, but one of great importance to functional age, concerns the requirement that the measures used to index the construct intercorrelate; a prediction common to both the strong and weak models of functional age is that age-dependent functions do intercorrelate. With the strong model one factor is predicted to contain the measures, whereas multiple factors are consistent with the weak model. Not surprisingly, factor analytic research has yielded major "aging" factors with loadings on such variables as vital capacity, sensory function, and timed cognitive and cognitive/motor performance (Dirken, 1972; Heron & Chown, 1967; Stones et al., 1985). But the important question of whether the correlations among the functions persist, after the variance attributable to chronological age has been partialed out, has been investigated infrequently.

The answer to the above question is critical because functional age, as a general concept, is rendered operationally meaningless unless some higher order and encompassing construct can be measured. A statement that Mr. X is functionally younger (or older) than his age peers has general meaning only if it applies across an array of psychological and physical functions. A related example can be drawn from intelligence testing: The concept of general intelligence has little utility if the subtests on IQ scales fail to intercorrelate. Some findings indicate that relationships do persist among physiological and cognitive functions with age partialed out (Birren & Cunningham, 1985, p. 20, Jalvisto, 1965), but more research on the question is required.

## Traditional Derivation of Functional Age Scores

Two types of regression procedure have been used to obtain functional age scores. The traditional procedure, pointedly criticized by Costa and McCrae

(1980), involves multiple regression of chronological age against a set of functions. The index of functional age is given by the discrepancy between chronological age and predicted age. This measurement model parallels the "mental age" notion in intelligence testing, but is not appropriate in the assessment of functional age for several reasons. For illustration purposes only, consider a hypothetical example such that chronological age can be predicted perfectly from the "true scores" on tests of forced vital capacity *(FVCt)* and digit symbol *(DSt)*, both of which are associated with random measurement error ($e_i$ and $e_j$, respectively). In this example, the age predicted from multiple regression can be shown to reduce to random error:

$$\text{Functional Age} = \text{Age} - \text{Predicted Age} = \text{Age} - u(FVCt + e_i) - v(DSt + e_j), \quad (1)$$

where $u$ and $v$ are regression weights; but since age was defined as an exact function of the true scores,

$$\text{Age} - u(FVCt) - v(DSt) = 0, \quad (2)$$

and

$$\text{Functional Age} = -u(e_i) - v(e_j). \quad (3)$$

Paradoxically, this example shows that the stronger the relationships between the true scores on the functions and chronological age, the less meaningful is the traditional functional age index.

The major pitfalls associated with the traditional procedure can be avoided by a revised procedure developed from one described in Borkan and Norris (1980a, 1980b). This procedure requires separate regressions of each function on age in order to obtain independent functional age scores for each measure taken. The revision we advocate requires an aggregation of the functional age scores over the full array of measures. We demonstrate formally in the following section why this procedure provides a major technical advance in functional age measurement.

## A Revised Procedure for an Aggregate Functional Age Index

Although Borkan and Norris (1980a, 1980b) opted for profile representation of functional age, their procedure allows an aggregate index to be computed. We will show that this aggregate index is relatively free from random error and, given that appropriate measures were selected, fairly represents overall functional capability.

The procedure of Borkan and Norris (1980a, 1980b) for obtaining a functional age score with a single measure (e.g., digit symbol) is as follows. The initial step involves conversion of raw scores on both the function and chronological age into $z$ scores. The next step is to obtain a correlation between the function and age (i.e., $r_i$ where $i$ denotes the function). Because both sets of scores were subjected to normal transformation, $r_i$ represents the regression coefficient of both $Y$ on $X$ and $X$ on $Y$. The final step that must concern us is the derivation of the functional age score. For person $j$ of age $A_j$, this score is the discrepancy between the obtained and predicted $z$ scores on the function:

$$\text{Functional Age} = z_{ij} - r_i \times zA_j. \quad (4)$$

To be consistent with our earlier criticism of the traditional functional age index, we must consider the effects of random measurement error. Based on classical psychometric theory (Nunnally, 1967), the $z$ score on function $i$ by person $j$ consists of a true score component ($zt_{ij}$) and a random error component ($e_{ij}$). Although the $z$ score of age may also contain measurement error, this error will be assumed to be negligible and therefore disregarded. The preceding functional age expression therefore is subject to random error effects as follows:

$$\text{Functional Age} = zt_{ij} + e_{ij} - r_i \times zA_j. \quad (5)$$

Random error effects are expected to nullify when measures are aggregated (i.e, when the functional age scores on tests of digit symbol, vital capacity, etc. are aggregated on a within subject basis). Consequently, an aggregate functional age index is anticipated to be less subject to random error effects than either the traditional index or the profile representation advocated by Borkan and Norris (1980a, 1980b). An aggregate index is also consistent with the denotation of functional age as general capability to function relative to age peers. It can be represented as follows:

$$\text{Aggregate Functional Age} = \sum_{i=1}^{i=n} (zt_{ij} - r_i \times zA_j). \quad (6)$$

## Selection of Measures

Another issue in functional age measurement concerns the selection of variables. The selection of appropriate measures for inclusion in a functional age battery has bearing on the construct validity of the index. Costa and McCrae (1980) pointed out that nonoverlap in the measures included in functional age batteries was normal in earlier investigations, with only a few measures being commonly selected across studies. Borkan and Norris (1980a, 1980b) used only age dependency as the selection criterion but aimed to include a diversified array of variables. Their approach readily lends itself to profile representation of functional age but can be criticized because (1) covariation among measures is not demonstrated beyond the correlation with age; (2) the relative reliabilities of functions are not considered, and (3) variables may be selected that have little or no bearing on a person's ability to function adequately.

## Construct Validity Criteria

We believe that the primary requirement for construct validity is the selection of variables that have direct bearing on *capability to function* in the environment. Failure to utilize this criterion may result in the selection of variables of trivial importance (e.g., hair greying). Its use narrows the selection of variables considerably from the ranges deployed in earlier investigations. Omitted are variables that (1) are irrelevant to functional capability, (2) may permit easy correction for impairment (e.g., sensory functions), and (3) have only indirect bearing on functional capability (e.g., blood pressure, since the effect of hypertension on capability to function can be appraised more directly from cognitive performance).

We can define capability to function as "fitness" in both the physical and psychological domains. This definition allows us to select from an array of relevant measures. A World Health Association monograph (Andersen, Shephard, Denolin, Varnauskas, & Masironi, 1971) defines physical fitness as "the ability to perform muscular work satisfactorily". Shephard (1984b) singled out two aspects of physical fitness that need to be assessed in older people: endurance potential and flexibility. Psychological fitness includes cognitive and cognitive/motor functions that can be measured by any number of standard tests.

Other selection criteria also are required if construct validity is to be attained. The first is that the measures exhibit age dependency; otherwise, the meaning of the construct (i.e., functional capability relative to age peers) is inadequately represented. The second is that the functional age index attain adequate reliability, both with respect to internal consistency and temporal stability. For an aggregate index to attain internal consistency, interrelationships among the measures over and above that resulting from age dependency is necessary. Consequently, the measures are required to exhibit significant partial correlations after effects from age are removed. The temporal stability criterion is intended to ensure that the functional age index represents a relatively stable characteristic that is resistant to transient environmental and intrapersonal disruptions.

## A Model of Functional Age

The preceding recommendations concerning measurement models for functional age can be summarized as follows:

> The meaning of the construct is functional capability relative to age peers. A construct validity perspective on the development of a functional age index requires that the measures incorporated should (1) be of direct relevance to functional capability, (2) be selected from both the physical and cognitive or cognitive/motor domains, (3) exhibit age dependency, (4) intercorrelate to an extent beyond that attributable to aging effects, and (5) possess temporal stability. Functional age scores can be derived for each measure separately by regression of standard scores of the function on standard scores of age and subtraction of the predicted from the ob-

tained scores. The single scores can be aggregated into an overall index that can be tested for reliability and ecological validity.

## The FAPA Study and Construct Validation of a Functional Age Index

We recently completed a multifaceted investigation that we term the Functional Age and Physical Activity (FAPA) study. Some of the findings have been published, presented as papers, or are in journal review (McNeil, Stones, Kozma, & Hannah, 1986; Stones & Kozma, 1985b, 1987; Stones et al., 1985; Stones, Kozma, McNeil, & Stones, 1986; Stones, Kozma, & Stones, 1987). In this section, we will use unpublished analyses from the FAPA study to evaluate the construct validity of a function age index developed according to recommendations contained in the preceding section. In a later section, we examine the relationship of chronic physical activity to levels on the index.

### Subjects

The analyses are based on 1984 data from 311 subjects aged between 50 and 86 years (mean, 62.8 years; *SD,* 6.7 years); 200 subjects were retested 1 year later. The subjects were divided into five groups: (1) 123 *exercisers* (mean age, 61.7 years; 30% male) who belonged to an exercise program for persons aged over 50 years that emphasizes both flexibility and endurance exercises (Stones et al., 1985); (2) 60 *registrants* for that program at the time of the 1984 assessment (mean age, 62.2 years; 32% male); (3) 92 *controls* who were matched with the exercisers and registrants on demographic distributions of age, gender, and occupational status (i.e., the higher of self or spouse) but who expressed no intention to participate in formal exercise (mean age, 62.9 years; 34% male); (4) 8 male Masters *athletes* (mean age, 60.1 years), all of whom had been active competitors for a number of years; and (5) 28 *Elderhostelers* who came to Newfoundland from various parts of Canada and the United States for a minimum 1-week period of study (mean age, 70.7 years; 36% male). We have indicated elsewhere that older athletes and Elderhostelers have much higher physical activity levels than their age peers, and we have discussed why these groups should be considered elite groups of successfully aging persons (Stones & Kozma, 1985b; Stones et al., 1987).

### Measures

The measures obtained were body mass (weight over height squared), blood pressures, vital capacity, trunk forward flexion (Standardized Test of Fitness, 1981), balance (Stones & Kozma, 1987), hearing loss (in the better ear at 4000 Hz), presbyopia (Morgan, 1981), reaction time (Jalvisto, 1965), the W.A.I.S.

Digit Symbol subtest, the Memorial Univeristy of Newfoundland Scale of Happiness (MUNSH; Kozma & Stones, 1980), trait anxiety (Spielberger, Gorsuch, & Lushene, 1970), a short psychological hardiness questionnaire (McNeil et al., 1986), and habitual activity level (Standardized Test of Fitness, 1981). Notable among measures not taken is aerobic power. Unfortunately, direct estimation of aerobic power is not feasible in field research, and indirect estimation lacks accuracy and sensitivity with older adults (Shephard, 1984b; Stacey, Kozma, & Stones, 1985).

## Measures Selected for Inclusion in the Functional Age Index

Four measures satisfied the construct validity criteria of (1) direct relevance to functional capability, (2) age dependency, (3) and temporal stability. We will comment later on their interrelationships. The measures selected are balance, digit symbol, flexibility, and vital capacity. The remaining measures failed to satisfy at least one criterion.

*Good balance* requires both cognitive and motor skills, such that central monitoring of feedback from multiple bodily systems is coupled with corrective muscular action. Good balance is important to all forms of locomotion, and poor skills contribute to falls. Myers and Huddy (1985) found balance to correlate at approximately .5 with activities of daily living (ADL) self-assessments, thereby providing concurrent validation of the measure against overall functional capability. The task we used involved balancing on the right foot and left foot, respectively, under eyes-open and -closed conditions. Each trial was timed until balance was lost (maximum, 60 seconds). The correlation with age was $-.325$ ($p < .001$) with our data, although higher age correlations have been reported in studies that utilized a wider age range (Era & Heikkinen, 1985; Potvin et al., 1980).

*Digit symbol* and similar cognitive/motor tests have been used widely in neuropsychological and functional age research (Dustman et al., 1984; Heron & Chown, 1967). Age dependency with the present data was $-.217$ ($p < .001$).

*Flexibility* and *endurance potential* are considered by Shephard (1984b) to be two aspects of physical fitness that are important to measure at the older age levels. Myers and Huddy (1985) report a correlation of approximately .5 between flexibility and activities of daily living (ADL), thereby evidencing the relevance of this measure to overall capability to function. In the FAPA study, flexibility was appraised from the best of three trials on the trunk forward flexion test. Although the age dependency was significant at a lower level than that of balance, digit symbol, and vital capacity (i.e., at $p < .05$), flexibility consistently has shown age dependency in studies with a wider age range (Rikli & Busch, 1986; Stephens et al., 1986b).

*Forced vital capacity* is a limiting factor for endurance potential; it is commonly used in functional age research, and low levels on the measure have been suggested to contribute to hypoxia (Borkan & Norris, 1980a, 1980b;

Dirken, 1972; Heron & Chown, 1967; Jalvisto, 1965). Age dependency for the best score on three trials was −.283 ($p < .001$).

## Findings Relevant to the Construct Validity of the Aggregate Index

The aggregate functional age index was obtained in the following manner. All raw data were transformed into $z$ scores (i.e., all the functions, age and gender). Predicted scores ($zF'$) were computed for each function separately by multiple regression against age ($zA$) and gender ($zG$) [i.e., $zF' = b(zA) + b'(zG)$]. Base functional age scores for each measure were obtained by subtracting the predicted scores from the obtained scores ($zF$) [i.e., $zF - zF'$]. Standardized functional age scores were obtained by dividing the base scores by the square root of $(1 - R^2)$, where $R$ is the corresponding multiple correlation coefficient. Finally, the aggregate functional age index was obtained by summation of the standardized functional age scores over measures. Both the aggregate index and the standardized functional age scores for the separate measures can be shown to be independent of chronological age and gender (i.e., they correlate at 0 with both), and they reflect the functional status of a subject relative to age peers.

*Temporal Stability.* The construct validity of the aggregate functional age index was evaluated with respect to temporal stability and internal consistency. One-year temporal stability was assessed using a subsample of 200 subjects from whom retest scores were collected. Table 9.1 shows that the standardized functional age scores for the separate measures retain stability. The stability of the aggregate index was .75.

*Internal Consistency.* The internal consistency of the aggregate index was assessed in three ways. First, the interrelationships among measures were appraised from corrected item-total correlations. The corrected item-total correlation is the correlation of the standardized functional age scores on any one measure with the aggregate of scores on the remaining measures. The values for the corrected item-total correlations shown in Table 9.2 uniformly

TABLE 9.1. 1-Year Temporal Stabilities of the Standardized Functional Age Scores and the Aggregate Index in the FAPA Study

| Measure | Stability Coefficient |
|---|---|
| Balance | .629 |
| Digit symbol | .766 |
| Flexibility | .528 |
| Vital capacity | .778 |
| Aggregate index | .748 |

TABLE 9.2. Finding Relevant to Internal Consistency: Factor Loadings and Corrected Item–Total Correlations for Standardized Functional Age Scores in the FAPA Study

| Measure | Factor Loading | Corrected Item–Total Correlation | |
|---|---|---|---|
| Balance | .743 | .322 | ($p < .01$) |
| Digit symbol | .618 | .231 | ($p < .01$) |
| Flexibility | .414 | .138 | ($p < .05$) |
| Vital capacity | .593 | .202 | ($p < .01$) |

achieve statistical significance, thereby evidencing significant interrelationships that are independent of effects of age and gender. Corrected item–total correlations also were computed on the standardized functional age scores for trials (i.e., since three of the measures contained multiple trials). The corrected item–total correlations all were significant at $p < .01$ and ranged from .21 to .51. The alpha coefficient corresponding to this analysis is .76.

Second, the interrelationships among the measure were appraised from factor analysis. A principal components analysis yielded only one factor with an Eigenvalue greater than 1.0; the factor accounted for 36% of variance. Table 9.2 shows that all four measures load highly on this factor.

Third, the reliability for a linear combination of four measures was evaluated (Nunnally, 1967, Eq. 7:14). This analysis is based on coefficient alpha reliabilities over trials for balance, flexibility, and vital capacity, and on the test-retest reliability for digit symbol. The coefficient for the linear combination was .90, indicating high reliability.

### Conclusions

We concluded that the attempt to construct an aggregate functional age index was successful from a construct validity perspective. The component measures are established markers of physical and cognitive/motor capabilities that are both age dependent and interrelated. The aggregate index was found to have high temporal stability and adequate internal consistency. It provides a useful measure of a person's overall capability to function relative to that of age peers.

## Research Findings: Intervention Effects

In this section and the two that follow (i.e., on undifferentiated and differentiated age trends), we evaluate the prediction, process, and functional age models in relation to research findings. The main hypothesis from the functional age model is that the generalized tonic effects from chronic exercise benefit overall functional capability. Our review of the existing literature will be selective, because not all findings have equal bearing on the evaluation of the respective models. The findings from the intervention studies bear primary relevance to the suppression and functional age models, because the durations of intervention typically are too short to permit a test of the mediation and moderation models.

Exercise intervention studies with older people were reviewed by Folkins and Sime (1981) and Olfman (1986). Folkins and Sime (1981) concluded that exercise intervention had been shown to improve cognitive functioning in geriatric mental patients (Powell, 1974, Stamford, Hambacher, & Fallica, 1974), but that no clear conclusions had emerged with respect to normal adults. However, more recent data are available. Many of the earlier studies with normal older adults possess major methodological limitations. These limitations include a small sample size (Barry, Steinmetz, Page, & Rodahl, 1966), unmotivated participants (Cape, 1983), an overly brief intervention (Cape, 1983; Gutman, Herbert, & Brown, 1977), and a high activity level before the intervention (Vanfraechem & Vanfraechem, 1977). In consequence, we restrict this review mainly to studies of healthy and motivated older adults that utilized an adequate sample size and a prolonged intervention period. Unpublished findings from the FAPA study will be reported in the relevant subsections.

The studies can be classified into those using a static comparison group design, a simple pretest-posttest design, and a quasi-experimental design or experimental design.

## The Static Comparison Group Design

This design includes a one-time assessment of physically active and physically inactive groups. The main confound associated with this design is that group differences may result from either self-selection or the effects of exercise. Attempts to differentiate between these two possibilities have included the use of a waiting-list group among the control conditions and the inclusion of experimental groups subjected to the intervention for different durations.

### Support for the Suppression Model

Evidence has accumulated about prior characteristics of persons self-selected for leisure-time physical activity. Hartung and Farge (1977) found that 84% of a sample of older runners and joggers were college graduates and, not surprisingly, had above-average intelligence. Stones et al. (1985) found the participants in an exercise program for older adults to be characterized by high occupational status. Stephens et al. (1986a) also found a positive relationship between occupational status and physical activity participation. We can infer from these findings that older exercisers are more likely to be drawn from the upper socioeconomic strata of their cohort. That this strata is associated with high cognitive proficiency provides support for the suppression model: People with higher cognitive abilities are more likely to exercise regularly than people with lesser abilities.

## Support for the Functional Age Model

In two studies, evidence in support of the functional model can be inferred that is not confounded by effects of socioeconomic status. The first findings were obtained from the FAPA study, which attempted to account for self-selection effects in two ways: A waiting-list control group was included (i.e., the registrants), and the control group was of occupational status comparable to all other groups. The five groups were found to differ significantly on one or both indexes from a physical activity questionnaire (Standardized Test of Fitness, 1981). The order, from lowest to highest activity, is as follows; controls, registrants, exercisers, athletes, Elderhostelers. Mean values on the aggregate functional age index and the standardized functional age scores for the component measures are presented in Table 9.3. Significant group effects ($p < .01$) were obtained from ANOVAs on all the indexes except vital capacity; the highest $F$ value was obtained for the aggregate index. Using Dunnett's test, significant differences from the control group means ($p < .05$ and beyond) were obtained for (1) the exerciser, athlete, and Elderhosteler groups on both the aggregate index and flexibility; (2) the athlete and Elderhosteler groups on balance; and (3) the Elderhosteler group on digit symbol.

These findings show that the groups with the higher levels of physical activity were higher also in functional capabilities. In fact, the order of means across groups is essentially the same for all of the functional indexes and the activity measure. This trend cannot be accounted for by prior differences from occupational status, since the groups all were high on this variable. We think a more probable interpretation is that physical activity has general

Table 9.3. Group Means on Standardized Functional Age Scores and the Aggregate Index for Five Groups From the FAPA Study

| | Groups | | | | |
|---|---|---|---|---|---|
| Measure | Control | Registrant | Exerciser | Athlete | Elderhosteler |
| Balance | −0.096 | −0.244 | 0.014 | 0.706 | 0.575 |
| Flexibility | −0.324 | −0.161 | 0.233 | 0.605 | 0.212 |
| Digit symbol | −0.195 | −0.028 | 0.021 | 0.041 | 0.596 |
| Vital capacity | −0.083 | 0.045 | −0.050 | 0.207 | 0.337 |
| Aggregate index | −0.698 | −0.387 | 0.218 | 1.559 | 1.719 |

benefits for functional capability, as reflected most sensitively by scores on the aggregate functional age index.

The second set of findings were reported by Myers and Hamilton (1985). Their study is interesting in that the length of time spent in an exercise program significantly predicted levels on recall and recognition tasks in multiple regression analysis. Because an index of total physical activity failed to predict memory performance, the authors reasoned that specific aspects of the program (i.e., flexibility and low-intensity aerobic exercises) facilitated memory performance.

## The Simple Pretest-Posttest Design

This design confounds intervention effects with effects of practice or time of measurement. Studies by Vanfraechem and Vanfraechem (1977) and Stacey et al. (1985) divided exercisers into subgroups in an attempt to disentangle the confound. Vanfraechem and Vanfraechem (1977) compared changes in balance and reaction time after an exercise intervention with elderly institution residents. The residents were classified as inactive or more active before the intervention. Because no significant intervention effects were obtained with the more active group, the significant and beneficial changes in the inactive group were attributed to program effects rather than practice effects.

Stacey et al. (1985) compared new and returning members of an ongoing exercise program at the beginning and end of a half-year session. The mean age of the entire sample was approximately 60 years. Groups and time of measurement main effects were obtained in an ANOVA of reaction time, suggesting that effects from the previous intervention period contributed to the superior performance by returning members. Significant improvements over time were obtained on flexibility, balance, and digit symbol. Although the magnitude of these changes were considerably greater than might be expected on the basis of practice effects alone (e.g., approximately 0.25 *SD*), the absence of an appropriate control condition precludes accurate determination of casual effects.

## The Experimental and Quasi-Experimental Design

Good designs in this category include pretest-posttest measurement and appropriate control conditions. Recent intervention studies with older community residents that meet these criteria include Dustman et al. (1984) and the FAPA project. Dustman et al. (1984) solicited 28 sedentary subjects, aged 55 to 70 years, who were alternately assigned to an aerobic exercise group or an exercise control group. The former group concentrated on fast walking and slow jogging, whereas the latter was exposed to strength and flexibility exercises. The intervention lasted 4 months. A nonexercise control group was obtained from a different source but was equivalent to the other groups in years of education and performance on a culture fair intelligence test; however, this group was younger than the other groups by 3 to 5 years.

The measures taken included aerobic power and a number of psychological tests. The psychological measures included sensory thresholds, visual acuity, and neuropsychological tests (i.e., critical flicker fusion threshold, culture fair intelligence, digit span, digit symbol, dots estimation, reaction time, and the Stroop test). The findings with respect to fitness indicated a gain in aerobic power by the aerobic exercise group (27%) that was significantly greater than by the exercise control group (9%). No evidence for significant intervention effects were obtained with respect to sensory thresholds or visual acuity. However, evidence for intervention effects was obtained with respect to the neuropsychological performances.

The strongest evidence for intervention effects in cognitive performance was obtained after the scores on the neuropsychological tests were standardized and aggregated. This aggregation procedure resembles that utilized in the construction of our aggregate functional age index. The findings showed that the improvement on the aggregate index was significantly greater for the aerobic Exercise group than for the exercise control group, whereas the nonexercise control group did not improve significantly. Within-group analyses revealed significant improvements by the Aerobic Exercise group on five neuropsychological tests, whereas significant improvement was limited to a single test in each of the other two groups.

The Dustman et al. (1984) study is noteworthy because the design used was experimental rather than preexperimental. The findings of improved endurance and cognitive performance after the aerobic exercise intervention provide qualified support for the model that chronic exercise benefits functional age. The support is qualified because lesser benefit was observed in the exercise control group. We pointed out previously that different types of physical exercise have different implications for physical fitness: the Dustman et al. (1984) findings indicate that the specificity principle also extends to cognitive performance. Dustman et al. (1984) suggest that the effects of aerobic exercise on neuropsychological performance stem from a reduction in the extent of hypoxia.

The FAPA study provides a further good example of a quasi-experimental design. As mentioned in the previous section (i.e., on the construct validation of the functional age index), 200 subjects from the exerciser, registrant, and control groups in the FAPA study were retested 1 year after initial testing. They were reclassified into four groups after the post test depending on their participation in formal exercise during the intervening period. The reclassification is as follows. The *stayins* were 76 long-time participants in the exercise program who retained membership throughout the study. The 80 *controls* were not participant in formal exercise at any time. The *drop-outs* were 29 members of the exercise program at the initial assessment who had dropped out by the final assessment. The 15 *enrollees* were not participant in formal exercise at the initial assessment but had joined the exercise program several months before the final assessment. The four groups did not differ significantly with respect to age (mean, 62 years), gender distribution (approximately one-third male), or socioeconomic status.

The measures obtained at the post test were the same as obtained at the initial assessment (i.e., the functional age measures, reaction time, sensory functions, personality measures, activity indexes, etc.). All the scores obtained from the 200 subjects were transformed into a standardized functional age format at the initial assessment and posttest separately (i.e., the transformation was not restricted to just those measures included in the aggregate functional age index). The standardized scores were aggregated over the balance, digit symbol, flexibility, and vital capacity measures to derive aggregate functional age indexes at each assessment.

Two main sets of analyses were computed. First, ANOVAs were computed on the initial test values. The indexes that yielded significant effects ($p < .025$) are presented in Table 9.4 (i.e., flexibility, psychological hardiness, the mean duration of physical activity bouts, and the aggregate functional age index). Multiple comparisons on these indexes revealed that only the stayins were significantly different from the controls. The favorable values for the stayins probably reflect effects of chronic exercise, rather than self-selection, since the enrollees did not differ significantly from the controls.

Second, ANOVAs were computed on the changes in values on the indexes from the initial assessment to posttest (i.e., change equals pretest minus posttest). These analyses provide an appropriate test for intervention effects. Significant *F*s ($p < .005$) were obtained only with respect to two indexes: the mean duration of activity bouts and the aggregate functional age index (Table 9.4). Tukey–Kramer pairwise comparisons of change scores were used to evaluate these differences. The results are as follows; (1) on the activity index, the enrollees and stayings differed significantly ($p < .05$) from the controls and drop-outs, and (2) on the aggregate functional age index, the en-

TABLE 9.4. Group Means on Standardized Functional Age Scores and the Aggregate Index Associated With Statistically Significant Effects in the FAPA Study

| | | Groups | | | |
|---|---|---|---|---|---|
| Type of Data | Measure | Stay-ins | Controls | Drop-outs | Enrollees |
| Initial assessment | Flexibility | 0.346 | −0.364 | −0.028 | 0.136 |
| | Hardiness | 0.188 | −0.259 | 0.089 | 0.255 |
| | Bout duration | 0.255 | −0.224 | −0.007 | −0.234 |
| | Aggregate index | 0.498 | −0.620 | 0.315 | 0.306 |
| Change scores (initial minus final) | Bout duration | −0.230 | 0.201 | 0.387 | −0.738 |
| | Aggregate index | 0.225 | −0.222 | 0.561 | −1.120 |

rollees evidenced significant gains relative to the drop-outs and stayins ($p < .01$).

An additional set of analyses was computed on the within-group changes (i.e., by *t* tests). Significant differences were obtained only with the enrollees, who gained significantly on the aggregate functional age index and digit symbol.

In summary, findings from the FAPA study provided support for a model that exercise intervention contributes to a net gain in both physical activity and improved functional age. With the initial assessment data, only the stayins had significantly elevated levels on these indexes. By the time of the post test, the enrollees had gained significantly on one or both the indexes relative to the other groups. In addition, the enrollees evidenced significant within-group improvements on the aggregate functional age index and digit symbol. We concluded that the exercise intervention led to a significant improvement in generalized functional capability, a construct that encompasses the gain in cognitive performance.

## Conclusions

The quality of evidence obtained from intervention research varies with the design of the study. A finding that emerged from studies using the static comparison group design is that people of higher cognitive abilities are much more likely to participate in leisure-time physical activity. This self-selection effect must be taken into account in the evaluation of other research findings. However, findings from the FAPA study and by Myers and Hamilton (1985) suggest that evidence for exercise effects can be obtained from the more sophisticated designs within this category. Findings from studies with the simple pretest-posttest design are suggestive of a generalized benefit to functional capability after exercise intervention (Vanfraechem & Vanfraechem, 1977; Stacey et al., 1985). However, these findings require a cautious interpretation because of the methodological limitations inherent even in the more complex designs.

The strongest evidence for effects from exercise intervention derives from the the experimental and quasi-experimental category of research. This type of design controls for possible confounds from self-selection, practice, and time of measurement. Findings from two recent studies provided strong evidence for an encompassing improvement in functional capabilities after an aerobic exercise intervention, such that the generalized effects include gains in cognitive performance (Dustman et al., 1984; the FAPA study).

Finally, the distinction between aerobic exercise and other forms of physical activity appears to have important implications for the outcome of research. All studies that evidenced beneficial effects on functional capability used an aerobic intervention. Some studies that evaluated other categories of activity failed to obtain a significant association with performance measures (Dustman et al., 1984; Myers & Hamilton, 1985). This differentiation is consistent with a model that the facilitation of cognitive performance as a result of exercise is attained through hypoxia reduction.

## Research Findings: Undifferentiated Cross-Sectional Age Trends

An undifferentiated age trend refers to that within the population as a whole (differentiated trend refers to trends within physically active and inactive subpopulations, respectively). Comparison of an undifferentiated trend across measures provides a test of the mediation model. Predictions from this model are that both physical activity and the functions affected by physical activity decrease monotonically with age, and that changes in physical activity "explain" the changes in function.

Some estimates of percentage deterioration between the thirties and the sixties cohorts, respectively, are presented in Table 9.5. The estimates all derive from large or composite data bases. The pattern across measures can be summarized as follows: (1) indices relevant to endurance fitness (forced expiratory volume, aerobic power) are associated with deterioration of approximately 30–35% over 30 years; (2) cognitive/motor performances are associated with similar or lesser deterioration; and (3) changes in energy expenditure (i.e., an index of total physical activity) are of a lower order of magnitude.

Closer examination of the age trend for activity fails to provide evidence of a monotonic trend, thereby failing to confirm a basic prediction from the mediation model. The trend is illustrated in Table 9.6 both with respect to total energy expenditure and the proportion of each cohort that is "adequately active" (i.e., participates in sufficienct physical activity to produce a cardiovascular training effect). After age 30 years, the trend is a U-shaped

TABLE 9.5. Percentage Deterioration From Ages 30–39 Years to 60–69 Years on Selected Indices

| Index | Deterioration (%) Males | Deterioration (%) Females | Source |
|---|---|---|---|
| Forced expiratory volume | 35 | 29 | Heron & Chown (1967) |
| Aerobic power | 35 | 32 | Stephens et al. (1986b) |
| Mazes correct | 35 | 23 | Heron & Chown (1967) |
| Coding | 19 | 16 | Heron & Chown (1967) |
| Digit symbol | 40 | | W.A.I.S. |
| Digit symbol | 30 | | W.A.I.S.-R. |
| Energy expenditure | 19 | 18 | I.C.R.P. (1975) |
| Energy expenditure | 9 | 7 | Stephens et al. (1986a) |

TABLE 9.6. Energy Expenditure and Proportion of People "Adequately Active" by Decade of Life[a]

| | Energy Expenditure (KKD) | | Adequately Active (%) | |
|---|---|---|---|---|
| Age | Males | Females | Males | Females |
| 20s | 3.1 | 2.1 | 31.5 | 21.4 |
| 30s | 2.3 | 1.5 | 23.4 | 14.6 |
| 40s | 1.9 | 1.5 | 17.2 | 14.6 |
| 50s | 1.7 | 1.5 | 17.4 | 16.1 |
| 60s | 2.1 | 1.4 | 23.4 | 15.8 |

[a]Adapted from Stephens et al. (1986a).

curve for males and essentially flat for females. Other findings tend to confirm this pattern of nonmonotonocity (Montoye, 1975; van der Sluiijs, 1972). Consequently, we must conclude that the population as a whole does not become progressively more slothful as it ages, and that sloth alone does not explain the deterioration in functional capability.

## Research Findings: Differentiated Age Trend

The moderation model is similar to the mediation model in that physical inactivity is assumed to promote functional deterioration, but differs from it in that not all people are assumed to reduce their physical activity with age. Specifically, functional capability is predicted to remain fairly stable in lifelong exercisers but to deteriorate with age among the physically inactive. This model implies that chronic exercise slows the *rate of aging* in psychological processes.

### Studies Using the Reaction Time Task

Several investigators have claimed that chronic exercise moderates age dependency in reaction time such that the slowing in performance with age is postponed or prevented by lifelong exercise habits (Rikli & Busch, 1986; Spirduso, 1980). The findings were all obtained from a design that contrasts two or more levels of physical exercise at two age levels (Clarkson & Kroll, 1978; Rikli & Busch, 1986; Spirduso, 1975; Spirduso & Clifford, 1978). However, we are not convinced that evidence to date supplies robust support for the moderation model because of design limitations, problems concerning statistical inference, and competing interpretations of the findings.

### Possible Effects From Self-Selection

One set of problems, which also worried Spirduso (1980), concerns self-selection. Active and inactive people at all ages are self-selected rather than randomly assigned to conditions. We previously cited evidence that people *very* active in leisure-time physical activities tend to be drawn from the upper socioeconomic strata (Hartung & Farge, 1977), rarely smoke cigarettes (Stones et al., 1986), and probably differ from inactive people in inherited physical traits (Suominen et al., 1980). The design clearly confounds physical activity effects with other individual difference dimensions. The critical question, to which no ready answer is available, is whether self-selection effects or physical activity effects are responsible for any differential age trend in reaction time.

### Problems Concerning Statistical Inference

The data from the studies of reaction time were all analyzed by ANOVA. Robust support for the moderation model requires a significant activity-by-age interaction followed by significant a posteriori multiple comparisons. Unfortunately, some studies reported nonsignificant *F*s for the interactions followed by significant a priori multiple comparisons (Rikli & Busch, 1986; Spirduso & Clifford, 1978). Analyses of the latter type do not follow the conventional procedures for statistical inference; multiple comparisons should not be computed when preceded by nonsignificant results from the ANOVA. Consequently, results based on a priori comparisons that are preceded by a nonsignificant interaction term cannot be considered to provide robust support for the moderation model.

### The Findings

The findings on the significance of the activity by age interactions are inconsistent across studies. Spirduso (1975) obtained significant age-by-activity interactions in three of four analyses of the reaction time and movement time components of simple and complex reaction time tasks. The main effects of activity level and age also were significant. An attempt at replication by Spirduso and Clifford (1978) resulted in significant main effects but no significant interactions in any of four similar analyses. Because Clarkson and Kroll (1978) did not test for interaction effects in their report, we computed *F* ratios from their published data. These analyses show significant main effects of age and activity on all four dependent variables (simple and complex reaction time and movement time) but a significant interaction only on simple movement time. Finally, Rikli and Busch (1986) reported a significant interaction on choice reaction time but not on simple reaction time, and significant main effects on both variables (for corrections of errors in this article, see Erratum, *Journal of Gerontology, 42,* p. 68, 1987).

## Alternative Interpretations of the Findings

In summary, the preceding findings indicate significant age-by-activity interactions in 5 of 14 analyses. In the studies that attempted to replicate Spirduso's (1975) findings, the interaction was significant in only 2 of 10 analyses. Clearly, support for the moderation model cannot be considered robust: The evidence is not very convincing that chronic exercise postpones or prevents the slowing of reaction time with age. However, one cannot dismiss lightly the fact that at least 1 interaction was significant in 3 of 4 studies. Can the other models account for these apparently weak interactions?

Alternative interpretations of the findings can be obtained from both the suppression and functional age models. First, an inference from the suppression model is that persons with fast reaction times self-select themselves for chronic exercise. The findings of a significant main effect of activity in all 14 analyses cited is consistent with this model. However, the suppression model does not permit a ready explanation for why the activity-by-age interaction was ever significant. On what basis do people differing in reaction time select themselves for life-styles charactized by greater or lesser levels of physical activity? Possible interpretations of a significant interaction based on self-selection are either that (1) among people with fast reaction times, more young persons than old opt for an inactive life-style, or (2) among persons with slow reaction times, more young persons than old persons adopt a physically active life-style. Neither possibility appears to be sufficiently compelling, especially when given evidence that reaction time is improved by exercise intervention (Dustman et al., 1984; Stacey et al., 1985; Vanfraechem and Vanfraechem, 1977).

Second, the inference from the functional age model is that chronic exercise benefits functional capability up to an asymptotic level, such that most inactive subjects should exhibit poor performance relative to active age peers. The uniform findings of significantly faster performances by active subjects are consistent with this model. But after demographic trends for activity are taken into account, this model can also predict a weak age-by-activity interaction effect on performance. A weak interaction translates into an expectation that only some of the corresponding $F$ values will be significant. The demographic evidence is as follows. All the studies cited earlier in this section contrasted either male groups (Clarkson & Kroll, 1978; Spirduso, 1975; Spirduso & Clifford, 1978) or female groups (Rikli & Busch, 1986) aged 20–29 years and 50–70 years, respectively. Normative data suggest that inactive subjects within the older range are physically less active than inactive subjects in their twenties: The proportion of older males falling within the lower of two inactivity categories exceeds the corresponding proportion for younger males by 20–30% (Stephens et al., 1986a). The trend is similar for females. Given that the benefit to performance reaches asymptote beyond a given level of activity, a weak activity-by-age interaction effect on performance is predicted because the old inactive males are less active than the young inactive males.

## Other Tasks

Evidence obtained with other cognition-relevant tasks failed to provide convincing support for the moderation model. Ramig (1983) examined speaking and reading rates at three age levels and two levels of "physiological condition," where the latter was appraised from resting heart rate, blood pressures, body fat, and vital capacity. Ramig (1983) reported significant effects of age on four dependent variables (speaking and reading rates with and without pause time), but a significant age-by-physiological-condition interaction only with one dependent variable. Suominen et al. (1980) compared age correlations and age regressions between physically active and inactive men on more than 30 measures. The cognition-relevant measures included reaction time, balance, auditory and vibratory perception, manipulative dexterity, and digit symbol. Age dependency on these measures differed significantly between the active and inactive males only with respect to auditory perception, with the regression slopes not differing significantly across groups.

## Conclusions

The findings from studies of differentiated age trends reveal significant main effects of activity level but fail to provide evidence of a robust activity-by-age interaction effect on performance, although some significant interactions were obtained. Consequently, the moderation model is not strongly supported by these findings: The main prediction from the moderation model is for a robust interaction. Neither can strong support be derived for the suppression model, since the trends in the data are unlikely to result entirely from self-selection.

The model receiving strongest support is the functional age model. This model predicts higher performance levels among active subjects, with the worst performance predicted for the least active subjects at all age levels. Evidence for age-by-activity interaction effects on performance are consistent with the functional age model to the extent that the findings are affected by age differences in activity level or that the young and old subjects are differentially susceptible to the tonic effects of chronic exercise.

# Study 1

The conclusions reached in the preceding sections are that support for the functional age model is convincing but that evidence for the moderation model is not robust. In other words, we think that chronic aerobic exercise has a generalized tonic effect on performance capability, but that exercise normally does not postpone or prevent the effects of aging on the respective functions. Instead, chronic exercise compensates for age deterioration in functional capability. However, acceptance of these conclusions ought not to lead to a premature cessation of the search for moderating effects from physical activity. It is possible that physical activity does moderate age dependency but on different categories of function and via different pathways from those previously investigated. The overuse principle provides one alternative pathway to guide this search.

### The Overuse Principle

The overuse principle dictates that overpractice provides protection against aging effects. An example was provided by La Riviere and Simonson (1965), who found that speed of handwriting did not slow with age among clerical workers who practiced the skill regularly, but that age deterioration was observed among other categories of workers. The relevance of the overuse principle at the cellular level was recognized by Spirduso (1980) " . . . cell aging is influenced to a large degree by the amount of activity in which the cell is involved" (p. 860). A hypothesis derived from the overuse principle is that age deterioration may be postponed in functions that are overpracticed during the habitual course of physical activity.

## The Tonic and Overpractice Effects (TOPE) Model

TOPE stands for the tonic and overpractice effects that we attribute to chronic physical activity. The Dustman et al. (1984) and FAPA studies provided strong evidence that the tonic effects on functional capability are maximized under conditions of chronic aerobic exercise. Other findings, reviewed under the sections on Intervention Effects and Differentiated Age Trend, are consistent with this conclusion. Elsewhere in this chapter, we have referred to the tonic effects of chronic exercise as a benefit to functional age.

The other hypothesis from the TOPE model is that age deterioration is postponed or prevented in overpracticed performance. Applied to physical activity, this hypothesis means that the skillful execution of familiar movement patterns remains relatively unimpaired by age. It is a risky hypothesis because we know of no investigation in the physical activity field that has directly addressed the issue. What we expect is that the more closely the experimental task mirrors the overpracticed skill, the less will be the evidence for age deterioration. Study 1 is an attempt to test the TOPE model.

### The Design, Task, and Hypotheses

The design is a conventional one that utilizes active and inactive groups at two age levels. However, we attempted to ensure comparability in activity across the respective age groups by the use of stringent selection criteria for both the active *and* inactive groups. The choice of task was determined by the necessity to include both overpracticed and unfamiliar forms of the same movement pattern. Because overpractice effects should be maximized in repetitive and cyclic movement forms, rather than discrete movement, we decided to use overpracticed and underpracticed versions of the tapping test. Simple foot-tapping can be considered an overpracticed task because the up-and-down pattern is highly overpracticed in normal walking. Up-and-down hand-tapping is much less familiar as a purposeful form of movement, being overpracticed only in select occupational groups (e.g., drummers). Both tasks requires low muscular effort, so it is probable that central factors contribute more to performance than peripheral factors (e.g., the central factors include the monitoring of limb position and changes to the direction of limb movement).

Tapping performance previously has been shown to exhibit reliability (Barry et al., 1966), age dependency (Borkan & Norris, 1980a, 1980b), and sensitivity to the effects of cardiovascular disorder (Simonson & Enzer, 1941). The versions used in Study 1 include independent trials with the hands and feet under both coupled and decoupled conditions.

*The Hypothesis Concerning Tonic Effects.* The relevant hypothesis from the TOPE model is that tonic effects from chronic exercise will result in faster movement by chronic exercisers than by inactive subjects, particularly under unconstrained conditions. An unconstratined condition, in this context, means an absence of any imposed work load or high demands on movement coordination. Under conditions of constraint by an external load (Welford, 1984) or by requirements such as interlimb coordination (Lofthus, 1981), movement speed has been shown to be attenuated. Consequently, alternate versions of the tapping test were included in Study 1 that require tapping with a single limb (i.e., decoupled tapping) or coordinated across lateral limbs (i.e., coupled tapping). An activity-by-coordination interaction was predicted: Any advantage in movement speed to the active subjects was anticipated to be greater with the decoupled task.

*The Hypothesis Concerning Overpractice Effects.* Specific protection against aging effects is hypothesized with familiar, overpracticed movement patterns. Compared to hand-tapping, up-and-down foot-tapping is overpracticed by exercisers and nonexercisers alike. Consequently, a limb-by-age interaction was predicted: Age differences were anticipated to be greater for hand-tapping than for foot-tapping.

## Methods

The design contrasted active and inactive groups at two age levels. The tapping tasks included hand-tapping and foot-tapping under decoupled and coupled conditions. In counterbalanced order, two trials were obtained for each task condition.

*Subjects.* Eighty subjects were divided into four groups, each containing 10 men and 10 women: Young Active, Young Inactive, Old Active, and Old Inactive. Group selection was based on age and physical activity level. The young active group contained physical education students of mean age 20.4 years. All these subjects exercised strenuously and for prolonged durations at least three times weekly (half exercised six or seven times per week). The young inactive group was of mean age 23.2 years, and no member exercised for more than 30 minutes total per week. The old active group was of mean age 61.3 years. All its members exercised at least twice weekly for 45 minutes as part of an exercise program that stressed flexibility and endurance. The endurance portion of each session lasted 30 minutes, during which time heart rate was self-monitored to maintain a level shown to promote endurance fitness safely. Most of the members of this group also exercised regularly outside the program, with half exercising four or more times weekly. The old inactive group was of mean age 61.5 years and was matched with the old active group with respect to the highest occupation attained by subject or spouse (i.e., usually managerial or professional). No subject in the old inactive group exercised for more than 30 minutes total per week.

*Apparatus.* The tapping apparatus consisted of two 35 × 40 cm tapping boards connected to two counters. Each board bore 31 conducting rods set into slots running its length, and each rod had a copper collar attached to one end with set screws. The collars were wired in two series, such that each rod was wired not to adjacent rods but to rods next-but-one on either side. Consequently, odd-numbered rods in series formed one side of the circuit and even-numbered rods the other. By applying a conductor across any two adjacent rods, the circuit could be closed. The rods were glued down and further secured by strips of heavy plastic across both end of the boards (i.e., 30 mm wide across the wired end of the rods and 15 mm wide at the other end, thereby reducing the length of the tapping space to 41 cm). The boards were attached to counters that accepted current from the main power source and stepped it down to 25 volts/1.5 amps. This secondary source fed into each tapping board. The boards in turn each were wired back to one of the two counters, such that the respective counter advanced one count each time the circuit was closed on that board.

For the hand-tapping task, paddles were built to close the circuit. Each paddle consisted of a 13-mm-thick, 7.5 × 7.5-cm block of plywood from which rose a perpendicular plywood handle (13 cm long, 2 cm diameter). The bottom surface of the paddle was covered with 1-cm-thick insulating foam, which was covered with metal foil tape to permit electrical conduction.

Electrically conducting slippers were designed for the foot-tapping task. The sole of each slipper was made from plastic covered by thin layers of foam rubber and adhesive felt. Metal foil conducting tape covered the bottom of the sole. Two long, narrow cloth tapes were sewn across the upper side of each slipper in the regions of the heel and ball of the foot, respectively.

Velcro strips were sewn to the end of the tapes so as to permit each slipper to be strapped to the subject's foot.

*Procedure.* Subjects were tested individually at the laboratory. Each practiced all the movement tasks for approximately 5 minutes in total before testing so as to become acquainted with the procedure. The tests were performed while seated on a hard chair 38 cm high.

The hand-tapping tasks were performed with the boards directly facing the subject and placed on a desk 63 cm high. In the decoupled task, the subject gripped the paddle around its vertical handle, rather as one would grip a video-game joystick, and tapped the board with the paddle, thereby activating the respective counter with each tap. The coupled task was performed with a paddle held in each hand, and each paddle tapped a separate board. The foot-tapping tasks were performed with the boards directly in front of the subject's chair, such that the subject's feet rested on them when seated comfortably. The subject wore the electrically conducting slippers when tapping in order to activate the counter at each foot-strike. The instructions were to tap as quickly as possible in the vertical plane (i.e., horizontal movement was not required.)

Cyclic frequency measures were obtained on two trials per task. For the upper and lower limbs, respectively, the three tasks were left-side and right-side tapping under the decoupled condition, and tapping under the coupled condition. In the decoupled tasks, the subject was told to tap the board as quickly as possible using up-and-down movements. The task was timed for 30 seconds, and the score was the number of taps during the interval. In the coupled condition, the instructions were to tap as quickly as possible for 30 seconds, with each lateral limb alternately striking its assigned board. In this way, movement frequency could be measured in each of the two limbs.

Order effects were controlled by varying the order in which tasks were presented across subjects. The first trial under any condition was designated Trial 1 for that condition and the second Trial 2. Under Trial 1, half the subjects performed all the hand-tapping tasks before the foot-tapping tasks, and this order was reversed for the remaining subjects. For half the subjects with each of the above orders, the decoupled tasks always preceded the coupled task in the same limb category (i.e., hands or feet), whereas this order was reversed for the remaining subjects. Four order conditions for Trial 1 were obtained via this procedure. The order of tasks for each subject on Trial 2 was the reverse sequence to that on Trial 1.

## Results

Preliminary analyses were computed with respect to subject ages and in order to determine whether tapping speed was affected by gender. The main analysis was concerned with movement speed in relation to the group and task conditions.

## Preliminary Analyses

The first analysis was computed to determine whether the groups differed with respect to chronological age. With chronological age as the dependent variable, the ANOVA design was age group (2) by activity group (2) by gender (2). The only significant effect was age group [$F(1,72) = 1915.51, p < .001$], indicating that age levels were comparable within each of the activity and gender classifications.

The second analysis was computed to determine whether movement speed varied as a main or interactive effect of gender. With mean movement speed as the dependent variable, the design was an age group (2) by activity group (2) by gender (2) ANOVA. Since the main effect of gender was nonsignificant [$F(1,72) = 1.44$] and interactions involving gender and the other independent group factors yielded $F < 1.0$, the groups were collapsed over gender in the main analysis.

## The Main Analysis

The main analysis was a six-way ANOVA design with repeated measures on four factors: age group (2) by activity group (2) by trials (2) by coordination (decoupled versus coupled) by limb (hands versus feet) by laterality (left limbs versus right limbs). The dependent variable was movement speed in hertz [taps per second (Hz)]. With respect to the main hypotheses, the predicted interactions were significant for activity by coordination [$F(1,76) = 6.84, p < .015$] and age by limb [$F(1.76) = 20.22, p < .001$]. The only other main effect or interaction that included an independent groups factor was a main effect of age group [$F(1,76) = 18.05, p < .001$].

Findings relevant to the two significant interactions above are presented in Table 9.7. With respect to the activity by coordination interaction, analysis of simple effects showed that the active groups were significantly faster than the

Table 9.7. Means for Movement Speed (Hz) Associated With Significant Age and Activity Group Interactions in Study 1

| | Group | |
|---|---|---|
| Task Condition | Young | Old |
| Hand-tapping | 5.46 | 4.74 |
| Foot-tapping | 4.45 | 4.25 |
| | Active | Inactive |
| Decoupled | 5.31 | 5.05 |
| Coupled | 4.25 | 4.28 |

inactive groups with decoupled movement [$F(1,76) = 5.97, p < .02$] but not with coupled movement [$F(1,76) < 1.0$]. With respect to the age by limb interaction, the young groups were significantly faster than the old groups on the hand-tapping task [$F(1,76) = 29.34, p < .001$] but not on the foot-tapping task [$F(1.76) = 3.32$]. Other analyses revealed the respective variances to be comparable across all four groups.

Significant main effects and first-order interactions also were obtained with respect to the repeated measures factors: No interactions were significant beyond the first-order level. The relevant means are presented in Table 9.8. Trial 2 was faster than Trial 1 [$F(1,76) = 27.21, p < .001$], indicating a practice effect. The hand-tapping task was performed faster than the foot-tapping task [$F(1.76) = 174.92, p < .001$]. Movement was faster under the decoupled than the coupled conditions [$F(1,76) = 250.71, p < .001$], reflecting the constraint imposed by the latter. Performance with the right limbs was faster than with the left limbs [$F(1,76) = 44.56, p < .001$]. The interactions among the repeated measures factors all included limb and/or laterality. A significant limb-by-coordination interaction [$F(1,76) = 112.90, p < .001$] indicated that the difference in performance under decoupled and coupled conditions was greater for hand-tapping than foot-tapping. A significant trial-by-limb interaction [$F(1,76) = 5.66, p < .02$] showed that practice benefited foot-tapping more than hand-tapping. A significant limb-by-laterality interaction [$F(1,76) = 19.27, p < .001$] indicated the advantage in performance of the right limb over the left limb to be greater with the hands than feet. Finally, the coordination by laterality interaction [$F(1,76) = 20.26, p < .001$] showed the discrepancy across right and left limbs to be greater under the decoupled than the coupled conditions.

TABLE 9.8. Means for Movement Speed (Hz) Associated With Repeated Measures Factors in Study 1

| | Factor | |
|---|---|---|
| Factor | Hand-Tapping | Foot-Tapping |
| Trial 1 | 5.0 | 4.2 |
| Trial 2 | 5.1 | 4.6 |
| Decoupled | 5.8 | 4.6 |
| Coupled | 4.4 | 4.1 |
| Right limb | 5.2 | 4.4 |
| Left limb | 5.0 | 4.3 |
| | Decoupled | Coupled |
| Right limb | 5.3 | 4.3 |
| Left limb | 5.1 | 4.2 |

## Discussion

The findings of Study 1 confirmed the hypotheses from the TOPE model. One hypothesis is that chronic exercise produces tonic effects that result in superior performance, particularly under task conditions of nonconstraint. This hypothesis is supported by the significant activity-by-coordination interaction. Movement was faster by chronic exercisers than by nonexercisers when no interlimb coordination was required, but did not differ significantly between groups when movement speed was constrained under the coupled conditions. The second hypothesis is that performance of overpracticed movement shows less age decrement than performance on a relatively unfamiliar task. The significant limb-by-age interaction supported this hypothesis: Significant age differences were obtained in hand-tapping but not foot-tapping. Both preceding sets of finding support the TOPE model that chronic exercise produces tonic effects with respect to movement speed, but that overpractice is necessary to postpone age deterioration. Before the model can be accepted with confidence, assumptions made that concern the tasks require further consideration and alternative interpretations of the findings require evaluation.

### The Activity-by-Coordination Interaction

We assumed in the preceding discussion that tonic effects from chronic exercise can be appraised more sensitively under task conditions of nonconstraint. However, other interpretations of the interaction can be proposed.

First, an interpretation derived from the suppression model appears to be implausible (i.e., that persons self-selected for chronic exercise are naturally fast at decoupled tapping). We can think of no good grounds to justify this interpretation. In fact, the traits that can be attributed to chronic exercisers are likely to include good coordination skills, anticipated to lead to superior performance under coupled conditions.

Second, the decoupled and coupled tasks differ on dimensions other than degree of constraint. Decoupled up-and-down tapping can be described as atypical because the synchronization that typifies normal bipedal locomotion is broken. Such synchronization usually extends over all four limbs, since the arms swing in time with the legs. Consequently, chronic exercise effects may be exhibited more strongly in the performance of atypical movement. Paradoxically, decoupled up-and-down tapping may require greater central processing than coupled tapping because movement in the contralateral limb must be actively suppressed. This interpretation provides an alternative to that of nonconstraint for the superior decoupled tapping performance by the active groups. Although both alternatives are consistent with the hypothesis from the TOPE model, that chronic exercise produces tonic effects, they specify different properties of the task that may be sensitive to such effects. With different tasks, differentiation between these alternative interpretations may be possible.

Before completing this subsection, we should point out that the distinction between atypical and typical movement should not be confused with that between unfamiliar and familiar movement. Familiarity refers to the movement pattern itself, whereas typicality refers to the context in which that pattern is performed. Foot-tapping, both decoupled and coupled, is familiar in that the movement pattern is approximated thousands of time daily by each limb in walking. However, the decoupled task is atypical because the movement in one limb typically is accompanied by synchronized movement in the other limb. Hand-tapping is less familiar as a purposeful form of movement, yet synchronization across limbs also is typical of this form.

### The Age-by-Limb Interaction

The significant age-by-limb interaction results from age differences in hand-tapping but not in foot-tapping. Based on the TOPE model, we attribute the absence of age differences in foot-tapping to overpractice. However, other interpretations are possible. The alternatives include the possibility that control of foot movement may suffer less from aging effects than control of hand movement (e.g., because of a restricted range of movement options in the lower limbs, a greater automaticity in lower limb movement, lower demands on processing from the higher brain centers, etc.). Although evidence that aging does appreciably affect foot movement is available (Clarkson and Kroll, 1978), further investigation is required to clarify the issue. An attempt to obtain appropriate evidence was made in Study 2.

## Study 2

Study 2 was a replication of Study 1 but for the task: back-and-forth tapping was utilized in Study 2. Back-and-forth tapping differs from up-and-down tapping in two ways. First, the back-and-forth pattern is overpracticed by neither feet nor hands during normal locomotion or other forms of habitual activity: It is unfamiliar to both limb categories. Second, the demands on central processing to monitor limb position are higher in back-and-forth tapping, since the limb moves continuously between target areas.

The hypotheses from the TOPE model translate into predictions of activity and age effects on performance, but not of an age-by-limb interaction. Specifically, the hypothesis that chronic exercising produces tonic effects yields a prediction of faster tapping speed by the active group under some or all the task conditions. Whether tonic effects are appraised more sensitively under conditions of nonconstraint or on tasks that place high demands on central processing is a secondary issue that the findings may help clarify. The hypothesis that overpractice attenuates age deterioration is not applicable in Study 2, since all forms of back-and-forth tapping are unfamiliar. Consequently, age and activity effects are predicted, but not an interaction between age and limb.

## Methods

The design was the same as in Study 1.

*Subjects.* Sixty-four subjects were divided into four groups, each containing 8 men and 8 women: Young Active, Young Inactive, Old Active, and Old Inactive. Subjects were recruited from sources similar to those in Study 1. Subjects in the both young active and old active groups exercised regularly, such that all exceeded a criterion level of three 30-minute bouts of strenuous activity three times per week. Subjects in the young inactive and old inactive groups fell far below this criterion level. Subjects in the two old groups were of mean age 63.3 years, and subjects in the two young groups were of mean age 22.3 years. Within each age level, the groups were comparable with respect to sociooccupational status.

*Apparatus.* The apparatus was the same as in Study 1.

*Procedure.* The procedure and design were the same as Study 1 except for the difference in the tapping task. The instructions in Study 2 were to tap as quickly as possible while alternating the position of limb strike between the front and back halves of the board (a horizontal displacement of approximately 20 cm). With the coupled task, the limbs moved in opposite directions such that the contralateral limbs simultaneously struck opposite ends of the respective tapping boards.

## Results

A preliminary analysis compared chronological age in an age group (2) by activity group (2) ANOVA design. The findings indicated only a significant main effect of age [$F(1,60) = 839.03$, $p < .001$], with all other $F < 1.0$.

The main analysis was an ANOVA restricted to just those factors of primary interest: age group (2) by activity group (2) by coordination (decoupled versus coupled) by limb (hands versus feet). Four main effects and a first-order interaction were significant. The most pertinent findings are shown in Table 9.9.

With respect to the predictions from the TOPE model, significant main effects were obtained for age group [$F(1,60) = 12.73$, $p < .001$] and activity group [$F(1,60) = 9.99$, $p < .002$]. The interaction between these factors was nonsignificant, as was the interaction between age and limb ($F < 1.0$). In fact, no interaction that involved an independent groups factor was significant. Consequently, the TOPE model was supported by the findings.

TABLE 9.9. Means for Movement Speed (Hz) Associated With Age and Activity Groups in Study 2

| Age | Active | Inactive |
|---|---|---|
| Young | 3.89 | 3.46 |
| Old | 3.41 | 3.07 |

With respect to the repeated measures factors, hand-tapping was faster then foot-tapping [$F(1,60) = 81.33$, $p < .001$], movement speed was faster under the decoupled condition than under the coupled condition [$F(1,60) = 204.16$, $p < .001$], and the significant limb-by-coordination interaction replicated that in Study 1 [$F(1,60) = 82.15$, $p < .001$].

## General Discussion of Studies 1 and 2

The TOPE model provides for tonic and overpractice effects associated with physical activity. As indicated, hypotheses from the TOPE model were supported in both studies. Since Study 2 was intended to test alternative interpretations of the findings in Study 1, we will discuss the evidence for the model by reference to both sets of findings.

### Evidence for Tonic Effects

Tonic effects from chronic exercise are evidenced by the faster performance by active groups over the inactive groups. With up-and-down tapping, this evidence was restricted to the decoupled task. With back-and-forth tapping, the evidence was generalized over all task conditions.

We suggested in the introduction to Study 1 that tapping tasks not constrained by the requirements of interlimb coordination might be more sensitive to the tonic effects of chronic exercise (i.e., the decoupled condition). However, an alternative suggestion was offered that interlimb synchronicity is normal in up-and-down tapping, with the implication that the the decoupled task provides an atypical context for movement. Furthermore, the deliberate suppression of synchronized movement in the contralateral limb may place extra demands on effortful processing during decoupled performance. This alternative interpretation suggests that tasks requiring effortful processing may be the more sensitive to the tonic effects of chronic exercise.

The findings of Study 2 are consistent with this alternative interpretation rather than that based on nonconstraint. Back-and-forth tapping requires effortful processing to ensure that the limb strikes within the designated target areas. The demands to monitor limb position carefully are high both in the decoupled and coupled conditions. Consequently, we suspect that the tonic effects from chronic exercise are manifested by a greater efficiency in purposeful processing.

### Evidence for Overpractice Effects

Evidence that age deterioration is attenuated in overpracticed movement was confined to Study 1, in which the up-and-down foot-tapping task was familiar but the hand-tapping task was unfamiliar. However, an alternative interpretation was offered that foot-tapping is less susceptible to aging effects than hand-tapping because of structural and functional differences between the upper and lower limbs. The findings from Study 2 enabled us to rule out this latter possibility. With back-and-forth tapping, age deterioration was exhibited equally in performance by the upper and lower limbs, respectively. Because back-and-forth tapping is unfamiliar to both limb categories, the interpretation supported by the combined findings from both studies is that overpracticed movement is more resistant to deleterious aging effects than its less familiar forms.

## Conclusions

Earlier in this chapter, we described several theoretical perspectives and models that predict beneficial effects from physical activity on age-dependent psychological performance. Some of these models do not fare well in the light of recent findings. Models that postulate a mediator variable function to physical activity are not supported, because physical activity shows a nonmonotic age trend after age 30 years. Models that incorporate chronic exercise as a moderator variable are not supported by robust evidence that age deterioration is postponed or prevented by chronic exercise: The few findings on reaction time that are consistent with this model are open to alternative interpretation, whereas the majority of studies yielded nonsignificant age-by-activity interactions. Models that emphasize effects from self-selection are supported by findings that exercisers possess traits that set them apart from nonexercisers. However, effects of self-selection fail to explain the findings of benefit from exercise from the better controlled intervention studies.

A model that is supported by recent findings is encompassed under the theoretical perspective of functional age. Costa and McCrae (1980) pointed out several problems with the historical understanding and measurement of this construct. One purpose of this chapter is to report on a reconceptualization of functional age and our subsequent attempt to provide meaningful measurement. When evaluated against construct validity criteria, this effort was judged to be successful. Functional age was defined to mean functional capability relative to age peers, such that functional capability implies fitness in both the physical and psychological domains. Four measures taken from the FAPA study satisfied all the criteria that we specified as bearing relevance to construct validition. The criteria are that the measures directly index functional capability and possess the properties of age dependency, temporal stability, and interrelatedness. The measures selected are balance, digit symbol, flexibility, and vital capacity. Although other measures might usefully be added to or substituted for measures in this array (e.g., aerobic power can be substituted for vital capacity), the present battery does possess content validity in that the major dimensions of physical and psychological fitness are encompassed. The construct validity of the aggregate index was evidenced by its high internal consistency and high temporal stability even after effects resulting from age and gender were partialed out.

Findings from the FAPA study support the hypothesis that chronic exercise benefits overall functional capability, as measured by the functional age index. Support was obtained both from a comparison of groups differing in level of physical activity and from a 1-year intervention design that included long-time exercise program participants, drop-outs, new enrollees, and controls. Findings from the well-controlled study by Dustman et al. (1984) also are consistent with the functional age hypothesis: The effects of an aerobic exercise intervention were of simultaneous benefit to endurance fitness and cognitive performance. An important implication of this model, that ought not to be overlooked in future research, is that the effects of chronic exercise were both predicted and found to be generalized across interrelated domains of physical and psychological function, such that an aggregate index was shown to provide for more sensitive assessment of such effects than a profile of unaggregated indices. Because the benefits of chronic exercise are generalized across domains, we can refer to them as tonic effects.

The probable locus of tonic effects on cognitive performance is increased oxygen transport, or a reduction in hypoxia. Studies that evaluated an aerobic intervention generally reported benefit to cognitive performance, whereas a nonaerobic intervention included in the Dustman et al. (1984) study failed to obtain such benefit. Although the precise nature of the psychological processes that gain from enhanced oxygenation are currently unknown, increased attentional prowess probably is included. Findings that both reaction time (Clarkson & Kroll, 1978; Rikli & Busch, 1986; Spirduso, 1975; Spirduso & Clifford, 1978) and tapping speed (Studies 1 and 2) are faster among chronic exercisers suggest that movements are initiated and monitored more effectively by exercisers than by nonexercisers.

Although an evaluation of earlier findings failed to convince us that chronic exercise prevents or postpones age deterioration in reaction time (i.e., as opposed to providing benefit via tonic effects), we obtained stronger evidence that performance on an overpracticed task is resistant to aging effects. One of the authors (MJS) was alerted to this possibility after an observation that his mother performed as quickly as himself on an up-and-down foot-tapping task. At that time, the author was competing internationally in track events and his mother was in her late seventies. The validity of this observation was confirmed in Study 1, in which up-and-down foot-tapping was not performed significantly faster by people in their twenties than by a cohort aged in their sixities. Since a comparable hand-tapping task yielded evidence of age deterioration, the absence of an age effect in foot-tapping was attributed to overpractice of this form of movement during the course of normal walking.

To test this interpretation, Study 2 was conducted in which the back-and-forth tapping task was equally unfamiliar to both hands and feet. The findings that age deterioration was of equivalent magnitude in both limb categories makes plausible the interpretation that overpractice contributed to the outcome with foot-tapping in Study 1.

In conclusion, the findings reviewed in this chapter are compatible with a model that physical activity is associated with both tonic and overpractice effects (i.e., the TOPE model). The tonic effects of chronic aerobic exercise are generalized across interrelated physical and psychological domains of function. Overpractice effects result in resistance to age deterioration in the performance of highly overpracticed tasks.

*Acknowledgments.* This chapter was assisted by grants from NSERC and SSHRC to the authors. The authors acknowledge the contribution by Rebecca Filyer, who collected and analyzed the data for Study 2 during a student fellowship. Thanks also to Pam Kipniss and Eric Larkin, and to all members of the Fun with Fellowship and Fitness (3F) program who so generously donated their time to our research.

## References

Adrian, M.J. (1981). Flexibility in the aging adult. In E.L. Smith and R.C. Serfass (Eds.), *Exercise and aging: The scientific basis.* Hillside, NJ: Enslow.

Andersen, K.L., Masironi, R., Rutenfranz, J., & Seliger, V. (1978). *Habitual physical activity and health.* Copenhagen: World Health Association.

Andersen, K.L., Shephard, R.J., Denolin, H., Varnauskas, E., & Masironi, R. (1971). *Fundamentals of exercise testing.* Geneva: World Health Organization.

Astrand, P.O. & Rodahl, K. (1977). *Textbook of work physiology.* New York: McGraw-Hill.

Barry, A.J., Steinmetz, J.R., Page, H.F., & Rodahal, K. (1966). The effects of physical conditioning on older individuals. II. Motor performance and cognitive function. *Journal of Gerontology, 21,* 192–199.

Benjamin, H. (1947). Biologic versus chronologic age. *Journal of Gerontology, 2,* 217–227.

Birren, J.E., & Cunningham, W. (1985). Research on the psychology of aging: Principles, concepts and theory. In J.E. Birren and K.W. Schaie (Eds.), *Handbook of the psychology of aging* (2nd ed.). New York: Van Nostrand Reinhold.

Borkan, G.A., & Norris, A.H. (1980a). Assessment of biological age using a profile of physical parameters. *Journal of Gerontology, 35,* 177–184.

Borkan, G.A., & Norris, A.H. (1980b). Biological age in adulthood: Comparison of active and inactive U.S. males. *Human Biology, 52,* 787–802.

Brown, K.S., & Forbes, W.F. (1976). Concerning the estimation of biological age. *Gerontology, 22,* 428–437.

Cape, E. (1983). Activity and independence: Issues in the implementation of activity programs for institutionalized elders. *Canadian Journal on Aging, 2,* 185–196.

Cardus, D. (1978). Exercise testing: Methods and uses. *Exercise and Sports Sciences Reviews, 6,* 59–104.

Clarkson, P.M., & Kroll, W. (1978). Practice effects on fractionated response time related to age and activity level. *Journal of Motor Behavior, 10,* 275–286.

Cornaro, L. (1979). *The art of living.* (Originally printed in 1225). New York: Arno Press.

Costa, P.T., Jr., & McCrae, R.R. (1980). Functional age: A conceptual and empirical critique. In S.G. Haynes and M. Feinleib (Eds.), *Procedings of the Second Conference on the Epidemiology of Aging* (pp. 23–50). Bethesda, MD: National Institute on Aging.

Del Rey, P. (1982) Effects of contextual interference on the memory of older females differing in levels of physical activity. *Perceptual and Motor Skills, 55,* 171–180.

deVries, H.A., & Adams, G.M. (1972). Electromyographic comparison of single doses of exercise and metrobamate as to the effects on muscular relaxation. *American Journal of Physical Medicine, 51,* 130–141.

Dill, D.B., Robinson, S., & Ross, J.C. (1967). A longitudinal study of 16 champion runners. *Journal of Sports Medicine, 7,* 4–27.

Dirken, J.M. (Ed.) (1972). *Functional age of industrial workers.* Groningen, Netherlands: Walters-Noordhalt.

Durin, J.V., & Passmore, R. (1967). *Energy, work and leisure.* London: Heinemann.

Dustman, R.E., Ruhling, R.O., Russell, E.M., Shearer, D.E., Bonekat, H.W., Shigeoka, J.W., Wood, J.S., & Bradford, D.C. (1984). Aerobic exercise training and improved neuropsychological function of older individuals. *Neurobiology of Aging, 5,* 35–42.

Eisdorfer, C., & Wilkie, F. (1977). Stress, disease, aging and behavior. In J.E. Birren and K.W. Schaie (Eds.), *Handbook of the psychology of aging* (1st ed.). New York: Van Nostrand Reinhold.

Era, P., & Heikkinen, E. (1985). Postural sway during standing and unexpected disturbance of balance in random samples of men of different ages. *Journal of Gerontology, 40,* 287–295.

Erber, J.T. (1986). Age-related effects of spatial contiguity and interference on coding performance. *Journal of Gerontology, 41,* 641–644.

Folkins, C.H., & Sime, W.E. (1981). Physical fitness training and mental health. *American Psychologist, 36,* 373–389.

Friedman, M., & Rosenman, R.H. (1974) *Type A behavior and your heart.* Greenwich: Fawcett.

Godin, G., Jobin, J., & Bouillon, J. (1986). Assessment of leisure time exercise behavior by self-report: A concurrent validity study. *Canadian Journal of Public Health, 77,* 359–362.

Gutman, G.M., Herbert, C.P., & Brown, S.R. (1977). Feldenkrais versus conventional exercise for the elderly. *Journal of Gerontology, 32,* 562–572.

Hartung, G.H., & Farge, E.J. (1977). Personality and physiological traits in middle-aged joggers and runners. *Journal of Gerontology, 32,* 541–548.

Heath, S.W., Hagberg, J.M., Ehsami, A.A., & Holloszy, J.O. (1981). A physiological

comparison of young and older athletes. *Journal of Applied Physiology: Respiratory, Environmental and Exercise Physiology, 51,* 634–640.
Heron, A., & Chown, S. (1967). *Age and function.* Boston: Little, Brown.
International Commission on Radiological Protection (I.C.R.P.). (1975). *Report of the task group on reference man.* Oxford: Pergamon.
Jalvisto, E. (1965). The role of simple tests measuring speed of performance in the assessment of biological vigour. In A.T. Welford & J.E. Birren (Eds.), *Behavior, aging, and the nervous system.* Springfield, IL: Thomas.
Kozma, A., & Stones, M.J. (1980). The measurement of happiness: Development of the Memorial University of Newfoundland Scale of Happiness (MUNSH). *Journal of Gerontology, 35,* 906–912.
La Riviere, J.E., & Simonson, E. (1965). The effects of age and occupation on speed of writing. *Journal of Gerontology, 20,* 415–416.
Lofthus, G.K. (1981). Sensorimotor performance and limb preference. *Perceptual and Motor Skills, 52,* 683–693.
McIntosh, P.C. (1968). *Sport in society.* London: Watts.
McNeil, J.K., Stones, M.J., Kozma, A., & Hannah, E. (1986). Measurement of psychological hardiness in older adults. *Canadian Journal on Aging, 5,* 43–48.
McPherson, B., & Kozlik, C. (1980). Canadian leisure patterns by age: disengagement, continuity or ageism? In V.W. Marshall (Ed.), *Aging in Canada.* Don Mills, Ontario: Fitzhenry and Whiteside.
Montoye, H.J. (1975). *Physical activity and health: An epidemiological study of an entire community.* Englewood Cliffs, NJ: Prentice-Hall.
Montoye, H.J., Van Huss, W.D., Olson, H., Pierson, W.R., & Hudec, A.J. (1957). The longevity and morbidity of college athletes. *Phi Epsilon Kappa Fraternity,* East Lansing, Michigan: Michigan State University.
Morgan, R.M. (1981). *Measurement of human aging in applied gerontology.* Toronto: Kendall/Hunt.
Moritani, T., & deVries, H.A. (1980). Potential for gross muscle hypertrophy in older men. *Journal of Gerontology, 35,* 672–682.
Morris, J.N., Chave, S.P., Adam, C., Sirey, C.F., & Epstein, L. (1956). Vigorous exercise in leisure time and the incidence of coronary heart disease. *Lancet ii,* 569–570.
Murray, I.M. (1951). Assessment of physiologic age by combination of several criteria—vision, learning, blood pressure and muscle force. *Journal of Gerontology, 6,* 120–126.
Myers, A.M., & Hamilton, N. (1985). Evaluation of the Canadian Red Cross Society's Fun and Fitness Program for Seniors. *Canadian Journal on Aging, 4,* 201–212.
Myers, A.M., & Huddy, L. (1985). Evaluating physical capabilities in the elderly: The relationship between ADL self-assessments and basic abilities. *Canadian Journal on Aging, 4,* 189–200.
Nunnally, J.C. (1967). *Psychometric theory.* New York: McGraw-Hill.
Nuttall, R.L. (1972). The strategy of functional age research. *Aging and Human Development, 3,* 149–152.
Olfman, S. (1986). Unpublished Ph.D. thesis, Concordia University, Montreal, Quebec.
Overstall, P.W. (1980). Prevention of falls in the elderly. *Journal of the American Geriatrics Society, 29,* 481–484.
Paffenbarger, R., Hyde, M.A., Wing, A.L., & Steinmetz, C.H. (1984). A natural history of athleticism and cardiovascular health. *Journal of the American Medical Association, 252,* 491–496.

Pollock, M.L., Foster, C., Rod, J., Hall, J., & Schmidt, D.H. (1982). Ten-year follow-up upon the aerobic capacity of champion Masters track athletes. *Medicine and Science in Sports, 14,* 105.

Potvin, A.R., Syndulko, K., Tourtellotte, W.W., Lemmon, J.A., & Potvin, J.H. (1980). Human neurologic functions and the aging process. *Journal of the American Geriatrics Society, 29,* 1–9.

Powell, R.R. (1974). Psychological effects of exercise therapy upon institutionalized geriatric patients. *Journal of Gerontology, 29,* 157–161.

Ramig, L.A. (1983). Effects of physiological aging on speaking and reading rates. *Journal of Communication Disorders, 16,* 217–226.

Rikli, R., & Busch, S. (1986). Motor performance of women as a function of age and physical activity level. *Journal of Gerontology, 41,* 645–649.

Schaie, K.W. (1977). Quasi-experimental research designs in the psychology of aging. In J.E. Birren and K.W. Schaie (Eds.), *Handbook of the psychology of aging.* (1st ed.). New York: Van Nostrand Reinhold.

Schaie, K.W., & Parr, J. (1981). Concepts and criteria for functional age. In J.E. Birren (Ed.), *Aging: A challenge for science and social policy* (Vol. 3). Oxford: Oxford University Press.

Schwartz, G.E., Davidson, R.J., & Goleman, D.J. (1978). Patterning of cognitive and somatic processes in the self-regulation of anxiety: Effects of mediation versus exercise. *Psychosomatic Medicine, 40,* 321–328.

Shephard, R.J. (1978). *Physical activity and aging.* Chicago: Yearbook Medical Publishers.

Shephard, R.J. (1984a). Critical issues in the health of the elderly: The role of physical activity. *Canadian Journal on Aging, 3,* 199–208.

Shephard, R.J. (1984b). Management of exercise in the elderly. *Canadian Journal of Applied Sports Sciences, 9,* 109–121.

Shute, G.E., Fitzgerald, S.G., & Haynes, S.N. (1986). The relationship between internal attentional control and sleep-onset latency in elderly adults. *Journal of Gerontology, 41,* 770–773.

Siconolfi, S.F., Tasater, T.M., Snow, R.D., & Carlton, R.A. (1985). Self-reported physical activity compared with maximal oxygen uptake. *American Journal of Epidemiology, 122,* 101–105.

Sidney, K.H., & Shephard, R.J. (1977). Activity patterns of elderly men and women. *Journal of Gerontology, 32,* 25–32.

Simonson, E., & Enzer, N. (1941). The state of the motor centers in circulatory insufficiency. *Archives of Internal Medicine, 68,* 498.

Smith, E.L., & Gilligan, C. (1983). Physical activity prescription for the older adult. *The Physician and Sportsmedicine, 11,* 91–101.

Spielberger, C.D., Gorsuch, R.L., & Lushene, R.E. (1970). *Manual for the State-Trait Anxiety Inventory.* Palo Alto, CA: Consulting Psychologists Press.

Spirduso, W.W. (1975). Reaction and movement time as a function of age and physical activity level. *Journal of Gerontology, 30,* 435–440.

Spirduso, W.W. (1980). Physical fitness, aging, and psychomotor speed. *Journal of Gerontology, 35,* 850–865.

Spirduso, W.W. (1982). Exercise and the aging brain. *Research Quarterly for Exercise and Sport, 54,* 208–218.

Spirduso, W.W., & Clifford, P. (1978). Neuromuscular speed and consistency of performance as a function of age, physical activity level and type of physical activity. *Journal of Gerontology, 33,* 26–30

Stacey, C., Kozma, A., & Stones, M.J. (1985). Simple cognitive and behavioral changes resulting from improved physical fitness in persons over 50 years of age. *Canadian Journal on Aging, 4,* 67–73.
Stamford, B.A., Hambacher, W., & Fallica, A. (1974). Effects of daily physical exercise on the psychiatric state of institutionalized geriatric mental patients. *Research Quarterly, 45,* 34–41.
Standardized Test of Fitness. (1981). Government of Canada (Fitness and Amateur Sport), Ottawa.
Stephens, T., Craig, C.L., & Ferris, BF. (1986a). Adult physical activity in Canada: Findings from the Canada Fitness Survey I. *Canadian Journal of Public Health, 77,* 285–290.
Stephens, T., Craig, C.L., & Ferris, B.F. (1986b). Adult physical fitness and hypertension in Canada. *Canadian Journal of Public Health, 77,* 291–295.
Stones, M.J., & Kozma, A. (1980). Adult age trends in record running performances. *Experimental Aging Research, 6,* 407–416.
Stones, M.J., & Kozma, A. (1981a). The Canadian origin of functional age research. *Canadian Psychology, 22,* 104–106.
Stones, M.J., & Kozma, A. (1981b). Adult age trends in athletic performance. *Experimental Aging Research, 7,* 269–280.
Stones, M.J., & Kozma, A. (1982a). Cross-sectional, longitudinal, and secular age trends in athletic performances. *Experimental Aging Research, 8,* 185–188.
Stones, M.J., & Kozma, A. (1982b). Sex differences in changes with age in record running performances. *Canadian Journal on Aging, 1,* 12–16.
Stones, M.J., & Kozma, A. (1984a). Longitudinal trends in track and field performances. *Experimental Aging Research, 10,* 107–110.
Stones, M.J., & Kozma, A. (1984b). In response to Hartley and Hartley: Cross-sectional age trend in swimming records; decline is greater at the longer distances. *Experimental Aging Research, 10,* 149–150.
Stones, M.J., & Kozma, A. (1985a). Physical performance. In N. Charness (Ed.), *Aging and human performance.* London: Wiley.
Stones, M.J., & Kozma, A. (1985b). Comparison of older athletes with nonathletes. Paper presented at the Canadian Association on Gerontology Annual Scientific and Educational Conference, Hamilton, Ontario.
Stones, M.J., & Kozma, A. (1986a). Age by distance effects in running and swimming records: A note on methodology. *Experimental Aging Research, 12,* 203–206.
Stones, M.J., & Kozma, A. (1986b). Age trends in maximal physical performance: Comparison and evaluation of models. *Experimental Aging Research, 12,* 207–215.
Stones, M.J., & Kozma, A. (1987). Balance and age in the sighted and blind. *Archives of Physical Medicine and Rehabilitation, 66,* 85–89.
Stones, M.J., Kozma, A., McNeil, J.K., & Stones, L. (1986). Smoking behavior and participation in organized exercise. *Canadian Journal of Public Health, 77,* 153–154.
Stones, M.J., Kozma, A., & Stones, L. (1985). Preliminary findings on the effects of exercise program participation in older adults. *Canadian Journal of Public Health, 76,* 272–273.
Stones, M.J., Kozma, A., & Stones, L. (1987). Fitness and health evaluations by older exercisers. *Canadian Journal of Public Health, 78,* 18–20.
Stones, M.J., Stones, L., & Kozma, A. (1987). Indicators of elite status in persons aged over 60 years: A study of Edlerhostelers. *Social Indicators Research, 19,* 275–286.
Suominen, H., Heikkinen, E., Parkatti, T., Forsberg, S., & Kiiskinen, A. (1980). Effects

of "lifelong" physical training on functional aging in men. *Scandanavian Journal of Social Medicine, 55,* 225–240.

Taylor, H.J., Jacobs, D.R., Jr., Schucker, B., Knudsen, A., Leon, A.S., & Debacker, G. (1978). A questionnaire for the assessment of leisure-time physical activities. *Journal of Chronic Disorders, 31,* 741–755.

Tomporowski, P.D., & Ellis, R.N. (1986). Effects of exercise on cognitive processes: A review. *Psychological Bulletin, 99,* 338–346.

Vanfraechem, A., & Vanfraechem, R. (1977). Studies of the effect of a short training period on aged subjects. *Journal of Sports Medicine and Physical Fitness, 17,* 373–380.

van der Sluiijs, H.A. (1972). A standard analysis of daily energy expenditure and patterns of actitivy. In J.M. Dirken (Ed.), *Functional age of industrial workers.* Groningen, Netherlands: Walters-Noordhalt.

Wechsler, D. (1958). *The measurement and appraisal of adult intelligence* (4th ed.). Baltimore: Williams & Wilkins.

Welford, A.T. (1977). Motor performance. In J.E. Birren and K.W. Schaie (Eds.), *Handbook of the psychology of aging* (1st ed.). New York: Van Nostrand Reinhold.

Welford, A.T. (1984). Between bodily changes and performance: Some possible reasons for slowing with age. *Experimental Aging Research, 10,* 73–88.

Wilkins, R., & Adams, O. (1983). Health expectancy in Canada, late 1970s: Demographic, regional and social dimensions. *American Journal of Public Health, 73,* 1078.

Woodruff, D. (1985). Arousal, sleep and aging. In J.E. Birren and K.W. Schaie (Eds.), *Handbook of the psychology of aging.* (2nd ed.). New York: Van Nostrand Reinhold.

# Author Index

Note: Consecutive page numbers that are not hyphenated indicate citation in a reference list as opposed to text.

# Subject Index

MIX
Papier aus verantwortungsvollen Quellen
Paper from responsible sources
FSC® C105338

If you have any concerns about our products,
you can contact us on
**ProductSafety@springernature.com**

In case Publisher is established outside the EU,
the EU authorized representative is:
**Springer Nature Customer Service Center GmbH**
**Europaplatz 3, 69115 Heidelberg, Germany**

Printed by Libri Plureos GmbH
in Hamburg, Germany